W9-AUR-418

# SCLEROTHERAPY

## Treatment of Varicose and Telangiectatic Leg Veins

# SCLEROTHERAPY

## Treatment of Varicose and Telangiectatic Leg Veins

**Mitchel P. Goldman**, M.D.

Assistant Clinical Professor
Division of Dermatology
Department of Medicine
University of California, San Diego
San Diego, California

*With 373 illustrations, including 161 in color*

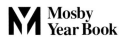 **Mosby Year Book**

St. Louis   Baltimore   Boston   Chicago   London   Philadelphia   Sydney   Toronto

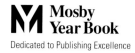

**Mosby Year Book**

Dedicated to Publishing Excellence

Editor: Eugenia A. Klein
Assistant Editor: Barbara S. Menczer
Project Manager: Karen Edwards
Production Editor: Gail Brower
Book and Cover Design: Gail Morey Hudson

**Copyright © 1991 by Mosby–Year Book, Inc.**

A Mosby imprint of Mosby–Year Book, Inc.

All rights reserved. No part of this publication may be reproduced, stored in a retrieval system, or transmitted, in any form or by any means, electronic, mechanical, photocopying, recording, or otherwise, without prior written permission from the publisher.

Permission to photocopy or reproduce solely for internal or personal use is permitted for libraries or other users registered with the Copyright Clearance Center, provided that the base fee of $4.00 per chapter plus $.10 per page is paid directly to the Copyright Clearance Center, 27 Congress Street, Salem, MA 01970. This consent does not extend to other kinds of copying, such as copying for general distribution, for advertising or promotional purposes, for creating new collected works, or for resale.

Printed in the United States of America

Mosby–Year Book, Inc.
11830 Westline Industrial Drive, St. Louis, Missouri, 63146

**Library of Congress Cataloging in Publication Data**

Goldman, Mitchel P.
    Sclerotherapy : treatment of varicose and telangiectatic leg veins
  / Mitchel P. Goldman
        p.      cm.
    Includes index.
    ISBN 0-8016-0251-3
    1. Varicose veins — Treatment.    2. Injections, Sclerosing.
  I. Title.
    [DNLM: 1. Sclerotherapy.   2. Telangiectasis — therapy.   3. Varicose
  Veins — therapy.     WG   620   G619s]
    RC695.G65      1991
    616.1'43 — dc20
    DNLM/DLC                                             91-8805
For Library of Congress                                  CIP

CL/WA   9   8   7   6   5   4   3

# Contributors

**JOHN J. BERGAN, M.D., F.A.C.S.**

Scripps Memorial Hospital
La Jolla, California;
Clinical Professor of Surgery
Department of Surgery
University of California, San Diego
San Diego, California

**HELANE S. FRONEK, M.D.**

Attending Physician
Department of Thoracic and Vascular Surgery
Scripps Clinic and Research Foundation
La Jolla, California;
Clinical Instructor in Medicine
University of California, San Diego
San Diego, California

*To my family*
**Hedy, Risa,** and **Melissa**

# Preface

Varicose and/or telangiectatic leg veins occur in up to 80 million adults in the United States alone. Contrary to the popularly held belief among physicians, they are not merely a cosmetic nuisance, since over 50% of patients who seek treatment do so because of pain and discomfort. In addition, varicose veins have a real association with underlying venous hypertension and its resulting manifestations on the skin, which end in ulceration. Varicose veins are a predisposing factor in the development of superficial thrombophlebitis. Therefore, the treatment of this abnormal vascular condition is warranted for both medical and cosmetic reasons.

Up until the last few years, surgical ligation and stripping procedures were the only commonly recognized modalities for treating varicose veins in this country. Sclerotherapy treatment, which has been used for decades in Europe, primarily by dermatologists, was thought of disparagingly or ignored completely. The treatment of varicose veins within vascular surgery departments was relegated to the intern or first year resident, with veins thought of only as a nuisance within the surgical field.

Patients, usually women, who sought treatment from dermatologists for telangiectatic vessels on the legs were told most often that these did not require treatment or that treatment was not efficacious. At times these vessels were treated with various laser modalities or electrodesiccation, all fraught with complications including scarring. Sclerotherapy techniques, which have been largely ignored in dermatology and vascular surgery training, were used inappropriately in the past. High concentrations of strong sclerosing solutions were used to treat extremely thin-walled, delicate telangiectasias. This produced a number of complications and served to discredit this procedure.

While American physicians were either mistreating or inappropriately treating leg veins in this country, our European colleagues were perfecting sclerotherapy and other nonsurgical treatments of varicose and telangiectatic leg veins. In an effort to bridge the gap between our European and American colleagues, the North American Society of Phlebology was founded in 1986. Educational symposia sponsored by the society were phenomenally successful. All across the country among physicians in various specialties there proved to be a tremendous interest in learning how to treat these conditions. This was probably spurred on by an increasing public interest in and awareness of nonscarring techniques available to eliminate unsightly veins.

In 1989 the American Society for Dermatologic Surgery recognized the importance of phlebology training and invited the North American Society of Phlebology to be a member of the *Journal of Dermatologic Surgery and Oncology*. Also in 1989, the American Venous Forum was formed as an offshoot of the American Vascular Surgery Society. In 1990 the American Academy of Dermatology established a task force on phlebology to better define the curriculum for dermatology residency programs. These three organizations established a framework for the development of a phlebology curriculum.

What has been lacking is a reference source in the English language encompassing sclerotherapy treatment of varicose and telangiectatic leg veins. Most of the available scientific papers were published decades ago or are scattered among many different subspecialty journals. This textbook was written in an effort to present in a coherent fashion all of the available information necessary for the physician to obtain a working expertise in the treatment of varicose and telangiectatic leg veins. I have tried to incorporate as much of the non-English literature as is appropriate so that this textbook truly assumes a "worldly" stature.

It is my hope that this textbook will serve as an impetus for future research in the field of phlebology. This book has been written to be a readable resource for medical students, residents, and those physicians just beginning their training in phlebology, as well as to advance the training of those more expert in sclerotherapy techniques.

**Mitchel P. Goldman, M.D.**

# Acknowledgments

Since this is the first medical textbook I have published, it seems appropriate to begin my acknowledgments with the person who had the most influence on my scientific development — my father. Since my earliest childhood days, my father instilled in me a love of science. This began with the usual set of father and son projects at school, but then extended beyond scholastic requirements. Our family always went exploring, in the Everglades, at the beach, or in our own backyard. My father's respect for life, whether it be animal or human, and his selfless caring for those around him led to my becoming a physician — what he had really wanted to be. Therefore, this first acknowledgment is to my father.

The influence of the late William Watson, Professor of Dermatology at Stanford University, led to my becoming a dermatologist. His contagious enthusiasm for dermatology and teaching helped me realize the great potential of this field. Even though it is an established specialty, dermatology, more than any other medical discipline, is at the dawn of an expansive age of development. I wanted to be a part of that growth.

While I was a dermatology resident at the University of California, Los Angeles, Peter Goldman and David Duffy introduced me to sclerotherapy. They gave of their time and talents without reserve to our residency program. Their teaching led to my first experimental and clinical studies concerning the mechanism of action of sclerosing agents. They have both continued to inspire me and many other dermatologists. Under the guidance of Professors Richard Bennett, Richard Strick, and Richard Kaplan, I developed and used the techniques for comparative experimentation. Further, Richard Bennett taught me to express my thoughts in writing based on a thorough understanding of the medical literature. He was and continues to be my mentor and close friend.

My postgraduate training in sclerotherapy included the in-depth teachings of Arnost Fronek and Anton Butie, who also shared their experience and knowledge freely. Anton Butie encouraged me in my research and was always available for consultation. I value his personal and professional friendship. More recently, I have had the privilege of growing from the shared experiences of Helane Fronek, John Bergan, Walter de Groot, and Paul Ouvry. These physicians, among many others who will go unmentioned, are all a credit to their profession.

In addition, much more was involved in the preparation of this manuscript. Patricia Cavander, Arnost Fronek, and Anton Butie translated all of the French and German literature. Janis Emmert and Esther Pusich at the Scripps Memorial Hospital Kinyon Medical Library assisted with literature retrieval. The Office of Medical Illustration and Medical Photography provided outstanding service in reproducing the many figures in the text. It was a pleasure working with Michelle Williamson, a superb medical illustrator, in developing the creative and often-times multiple redrawings of the diagrams and figures.

The nature of this text, in regard to the rapidly expanding discipline of phlebology, required the input of many of my colleagues. In particular, I would like to thank the following reviewers: Helena Igra-Serfaty (Chapters 1, 2, 3, 4, 7, 9, and 11), the best editor and reviewer any writer could have; Anton Butie and

Dale Martin (Chapters 1, 2, 3, and 8); Kim Butterwick (Chapters 1, 2, 3, 8, and 11); John Bergan (Chapters 1, 2, 3, and 8); Helane Fronek (Chapter 9); Hugo Partsch and the technical staff at Medi USA, Julis Zorn Inc., Sigvaris, the Jobst Institute, and Freeman Manufacturing Company (Chapter 6); and Jerry Garden (Chapter 12) all contributed to the accuracy and comprehensibility of the text. A special thanks goes to Jutta Kerner who assisted in researching and writing the section on Variglobin in Chapters 7 and 8.

I would like to thank my partners in Dermatology Associates of San Diego County, Inc., Drs. Richard Fitzpatrick, Javier Ruiz-Esparza, and Nancy Satur, for their encouragement and understanding and for giving me the latitude to prepare this manuscript. They also assisted me with the numerous experimental and clinical studies that are sited in the text.

Finally, I would like to thank my wife Hedy and daughters Risa and Melissa for their patience during this seemingly never-ending project. It is to my devoted and loving family that this book is dedicated.

                                                                              **M.P.G.**

# Contents in Brief

# Contents in Detail

# SCLEROTHERAPY

## Treatment of Varicose and Telangiectatic Leg Veins

# Introduction

Varicose and telangiectatic veins have affected humankind during all recorded history. Although the occurrence of varicose veins in a four-legged animal has been rarely noticed (Fig. A),[1] the species *Homo sapiens* is known to develop varicose veins in a significant percentage of the population. This fact emphasizes the great importance of the erect stance in the development of varicose veins.

The primary therapeutic procedure for all stasis complications except malignant degeneration is to normalize the underlying pathologic physiology that gives rise to cuticular venous hypertension—increased interstitial fluid and resultant decreased oxygenation and defective nutrition of the skin. Ideally, first treatment should be directed toward correcting cuticular venous hypertension. However, surgeons are understandably loathe to operate through eczematous skin potentially contaminated with bacteria. Thus dermatologic treatment is extremely important in providing the optimal operative field. Alternatively, direct sclerotherapy of an underlying incompetent communicating vein through the ulcer may be performed. Sclerotherapy in this setting has been shown to markedly enhance ulcer healing.[2]

## HISTORICAL ASPECTS OF TREATMENT

As with most physical diseases, offerings to the Gods for help comprised the earliest method for treating varicose veins as shown from a votive relief found at the Greek Temple of Aesculapius in 400 BC (Fig. B). Physicians of the day, however, attempted to formulate more terrestrial treatments. Egyptian papyrus scrolls have been found that contain instructions for the treatment of leg disorders. Ebers, in his papyrus of 1550 BC, avised that surgery should not be performed on varicose veins.[3] The humoral theory of Hippocrates dictated bloodletting as a form of treatment for varicose veins, which was the treatment of choice into the Middle Ages. The first description of medical treatment appears in the writings of Hippocrates in the fourth century BC. He describes treating varicose veins by traumatizing them with "a slender instrument of iron" to cause thrombosis.[4] Surgeons as well were developing various treatments for varicose veins. Stripping and cauterization was practiced by Celsus (30 BC to 30 AD). Antillus was the first to mention ligation of the vessels. In the second century AD, Galen recommended that varicose veins be torn out by a hook. Paulus of Aegina (around 660 AD in Alexandria) performed ligation and stripping of segments of the varicosity. After William Harvey's discovery of the true nature of the circulation, surgical removal of the affected veins was rejected because the procedure could cause complications that were more dangerous than the disease itself. The modern history of surgical treatment began after the introduction of anesthesia and sterile techniques in the late nineteenth century. This is reviewed in Chapter 10.

Compression therapy was recognized very early on as an effective form of therapy (see Chapter 6). Marianus Sanctus Barolitanus (1555), Pare Johnson (1678), and de Marque (1618) recommended the use of plaster bandages, but firm support was not widely used until Wiseman (1676) introduced the laced leather stocking.[5] Compression therapy alone is associated with a high rate of ulcer recurrence,[6] but it may be quite effective in patients with limited venous dis-

1

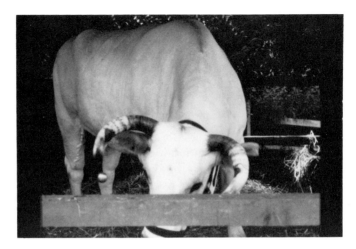

**Fig. A** Brahma bull with a varicose vein on the right posterior medial leg. (Courtesy A. Butie, M.D.)

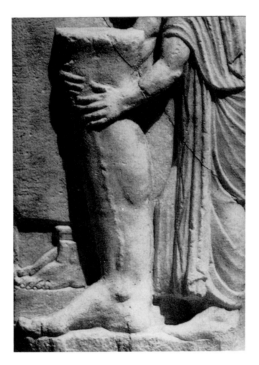

**Fig. B** According to the inscription, this tablet found on the west side of the acropolis in Athens was dedicated to Doctor Amynos by Lysimachidis of Archarnes. This represents the earliest known depiction of varicose veins from the end of the fourth century BC. (From National Archaeological Museum of Greece.)

ease.[7] To be effective, a compression bandage must generate 40 to 70 mm Hg.[8] This means that the toes of a correctly bandaged leg must become slightly cyanotic when the leg is horizontal and return to a pink color on standing.

The first use of an intravenous injection in a human has been attributed to Sigismund Eisholtz (1623-1688). He used an enema syringe to inject distilled plantain water into a branch of the crural vein to irrigate an ulcer by means of a small syphon.[12] In 1682, D. Zollikofer of St. Gallen, Switzerland, reported on the injection of an acid into a vein to create a thrombus.[12]

Intravascular sclerotherapy of varicose veins was first performed in 1840 with a solution of absolute alcohol.[15] In 1851 a solution of ferric chloride was used for sclerotherapy,[16] shortly after the introduction of the hypodermic syringe in 1845 by Rynd.[17,18] The syringe of Rynd and the subsequently modified syringe of Pravaz were both modifications of the lachrimal syringe developed by Anel in 1713.[19] In the early part of this century, many different compounds were tried as sclerosing agents (see box below). These included the following: 50% grape sugar,[20] mercury biiodide,[21] 20% and 30% sodium salicylate,[22,23] sodium citrate,[24] 20% to 30% sodium chloride,[24] 1% bichloride of mercury,[25] 50% to 60% calorose (75% invert sugar with 5% saccharose),[26] and 12% quinine sulfate with 6% urethane.[26] These substances were widely used but resulted in unacceptable levels of allergic reactions, necrosis, pain, and even fatalities.[27-29] It was not until the advent of new sclerosing agents in the 1930s to 1950s that sclerotherapy treatment was reestablished (primarily in Europe) as a viable form of treatment

---

### HISTORICAL INTRODUCTION OF SCLEROSING AGENTS

| | |
|---|---|
| 1840 | Absolute alcohol (Monteggio, Leroy D'Etiolles) |
| 1851-1853 | Ferric chloride (Pravaz) |
| 1855 | Iodo-tannic liquer (Desgranges) |
| 1880 | "Chloral" (Negretti) |
| 1904 | 5% Phenol solution (Tavel) |
| 1906 | Potassium iodo-iodine (Tavel) |
| 1910 | "Sublime" (Scharf) |
| 1917 | Hypertonic glucose/calorose (Kausch) |
| 1919 | Sodium salicylate (Sicard and Gaugier) |
| 1919 | Sodium bicarbonate (Sicard and Gaugier) |
| 1920 | Bichloride of mercury (Wolf) |
| 1922 | 12% Quinine sulfate with 6% urethane (Geneurier) |
| 1922 | Biiodine of mercury (Lacroix, Bazelis) |
| 1926 | Hypertonic saline with procaine (Linser) |
| 1927 | 50% Grape sugar (Doerffel) |
| 1929 | Sodium citrate (Kern and Angel) |
| 1929 | 20%-30% Hypertonic saline (Kern and Angel) |
| 1930 | Sodium morrhuate (Higgins and Kittel) |
| 1933 | Chromated glycerine (Sclermo) (Jausion) |
| 1937 | Ethanolamine oleate (Biegeleisen) |
| 1946 | Sodium tetradecyl sulfate (Sotradecol) (Reiner) |
| 1949 | Phenolated mercury and ammonium (Tournay and Wallois) |
| 1959 | Stabilized polyiodated ions (Variglobin) (Imhoff and Sigg) |
| 1966 | Polidocanol (Aetoxisclerol) (Henschel and Eichenberg) |
| 1969 | Hypertonic saline/dextrose (Sclerodex) |

Modified from Goldman MP and Bennett RG: Treatment of telangiectasia: a review, J Am Acad Dermatol 17:167, 1987.

for varicose veins. However, clinical results of sclerotherapy treatment were less optimal than those obtained with surgical approaches.

Although Orbach[30] points out that the use of compression therapy for treatment of venous disease is mentioned in the Old Testament and was performed by Hippocrates in the fourth century BC, it has been used in sclerosing treatment of varicose veins only within the last 30 years. Postsclerosis compression, initially described by Sigg[31] and Orbach[32] in the 1950s and Fegan in the 1960s,[33] is perhaps the most important advance in sclerotherapy treatment of varicose veins since the introduction of relatively safe synthetic sclerosing agents in the 1940s. With the advent of "compression" sclerotherapy, clinical results equal to surgical procedures are now reported.

Hobbs,[2] Lofgren,[9] and Beninson[10] have pointed out that the treatment of varicosities per se may have no effect on alleviating superficial venous pressure. It is the treatment of the underlying communicating or perforating veins draining the gaiter area that is important.[2,6,11-13] These vessels may be either surgically ligated[6,11-13] or sclerosed.[2] Only then will the retrograde flow under high pressure via the calf muscle pump be diverted upstream and away from the skin. This will succeed in a lowering of the cuticular venous pressure and decreased capillary permeability and edema, thus increasing tissue oxygenation and nutrition.

## PRESENT DAY TREATMENT

Sclerotherapy, as practiced today, has been shown to be as effective as comparable surgical procedures (ligation and stripping) in long-term follow-up studies for most types of varicose veins excluding those with significant saphenofemoral incompetence.[34-37] Modern sclerotherapy has also been demonstrated to result in a relief of symptoms in up to 85% of patients with both varicose[38] and telangiectatic veins.[39] In addition, sclerotherapy treatment has been demonstrated to be a more physiologic approach to eliminating the abnormal varicose veins. One study of dissected cadaver legs demonstrated that over 50% of the patients with significant varicose veins had a normal greater saphenous system, suggesting that vein stripping may be an inappropriate procedure in a significant percentage of patients.[40]

Perhaps even more significant in this age of cost control, sclerotherapy treatment has been demonstrated to be much less costly than surgical procedures in the treatment of varicose veins.[41-44] In lieu of the inpatient hospital ligation and stripping operation, sclerotherapy treatment is performed on an outpatient basis with the patient able to return to work immediately after the procedure. At times, however, when saphenofemoral incompetence is present, a limited ligation and stripping procedure followed by sclerotherapy 3 to 6 weeks later may be necessary. Because of the "limited" nature of the procedure (as described in Chapter 10), hospitalization is usually not required, and the procedure is performed instead in an outpatient surgical facility. In addition to the cost savings, patient preference for outpatient sclerotherapy has been a major reason for the modernization of varicose vein treatment.[41] This preference has even occurred despite the recurrence of varicose veins (usually to a minor degree) in 88% of patients in whom sclerotherapy alone was performed.[41]

Most importantly, treatment of "early" varicose veins is thought to halt the progression into larger, more severe varices.[45,46] Early treatment may prevent the development of valvular incompetence. Also, treatment is easier to perform on early varicosities.

Patients seek therapy for telangiectasias or varicose veins principally because of their unsightly appearance. However, proper treatment is frequently difficult to find because correct surgical intervention and sclerotherapy are largely untaught in medical school or in residency programs. Frequently, patients with telangiectasias of the legs are told that they must live with the problem. Treatment options, including sclerotherapy, are either not discussed or are mentioned disparagingly. However, available evidence indicates that safe, effective forms of treatment other than surgery are possible and quite successful. In addition to the cosmetic benefits of sclerotherapy, studies have demonstrated that sclerotherapy treatment of incompetent perforating veins increases the efficacy of the calf muscle pump, resulting in an improved clearance of extravascular fluid.[14] Today, fortunately, physicians specializing in the treatment of venous disease (phlebologists, dermatologists, and vascular surgeons) can offer relatively simple treatments for this widespread medical ailment.

In summary, the presence of varicose and telangiectatic veins is not a normal physical finding but a medical disease deserving of treatment. Varicose and telangiectatic veins may be symptomatic, representing an obvious manifestation of venous disease with its resultant complications, and may pose medical risks and complications in and of themselves. The only advantages to having varicose veins according to Hippocrates are that "The bald are not subject to varicose veins; but should they occur, the hairs are reproduced," and "If varicose veins or hemorrhoids occur during mania, the mania is cured."[47]

Fortunately, the majority of patients with varicose and telangiectatic veins do not have a life-threatening problem. Therefore, treatment should be as simple as possible, with the least risk of significant side effects. Modern sclerotherapy treatment has been demonstrated to fulfill these requirements with efficacy comparable to operative procedures. This text examines the pathophysiology and practical application of sclerotherapy treatment for varicose veins and telangiectasias through a review of the world literature, presentation of experimental studies, and recommendations derived from my clinical practice and the practices of the contributing authors.

## REFERENCES

1. Butie A: Personal communication, 1989.
2. Hobbs JT: The problem of the post-thrombotic syndrome, Postgrad Med (Aug Supp):48, 1973.
3. Strandness DE Jr and Thiele BL: Selected topics in venous disorders, Mt Kisco, NY, 1981, Futura Publishing Co.
4. Benton W: Hippocratic writings on ulcers, Chicago, 1970, Brittanica Great Books.
5. Browse NL, Burnand KG, and Thomas ML: Diseases of the veins: pathology, diagnosis, and treatment, London, 1988, Edward Arnold.
6. Negus D and Friedgood A: The effective management of venous ulceration, Br J Surg 70:623, 1983.
7. Morris WT and Lamb AM: The Auckland Hospital varicose veins and venous ulcer clinic: a report on six years work, NZ Med J 93:350, 1981.
8. Leu HJ: Differential diagnosis of chronic leg ulcers, Angiology 14:288, 1963.
9. Lofgren EP: Leg ulcers: symptoms of an underlying disorder, Postgrad Med 76:51, 1984.
10. Gravatational eczema. In Rook A et al (editors): Textbook of dermatology, ed 4, Cambridge, Ma, 1986, Blackwell Scientific Publications Inc.
11. Cockett FB and Thomas ML: The iliac compression syndrome, Br J Surg 52:816, 1965.
12. Kwaan JHM, Jones RN, and Connolly JE: Simplified technique for the management of refractory varicose ulcers, Surgery 80:743, 1976.
13. Lim LT, Michuda M, and Bergan JJ: Therapy of peripheral vascular ulcers: surgical management, Angiology 29:654, 1978.
14. Raso AM et al: Studio su 357 casi di flebite degli arti inferiori su due campioni interregionali, Minerva Chir 34:553, 1979.
15. Schneider W: Contribution to the history of the sclerosing treatment of varices and to its anatomo-pathologic study, Soc Fran de Phlebol 18:117, 1965.

16. Charles-Gabriel Pravas: Compt Rend Acad Sc 236:88, 1953.
17. Garrison FH: An introduction to the history of medicine, Philadelphia, 1929, Saunder Co.
18. Rynd F: Neuralgia: introduction of fluid to the nerve, Dublin Med Press 13:167, 1845.
19. Anel D: Nouvelle methode de guerir les fistules lacrimales, on recueil de defferentes pieces pour et contre, et en faveur de la meme methode nouvellement inventee, Turin Zappatte, 1713.
20. Doerffel: Klinisches und Experimentelles uber Venenverodung mit Kochsalzlosung und Traubenzucker, Deutsche Med Wohnschr 53:901, 1927.
21. Bazelis R: Thesis de doctorate, Paris, 1924.
22. Schwartz E and Ratschow M: Experimentelle und Klinische erfahrungen bei der Kunstlichen Verodung von Varicen, Arch Klin Chir 156:720, 1929.
23. Meisen V: A lecture on injection-treatment of varicose veins and their sequelae (eczema and ulcus cruris), clinically and experimentally, Acta Scand 60:435, 1926.
24. Kern HM and Angle LW: The chemical obliteration of varicose veins: a clinical and experimental study, JAMA 93:595, 1929.
25. Wolf E: Die histologischen Veranderungen der Venen nach intravenosen sub limatein Spritzungen, Med Klin 16:806, 1920.
26. Lufkin NH and McPheeters HO: Pathological studies on injected varicose veins, Surg Gynecol Obstet 54:511, 1932.
27. D'Addato M: Gangrene of a limb with complete thrombosis of the venous system, J Cardiovas Surg (Torino) 7:434, 1966.
28. Hohlbaum J: Todliche Embolie nach Varicenbehandlung mit Preglosung, Zentralbl Chir 7:218, 1922.
29. Hempel C: Erfahrungen mit Sublimatinjektichen bei Varizen, Deutsche Med Wochenschr 71:900, 1924.
30. Orbach EJ: Compression therapy of vein and lymph vessel diseases of the lower extremities, Angiology 30:95, 1979.
31. Sigg K: The treatment of varicosities and accompanying complications, Angiology 3:355, 1952.
32. Orbach EJ: A new approach to the sclerotherapy of varicose veins, Angiology 1:302, 1950.
33. Fegan WG: Continuous compression technique of injecting varicose veins, Lancet 2:109, 1963.
34. Hobbs JT: The treatment of varicose veins: a random trial of injection/compression versus surgery, Br J Surg 55:777, 1968.
35. Hobbs JT: Surgery and sclerotherapy in the treatment of varicose veins: a random trial, Arch Surg 109:793, 1974.
36. Chant ADB, Jones HO, and Wendell JM: Varicose veins: a comparison of surgery and injection/compression sclerotherapy, Lancet 2:1188, 1972.
37. Henry MEF, Fegan WG, and Pegum JM: Five-year survey of the treatment of varicose ulcers, Br Med J 2:493, 1971.
38. Fegan G: Varicose Veins, London, 1967, William Heinemann Medical Books, Ltd.
39. Weiss R and Weiss M: Resolution of pain associated with varicose and telangiectatic leg veins after compression sclerotherapy, J Dermatol Surg Oncol 16:333, 1990.
40. Schwartz SI: Year book of surgery, Chicago, 1979, Year Book Medical Publishers.
41. Kistner RL et al: The evolving management of varicose veins, Postgrad Med 80:51, 1986.
42. Piachaud D and Weddell JM: Cost of treating varicose veins, Lancet 2:1191, 1972.
43. Doran FSA and White M: A clinical trial designed to discover if the primary treatment of varicose veins should be by Fegan's method or by operation, Br J Surg 62:72, 1975.
44. Beresford SAA et al: Varicose veins: a comparison of surgery and injection/compression sclerotherapy five year follow-up, Lancet 1:921, 1978.
45. Gallagher PG: Major contributing role of sclerotherapy in the treatment of varicose veins, Vascular Surgery 20:139, 1986.
46. Ludbrook J: Valvular defect in primary varicose veins: cause or effect? Lancet 2:1289, 1963.
47. Coar T: The aphorisms of Hippocrates: with a translation into Latin and English, London, 1822, Longman and Co.

# 1   Anatomy and Histology of the Venous System of the Leg

The venous system of the lower extremities functions as a conduit for carrying deoxygenated blood from the muscles and cutaneous and subcutaneous tissues to the heart and also functions as a reservoir of blood. Although all veins have a similar structure, the particular functions of the venous system of the leg are imposed by their surroundings. When covered by muscle and fascia, the deep veins serve as a transport system. Depending on the tension of the perivenous tissues, deep veins may either draw blood from the superficial veins or pump blood towards the heart. External to the fascia and muscles, superficial veins serve primarily as reservoirs with limited transport capability.

## ANATOMY

The venous system of the lower limbs consists of two channels: one within the muscular system and one superficial to it (Fig. 1-1). Along most of their course, veins are intimately associated with both arteries and nerves. In certain locations this association assumes clinical and therapeutic importance. The short saphenous vein (SSV) is intimately connected with the tibial and sural nerves that are located equidistant either medial or lateral to the vein. This may explain the pain that occurs when this vein is varicose (Fig. 1-2).[1] When the SSV terminates into the long saphenous vein (LSV) in the midthigh, it lies very close to the sciatic nerve. This is important because varicose veins in this location may press on the nerve and cause a "sciatica"-like pain.[1]

Careless surgical exploration or excessive perivascular inflammation may cause a neuralgia to nearby nerves and damage to adjacent arteries. The saphenous nerve is intimately associated with the LSV or the SSV at the level of the knee joint after it emerges from the subsartorial canal (Fig. 1-3). It lies along the vein anteriorly through the leg to the medial aspect of the dorsum of the foot before dividing into branches that supply the medial toes.[2] The superficial external pudendal artery is intimately associated with the LSV at the saphenofemoral junction where it may bifurcate to enclose the LSV (Fig. 1-4). Twin gastrocnemius arteries and a smaller lesser saphenous artery also occur in intimate association with the LSV within the calf.

The principal deep veins are the femoral and popliteal/tibial veins. These begin in the foot as plantar digital veins. These veins as well as other deep veins in the body contain one-way valves, located every few centimeters, which direct blood flow towards the heart (see Fig. 1-1). If the valve cusps do not meet and therefore the blood flows away from the heart as well as towards it, the valve is defined as being incompetent. In addition, within the soleal muscle are thin-walled venous reservoirs that are valveless and number from 1 to 18. They are usually linked to one another by venous channels (which contain valves) and empty high in the calf into the posterior tibial veins.[6] It should be emphasized that through the action of muscular compression almost 90% of all venous blood leaves the legs by the deep veins (Fig. 1-5).[1,3] Fluoroscopic study has demonstrated that with muscular exercise, blood is drawn from the superficial veins

*Text continued on p. 12.*

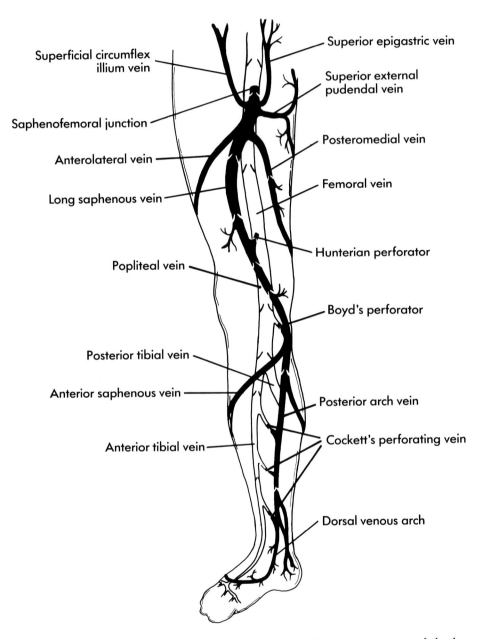

**Fig. 1-1** Simplistic diagram of the major veins within the venous system of the lower limbs.

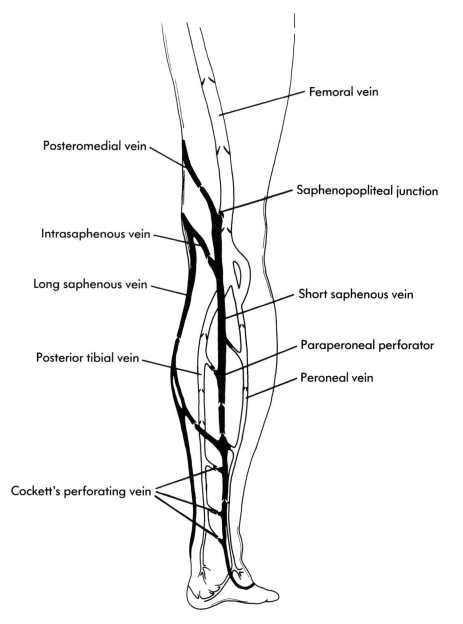

**Fig. 1-1 cont'd.**    For legend see opposite page.

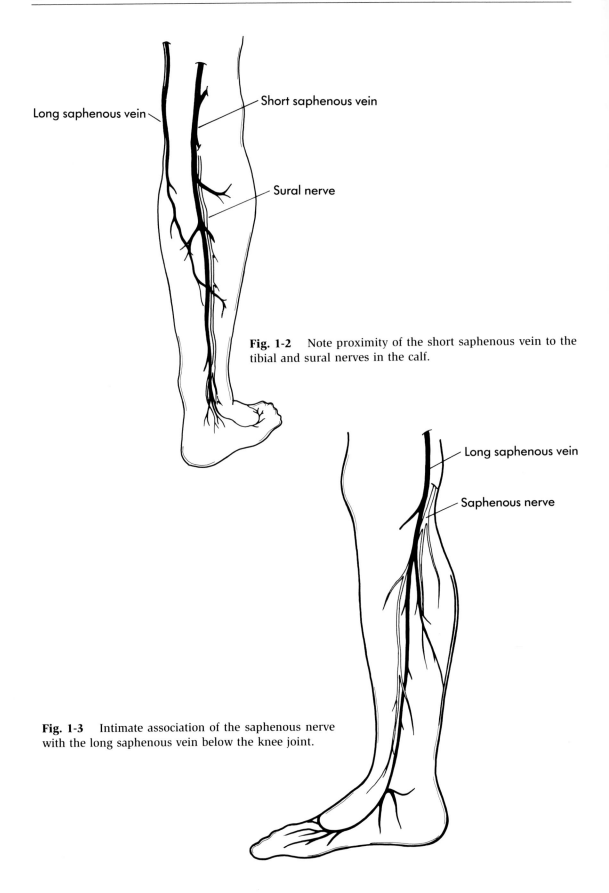

Long saphenous vein

Short saphenous vein

Sural nerve

**Fig. 1-2** Note proximity of the short saphenous vein to the tibial and sural nerves in the calf.

Long saphenous vein

Saphenous nerve

**Fig. 1-3** Intimate association of the saphenous nerve with the long saphenous vein below the knee joint.

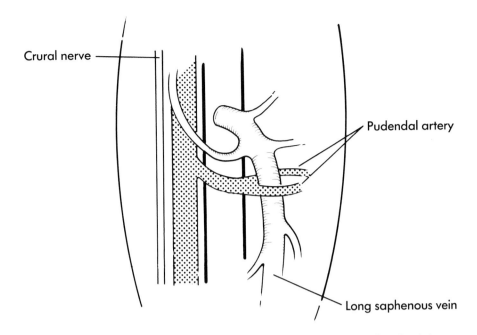

**Fig. 1-4**    Illustration of a possible association of a bifurcated external pudendal artery at the saphenofemoral junction.

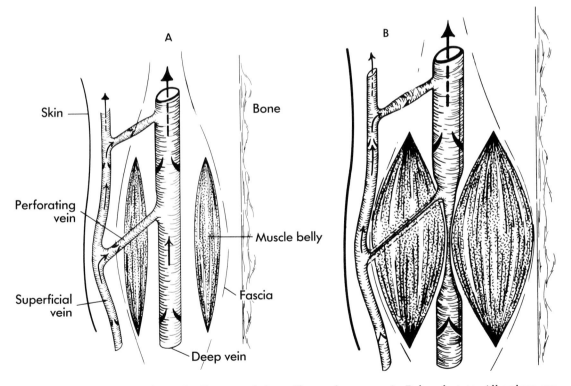

**Fig. 1-5**    Schematic diagram of the calf muscle pump. **A,** Relaxed state. All valves are open, allowing blood to flow in a proximal direction. Blood flows proximal in both the superficial vein and through the perforating vein into the deep veins. Note the fascial covering of the "deep system." **B,** With muscle contraction, the perforating veins are squeezed closed. Valves distal to the compression are closed to prevent distal blood flow.

through the communicating veins into the deep venous system (Fig. 1-6).[4] The only exception to the inward direction of blood flow is in the foot where the perforating vein valves allow flow from the deep to the superficial veins.[5] In addition, the majority of pedal perforating veins usually do not contain valves. Finally, occlusion of the superficial veins of the leg produces a flow of blood from the superficial to the deep pedal veins.[6] Thus a muscle pump in the foot also provides an important mechanism for venous return. This has been demonstrated using video-phlebography[7] and duplex scanning[8] to be activated by weight-bearing even in patients with underlying venous insufficiency. Therefore, except for the unique anatomic arrangement of the deep and superficial veins of the foot, the deep venous system is important in maintaining the functional cardiovascular system. This system is correctly termed the *calf muscle pump* or *peripheral heart*.[9]

## Venous Valvular System

Fabricius of Aquapendente (1533-1620) was the first to detail the anatomy of veins and their valves. He suggested that valves " . . . ensure a fair distribution of the blood . . . prevent distention . . . and stop blood from flooding into the limb. . . ."[10] Since venous valves comprise the weakest link in the calf muscle pump, an understanding of the pathophysiology of normal and diseased valves is crucial. Studies of the embryologic development of veins show that the number of venous valves decreases in utero with fetal maturity. It has been suggested that this disappearance continues, albeit at a reduced but variable rate, during childhood, adolescence, and adult life.[11-13] However, an autopsy study of 178 subjects without venous disorders and 70 subjects with primary varicose veins failed to demonstrate a decreased number of venous valves in advanced-age groups.[14] This was confirmed in a study of 50 cadaver long saphenous veins.[15] Here, the mean number of valves (7.0) in 23 veins at ages from 17 to 59 years was not significantly different from the mean number of valves (7.2) in 27 veins at ages 60 to 90 years. Therefore, aging in itself does not appear to produce a decrease in

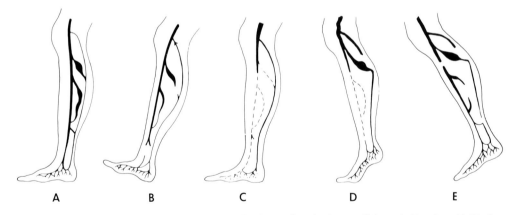

| A | B | C | D | E |

**Fig. 1-6** Sequence of blood flow within the lower leg during walking. **A,** Resting. **B,** Early contraction with the heel pressed and gastrocnemius muscle beginning contraction. **C,** Full contraction of all muscles. **D,** Knee flexion with contraction of the soleus muscle and relaxation of the gastrocnemius. **E,** Relaxation of all muscles. (Redrawn from Almen T and Nylander G: Serial phlebography of the normal leg during muscle contraction and relaxation, Acta Radiol 57:264, 1962.)

venous valves of the leg. There also does not appear to be a difference in the number of venous valves between men and women.[1]

The number of venous valves has been found to be decreased in varicose veins as compared to normal veins. Since age and sex in themselves do not decrease valvular number, other factors must contribute to the loss of venous valves. Two potential causes of valvular dysfunction are fibrosis caused by turbulent high pressure blood flow and a hereditary defect in vein wall and/or valvular support.

When competent, venous valves can withstand pressures of up to 3 atmospheres.[16] Therefore, for valvular damage to occur, the vein diameter must first dilate to render the valves incompetent (Fig. 1-7). This is supported by investigations that show that there is no difference in visoelastic behavior in perivalvular vein wall tissue.[17] Chronic venous dilation may produce a strain on valves leading to their sclerosis. This is postulated to occur through the production of turbulent blood flow. Fegan[18] reasons that turbulence, once established, interferes with the blood supply to the vein wall via the vasa vasorum or subjects the collagen fibers to an abnormal stress. Either or both of these changes lead to atrophic changes of the valves. This theory is supported by a study of 75 cadaver veins and 75 stripped veins from the medial malleolus to the saphenofemoral junction that demonstrated a statistically significant decrease in the number of valves in varicose veins (6.0 +/− 1.7) compared to normal veins (7.3 +/− 2.3).[15] Although 33 of 156 valves in varicose veins were sclerosed on examination after removal or autopsy, no evidence of sclerosis of the venous valves of normal veins was apparent.[15] However, sinus wall and valvular defects have been found in autopsy studies of up to 90% of adults without apparent varicosities.[19] Therefore, valve and valvular sinus abnormalities at best comprise only one factor in the development of varicose veins. A full explanation of the pathophysiologic significance of valvular deficiency and dysfunction is addressed later in Chapter 3 in the section on primary valvular incompetence.

The deep venous system is connected through multiple channels to superfi-

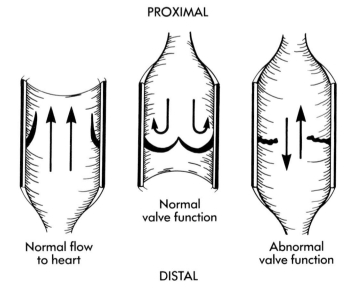

**Fig. 1-7**   Diagram of normal and abnormal valvular function caused by venous dilation.

cial veins. Thus many alternate routes are available for blood to return to the heart after blockage of any main vein such as the femoral vein. Superficial veins provide a pathway for venous return from the cutaneous and subcutaneous systems through the action of their one-way valves.[20] An anatomic study of the superficial venous system in 60 cadaveric limbs disclosed a marked diversity in the anatomy. No two limbs exhibited the same superficial venous arrangement.[21] However, some consistent patterns do exist as described next.

**Long saphenous vein.** The most prominent superficial vein is the long (great) saphenous vein (LSV). (The term saphenous is derived from the Greek word for visible.) This vein begins on the dorsum of the foot as a dorsal venous arch. It passes anterior to the medial malleolus and crosses the tibia obliquely, continuing along the medial aspect of the leg across the anteromedial thigh to empty into the common femoral vein (Fig. 1-8). There are many variations in the termination of the LSV into the femoral vein, which are discussed in Chapter 10. In over 80% of cases, the LSV lies on the deep fascia enclosed by a loose compartment of fat and areolar tissue.[21] Detailed dissection has noted only two perforating veins above the posterior tibial perforator connecting the LSV to the deep system.[21] Therefore, ligation at the saphenofemoral junction with a limited stripping (above the knee) is more anatomically correct than complete ligation and stripping to the ankle as formerly practiced (see Chapter 10).

The LSV receives multiple tributaries along its course. These may lie in a less supported, more superficial plane to the membranous fascia. The posterior arch vein, the anterior superficial tibial vein, and the medial superficial pedal vein join it in the lower leg. Two large tributaries from the posteromedial and anterolateral thigh join it proximally. These veins usually enter the LSV before it pierces the deep fascia. Both the medial and lateral superficial thigh veins may be so large as to be mistaken for the LSV itself.[22] A parallel, more superficial, thin-walled vein is seen frequently directly over or just posterior to the LSV. Finally, in the thigh the LSV may be duplicated, with the length of the duplication being variable.

The most constant perforating vein in the thigh connects the LSV to the femoral vein in the adductor (Hunter's) canal. A variable number of perforators connect the LSV to the posterior tibial, gastrocnemius, and soleal veins.[23]

**Short saphenous vein.** The most prominent and physiologically important superficial vein below the knee is the short (lesser) saphenous vein (SSV). This major tributary begins at the lateral aspect of the foot and ascends posterior to the lateral malleolus as a continuation of the dorsal venous arch. It continues up the calf between the gastrocnemius heads to the popliteal fossa, ending in the popliteal or great saphenous veins (Fig. 1-9).

The termination of the SSV is quite variable. Dodd and Cockett[24] were among the earliest to study the termination of the SSV. In the majority of patients evaluated, the SSV ended in the popliteal vein. In 33% it terminated above the level of the popliteal fossae, either directly with the LSV or with other deep veins. In 15.3% the SSV communicated with the popliteal vein, then continued on to terminate in the LSV. And in 9.7% the SSV emptied into the LSV or the deep veins below the popliteal fossae. The SSV, like the LSV, runs on or within the deep fascia. It usually pierces the deep fascia just below the flexor crease of the knee as it passes into the popliteal fossa. Gross incompetence of the SSV usually occurs only in areas where the SSV and its tributaries are superficial to the deep fascia, on the lateral calf and lower third of the leg behind the lateral malleolus.

The SSV often receives substantial tributaries from the medial aspect of the

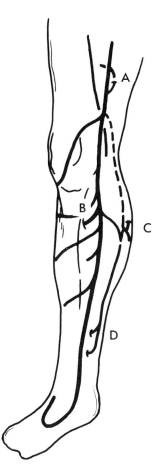

**Fig. 1-8** Typical course of the LSV including its common tributaries and perforating veins. *A,* Hunterian perforating vein; *B,* posterior tibial perforating vein; *C,* calf perforator in location of the intrasaphenous vein; *D,* medial ankle or Cockett perforators. (Redrawn from Thompson H: The surgical anatomy of the superficial and perforating veins of the lower limb, Ann R Col Surg (Eng) 61:198, 1979.)

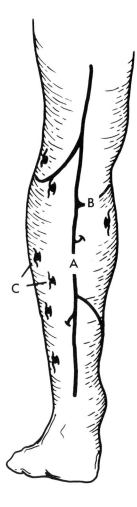

**Fig. 1-9** Typical course of the short saphenous vein with termination above the popliteal fossae and associated perforator veins. *A,* SSV; *B,* intersaphenous vein with calf perforator; *C,* paraperoneal perforating veins. (Redrawn from Thompson H: The surgical anatomy of the superficial and perforating veins of the lower limb, Ann R Col Surg (Eng) 61:198, 1979.)

ankle, thereby communicating with the medial ankle perforators.[20] It may also connect directly with the LSV.

**Other superficial veins.** Other prominent and consistent superficial veins are the accessory saphenous vein, which runs from the lateral knee to the saphenofemoral junction; the anterior crural veins, which run from the lower lateral calf to the medial knee; and the infragenicular vein, which drains the skin around the knee. In addition, there are many unnamed tributaries to the saphenous vein that may become dilated and tortuous through an increase in venous pressure. These reticular or connecting branch veins are apparent clinically, especially in patients with light-colored skin. They may merely represent a normal "reticular" network of subcutaneous veins or, when under high pressure, they may be grossly varicose. As they bulge out from the cutaneous surface they darken in color. Otherwise, infrared photography may be necessary to visualize their presence.[25] Their differentiation from the major venous system is critical when planning treatment.

**Perforating/communicating veins.** Perforating/communicating veins were first described in 1803 by Van Loder.[26] They occur from the ankle to the groin, connecting the deep veins to the superficial veins. The average number per leg has been found to be as much as 155[27] or as few as 64.[21] They usually contain one to three one-way valves depending on their length. The one-way valves serve to prevent the high venous pressure (from muscle contraction) from being transmitted to the superficial veins. Normally, perforating veins are thin-walled, varying in diameter from less than 1 mm to 2 mm in diameter.[26] They are invariably accompanied by an artery.

Anatomically, there are two types of perforating veins: direct and indirect. Direct perforators connect the superficial and deep veins without interruption. Indirect perforators connect the deep and superficial veins via muscular venous channels. Perforator veins usually run an oblique course through the deep fascia between muscle bundles. They are commonly located on either side of the sartorius and peroneal muscles and between the vastus lateralis and hamstrings. However, their course beneath the deep fascia may be variable (Fig. 1-10).[28] With muscular movement, the deep fascia is tightened. This puts the perforator veins under tension, which closes the veins and prevents blood from escaping from the deep veins of the calf muscle pump into the superficial veins (see Fig. 1-5). Although variable in exact location, a number of perforating veins occur with marked regularity (Table 1-1).

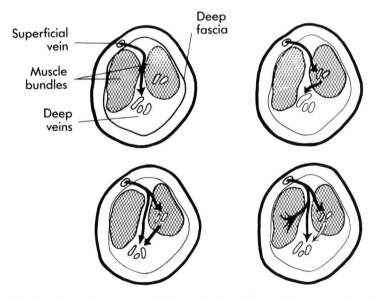

**Fig. 1-10** Perforating veins can travel through the calf muscles connecting the deep to the superficial veins in various paths.

**Table** 1-1    Distribution of incompetent perforator veins on 901 lower limbs

| | Percent of limbs with incompetent veins | |
| --- | --- | --- |
| **Perforator veins** | **Right limbs** | **Left limbs** |
| Saphenofemoral junction | 100 | 100 |
| Saphenopopliteal junction | 15 | 15.5 |
| Mid-Hunterian perforator | 7 | 6.7 |
| Genicular perforator | 2.9 | 1.6 |
| Lateral thigh perforators | 1.8 | 1.3 |
| 13.5-cm midcalf Cockett | 15.9 | 17.3 |
| 18.5-cm midcalf Cockett | 34.3 | 35.2 |
| 24-cm midcalf Cockett | 20 | 19.6 |
| 30-cm midcalf Cockett | 13 | 12.7 |
| 35-cm midcalf Cockett | 6.6 | 7 |
| 40-cm midcalf Cockett | 4.2 | 3.1 |
| Calf perforators (other) | 12 | 11.2 |
| Gastrocnemius/peroneal muscle perforator | 25 | 24 |
| Anterior tibialis/peroneal perforator | 3.1 | 2.9 |
| Lateral tibial perforators | 0.02 | 0.04 |
| Lateral foot perforators | 2 | 2.4 |
| Medial foot perforators | 3.5 | 2.9 |

Modified from Sherman RS: Varicose veins: further findings based on anatomic and surgical disections, Ann Surg 130:218, 1949.

**Table** 1-2    Clinically important communicating veins

| Name | Location |
| --- | --- |
| Submalleolar | Medial; retromalleolar |
| Cockett's | Medial; 7, 12, and 18 cm above medial malleolus |
| Boyd's | Medial; 10 cm below knee joint |
| Lateral leg | Lateral; variable in location |
| Midcalf (soleus and gastrocnemius points) | Posterior, 5 and 12 cm above os calcis |
| Dodd's (Hunterian) | Medial thigh (mid or distal) |

Perforator veins are presumed to play a fundamental role in the production of varicose veins.[29] An anatomic examination of 901 limbs found that the number of incompetent perforators in patients with varicose veins varied from 1 to 14.[29] The distribution of these perforators is detailed in Table 1-1, with clinically important communicating veins listed in Table 1-2. When perforator veins are incompetent, the resulting high pressure is transmitted directly from the deep veins of the calf muscle pump to the superficial veins. This causes dilation of the associated superficial veins (Fig. 1-11).[26,30] When incompetent, perforating veins become thick-walled and may reach a diameter of 5 mm or more.[31] They also have a larger central diameter than peripheral diameter. This causes the reflux blood flow to enter the superficial veins at high velocity and may contribute to the development of localized fascial defects and bulging varicosities.[32]

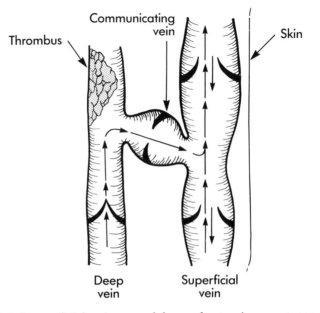

**Fig. 1-11**   Dilated superficial vein caused by perforator incompetence resulting from deep vein thrombosis blocking proximal flow of blood in the deep venous system. Note that with dilation of the superficial vein the valves are no longer competent.

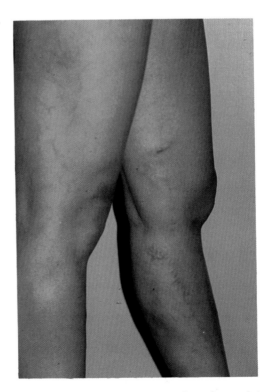

**Fig. 1-12**   Incompetent LSV with a competent saphenofemoral junction via incompetence of a Hunterian perforating vein demonstrated by venous Doppler examination.

There are one or two relatively constant perforating veins in the thigh associated with the medial intramuscular septum known as the Hunterian or Dodd's perforator(s). These connect the LSV to the femoral vein in the middle medial thigh and the middle lower third of the thigh.[33] These perforators are found in about 50% of dissected limbs. Many other perforators exist, but with the exception of the Hunterian perforator, they pierce muscles. The protection afforded by these muscles seems to preclude the possibility of these veins becoming incompetent.[34] Incompetence of the Hunterian perforator is a common cause for medial thigh varicose veins in patients with a competent saphenofemoral junction (Fig. 1-12).

Multiple smaller perforating veins may be present in the middle third of the lateral aspect of the thigh and the midline of the posterior thigh. These connect the LSV and its tributaries to the profunda femoris vein.

The posterior tibial perforator occurs in almost all limbs and connects the LSV to the posterior tibial veins. It is found approximately 5 to 10 cm distal to the knee on the medial calf.

Multiple perforating veins are also found with regularity along the medial calf. These connect the SSV to the gastrocnemius veins. When they occur adjacent to the peroneal muscles, they are referred to as paraperoneal perforators. Some authors state that there are 16 constant perforating veins that may become incompetent. Eight of these drain into the posterior tibial vein and four into the gastrocnemius and soleal veins. It is thought that other smaller perforating veins that connect to the tibial vein rarely become incompetent because they are supported by muscles that take their origin from the deep surface of the fascia.

A group of perforating veins located from the medial ankle to the calf has been reported to occur 6 to 10 cm, 13.5 to 15 cm, 18.5 to 20 cm, and 24 to 25 cm above the sole of the foot along Linton's line.[29] This group is referred to as Cockett's perforators (Fig. 1-13). They serve to connect the posterior arch vein with the posterior tibial veins but do not drain directly into the LSV.[35] Recently, a radiographic and surgical study found no predilection for their occurrence at any height.[36] In addition, it was found that these perforators did not occur at the level

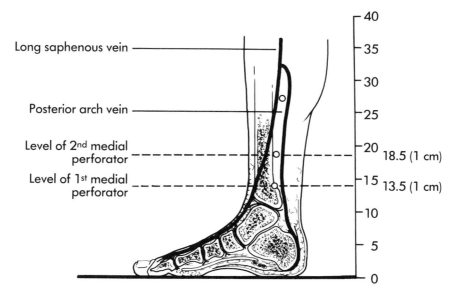

**Fig. 1-13**   Idealized illustration of the major Cockett perforating veins.

of Linton's line, but on a "lane" with a width of up to 3 cm. This latter study has dispelled some of the phlebologic dogma for predilection sites of perforating veins.

Perforating veins have also been described in the foot. Raivio has documented over 40.[37] One is situated about 2.5 cm below the inferior tip of the medial malleolus. A second one occurs about 3.5 cm below and anterior to the medial malleolus. The other two are on an arc about 3 cm anterior and below the medial malleolus. As previously mentioned, perforating veins in the foot have one-way valves that are reversed to allow blood to flow from the deep to the superficial veins.

## Fascial Envelope

The lower limb has a deep and a superficial fascia to contain the high-pressure calf muscle pump and support the deep venous system. The deep fascia is a dense fibrous membrane investing the entire lower limb like an elastic stocking and serves as a functional boundary between deep and superficial veins. The deep fascia is attached to the superficial fibers of the muscles it covers. The deep fascia is normally thin over the gastrocnemius muscles and is absent only over the perforating veins and fossa ovalis, the latter being protected by the cribriform fascia. Since the deep fascia surrounds the muscles of the limb and is relatively inextensible, contraction of the muscles causes a rise in pressure to all structures within its compartment.

The superficial fascia is composed of two layers: a superficial layer of loculated fatty tissue (Camper's fascia) and a deep layer of collagen and elastic tissue providing stronger support (Scarpa's fascia).[18] The superficial fascia covers the saphenous trunks[38] (Fig. 1-14), and tributaries to the saphenous veins are superficial to this. Since they are not within its support, tributaries to the great saphenous vein are usually more grossly dilated than the great saphenous vein itself, even when proximal high venous pressure produces the varicosity.[39] The super-

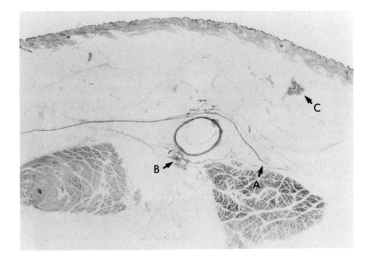

**Fig. 1-14**  Transverse section from the medial aspect of the thigh showing the fibrous envelope that ensheaths the LSV (*A*) and holds it against the deep fascia (*B*). A superficial tributary vein external to the fascia is visible (*C*). (Reproduced with permission from Thompson H: The surgical anatomy of the superficial and perforating veins of the lower limb, Ann R Col Surg (Eng) 61:198, 1979.)

ficial fascia is homologous with Scarpa's fascia of the anterior abdominal wall and may be considered as a single unit.[18] The superficial fascia in four-legged animals is said to provide a firmer support than that found in bipeds.[40] The support of the superficial fascia may partly explain why varicose veins affect humans and not quadrupeds.

Although the preceding description seems simple, connections between the superficial and deep venous systems and their fascial coverings are actually much more complicated. Detailed anatomic studies by Raivio[37] provide some explanation for this variability, but the importance of the knowledge of the variations in the system explains the need for individualization of treatment in a given patient.

# HISTOLOGY
## Vein Walls

The first part of the venous system consists of the venule, which serves as a collecting tube for capillaries. The venule is about 20 microns ($\mu$m) in diameter and consists of an endothelium surrounded by a fibrous tissue composed of a thin layer of collagenous fibers. The venule increases in diameter, with smooth muscle cells appearing within the fibrous sheath when the diameter is about 45 $\mu$m. At a diameter of 200 $\mu$m, the muscular layer becomes better defined. At a clinically recognizable diameter consistent with small venectasia, the vessels are composed of a thick media with myocytes. Collagenous fibers are clearly organized into bundles, and elastic fibers can be observed (see Chapter 3).[41] Larger diameters contain elastic fibers and a more organized structure (Fig. 1-15).

Microscopically, the normal young internal saphenous vein is a musculofibrous conduit with both passive and active function. The normal vein is slightly oval, with the short axis perpendicular to the skin. In response to an increase in intraluminal pressure, the diameter increases and the vein loses its oval appearance. Veins tend to assume an elliptical shape, particularly at low transmural pressures (Fig. 1-16). These qualities of shape deformability allow veins to change volume with very little force, thus aiding their role as a high capacitance system.[42,43] With continued increases in venous pressure or progression of varicose disease, the vein increases in both length and diameter and becomes tortuous. Whether normal or varicose, the saphenous vein is composed of three tunicas: intima, media, and adventitia (Fig. 1-17).

**Intima.** The intima is a thin structure consisting of a layer of endothelial cells and a deep fenestrated basement membrane bounded by a thin fragmented elastic lamina (Fig. 1-18).[9] The central portion of the cell containing the nucleus

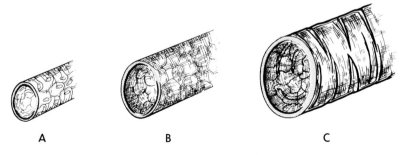

A                      B                      C

**Fig. 1-15**  Schematic illustration showing the walls of the blood vessels from capillary to vein. **A,** Capillary; **B,** venule; **C,** vein.

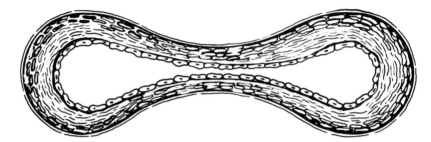

**Fig. 1-16**   Cross section of venous lumen. At high external pressures the vein collapses into an elliptical configuration. At low external pressures the vein assumes a circular to oval shape. (Modified from Moreno AH et al: Mechanics of distention of dog veins and other thin-walled tubular structures, Circ Res 27:1069, 1970. Permission granted by the American Heart Association, Inc.)

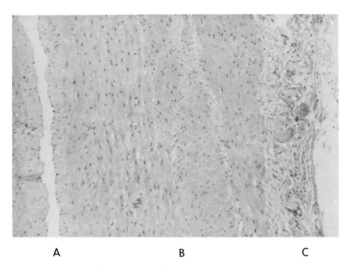

A                          B                          C

**Fig. 1-17**   Cross section of a fairly normal section from a varicose LSV from a 64-year-old man at the proximal thigh level. Three distinct layers are present. *A,* Intima; *B,* media; *C,* adventitia. (Hematoxylin-Eosin ×100.)

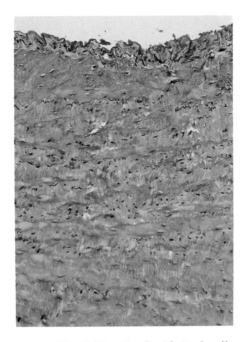

**Fig. 1-18**  Same specimen as Fig. 1-17 stained with Verhoeff-van Gieson (×150). Note some fragmentation of elastin fibers interspersed between muscle bundles with irregularity at the intima border. Elastic fibers stain black; collagen: red; muscle: brown-yellow.

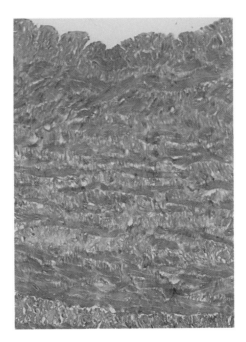

**Fig. 1-19**  Same specimen as Fig. 1-17 stained with Masson's trichrome (×150). Note the multiple layers of muscle bundles *(red)*.

bulges into the lumen and on its free surface exhibits multiple small microvilli. Although endothelial cells are easily destroyed by chemical and physical insults, they demonstrate a marked capacity for regeneration (see Chapter 7).[2]

**Media.** The media is composed of three layers of muscle bundles (Fig. 1-19). The inner layer consists of small bundles of longitudinally arranged muscle fibers. Loose connective tissue and small elastic fibrils separate the muscle bundles.[9] The middle layer is composed of wide bundles of smooth muscle in a circular orientation. The muscle bundles may be separated by thin or thick layers of elastic fibrils.[9] In addition, the outer layer is quite variable, being composed of longitudinal muscle bundles spread out through thick fibrous tissue. The outermost cells of the circular layer interdigitate with the innermost cells of the longitudinal layer to improve contractile efficiency.[44] The greatest extent of circular muscle occurs at the level of insertion of the valve leaflets; this region is the last to dilate in a varicose vein.[45] But this area is known to be dilated in primary valvular insufficiency.

**Adventitia.** The adventitia is the thickest portion of the vein wall. It is primarily composed of collagen whose interlacing fibers are oriented in a longitudinal, spiral, and circular fashion.[2] In larger vessels of the thigh, a considerable network of elastic fibers occurs and stretches from valve to valve.[18] The collagen layer merges with the perivenous connective tissue and contains the vasa vasorum and adrenergic nerve fibers.[46,47] The vasa vasorum composes the arteriovenous circulation in the wall of the blood vessel. As discussed later, alterations of the vasa vasorum may lead to the development of arteriovenous fistulas.

**Venous valves.** Venous valves are composed of a thin layer of collagen and a variable amount of smooth muscle covered on both surfaces by endothelium (Fig. 1-20).[48] An increase in muscle fibers is found at the base of the valve cusp running cicumferentially and longitudinally for a variable distance along the length of the valve cusp.[18] Elastic fibers extend along the whole length of the cusp and lie close to the endothelium. Collagen fibers are concentrated at the base, thinning out toward the free edge of the cusp. Fegan[18] proposes that the muscle fibers play an active role in regulating blood flow. Through performing anatomic dissection of multiple valves, he has come to believe that contraction of the circular muscles at the base of the valve reduces the vein diameter and contraction of the longitudinal fibers shortens and thickens the cusp. This type of coordinated muscle action maintains tone in the vein wall in the face of increased pressure from retrograde blood flow.

## Vein Wall Variations

The preceding description of the composition of vein walls is quite variable among various types and locations of veins. Depending on their location, veins assume many different functions. They are used as pumps and reservoirs and must withstand variations in gravitational and intravascular pressure demands. The muscular content of the vein wall also varies depending on the location of the vein. The percentage of smooth muscle increases with distal locations. Veins in the lower extremities are the only veins that are composed of greater than 40% smooth muscle, with veins in the foot having 60% to 80% smooth muscle as compared to 5% in axillary veins.[49] However, the hydrostatic pressure within the vein also correlates with smooth muscle content, with superficial veins having more smooth muscle than deep veins.[50] The differences in vein wall content may affect sclerotherapy treatment.

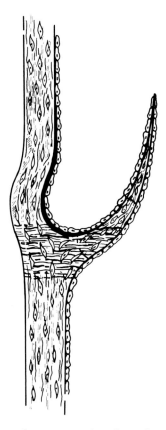

**Fig. 1-20**   Illustration of a cross section through a normal venous valve.

The function of vein wall collagen is to prevent overdistension, whereas elastin provides elastic recoil. With advancing age, multiple changes may occur in the vessel wall. The intima thickens increasing and disorienting elastic fibers.[9] The media develops a more disorganized arrangement of muscle bundles and hypertrophy of the outer muscular layer. Elastic fibers become more irregular and dystrophic. The elastic lamina becomes more fragmented, atrophic, thin, and irregular.[9] The adventitia becomes increasingly fibrous. Thus the lack of an organized elastic support and smooth muscle degeneration in an aged vein renders it more susceptible to pressure-induced distention.

Some histologic studies demonstrate that fibrotic wall changes are a common finding in the LSV in all age groups without venous disorders.[50] The incidence of fibrotic change increases from 25% to 50% in the population under 40 years of age to 100% in those over 70 years of age.[50]

## Venules

The venules in the upper and middermis usually run in a horizontal orientation. The diameter of the postcapillary venule ranges from 12 to 35 μm.[51] Collecting venules range from 40 to 60 μm in the upper and middermis and enlarge to 100 to 400 μm in diameter in the deeper tissues.[52] One-way valves are found at the subcutis (dermis)-adipose junction on the venous side of the circulation.[53] Valves are usually found in the area of anastomosis of small to large venules and also within larger venules unassociated with branching points. The free edges of the valves are always directed away from the smaller vessel and towards the larger and serve to direct blood flow towards the deeper venous system. The structure of these valves is identical to the valves found in deep and larger veins (Fig. 1-21).

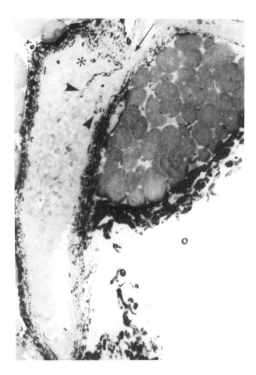

**Fig. 1-21** Valve-containing venule at the dermal-fat interface. Arrow indicates presumed direction of blood flow. Arrowheads indicate valve leaflets. Asterisk indicates open valve sinus; other sinus is closed because valve leaflet is in contact with vessel wall (1 μm section, ×485). (Reproduced with permission from Braverman IM and Keh-Yen A: Ultrastructure of the human dermal microcirculation. IV. Valve-containing collecting veins at the dermal-cutaneous junction, J Invest Dermatol 81:438, © by Williams & Wilkins, 1983.)

Postcapillary venules are composed of endothelial cells covered by a basement membrane, some collagen fibers, and, rarely, smooth muscle cells. Collecting veins in the deep dermis gradually receive more muscle cells until they become veins with a continuous muscle coat (see Fig. 1-15).[54,55] The schematic representation of the normal vascular structure of the skin and subcutaneous tissues in Fig. 1-22 details the intimate connections between the cutaneous veins and their underlying drainage pathways.

## Telangiectasias

Histologic examination of simple telangiectasias demonstrates dilated blood channels in a normal dermal stroma with a single endothelial cell lining, limited muscularis, and adventitia (Fig. 1-23).[56] Therefore, such vessels probably evolve from capillaries or early venules.

Blue-to-red arborizing telangiectasias of the lower extremities are probably dilated venules, possibly with intimate and direct connections to underlying larger veins of which they are direct tributaries (Fig. 1-24).[57-59] Electron microscopic examination of "sunburst" varicosities of the leg has demonstrated that these vessels are widened cutaneous veins.[60] They are found 175 to 382 μm below the stratum granulosum. The thickened vessel walls are composed of endothelial cells covered with collagen and muscle fibers. Elastic fibers are also present. Electron microscopy reveals an intercellular collagenous dysplasia, lat-

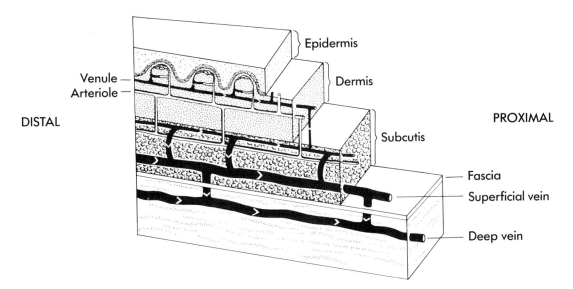

**Fig. 1-22**    Schematic diagram of the cutaneous and subcutaneous vascular plexus.

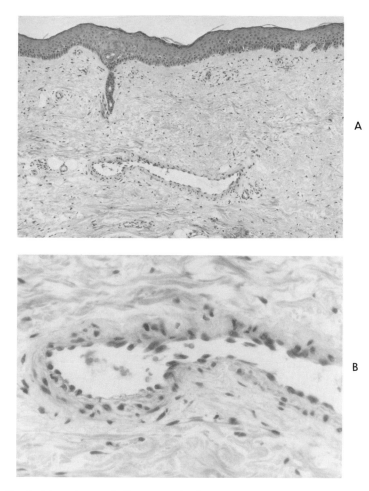

**Fig. 1-23**    Typical location and diameter of a linear telangiectasia on the thigh of a 45-year-old woman (hematoxylin − eosin; **A,** ×100; **B,** ×400).

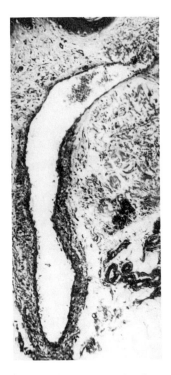

**Fig. 1-24** Leg telangiectasia arising from a venule. (Reproduced with permission from de Faria JL and Moraes IN: Histopathology of the telangiectasias associated with varicose veins, Dermatologia 127:321, 1963.)

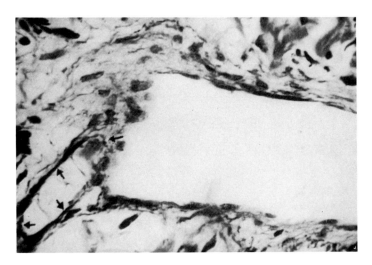

**Fig. 1-25** Leg telangiectasia arising from an arteriole. (Reproduced with permission from de Faria JL and Moraes IN: Histopathology of the telangiectasias associated with varicose veins, Dermatologia 127:321, 1963.)

tice collagen, and some matrix vesicles. These findings suggest that telangiectatic leg veins, like varicose veins, have an alteration of collagen metabolism of their walls. Therefore, like varicose veins, these veins are dysplastic.

Alternatively, arteriovenous anastomoses may result in the pathogenesis of telangiectasias. Faria and Moraes[59] demonstrated arteriovenous anastomoses in 1 of 26 biopsy specimens of leg telangiectasia (Fig. 1-25).

Skin biopsy of more unusual forms of telangiectasia such as unilateral nevoid telangiectasia may show an accumulation of mast cells.[61] In these cases the permanent vasodilation may be induced by the chronic release of one or more products of mast cells, particularly heparin.[62,63]

## Innervation

Innervation of the vein plays an important part in the regulation of venous tone. Different stimuli are known to produce venous constriction: pain, emotion, hyperventilation, deep breathing, Valsalva maneuver, on standing, and muscular exercise.[64] Although muscular veins have little or no sympathetic innervation, cutaneous veins are under hypothalamic thermoregulatory control and have both alpha- and beta-adrenergic receptors.[65] Since the outermost media and adventitia contain the nerve endings, myogenic conduction contributes to the neurogenic activation by coordinating venous contraction.[66] Even in the outer layers of the media, the separation of muscle cells from nerve endings is rarely less than 1000 Å.[67] Therefore, an intact smooth muscle layer is important in vein physiology.

Venous constriction and dilation occurs through both central and local nervous stimuli. Localized cooling provides both a potentiation of adrenergic stimulation and a direct stimulus for venous smooth muscle contraction.[68,69] Venoconstriction is reduced by warming.[69] Venoconstriction also occurs with infusions of norepinephrine,[70] epinephrine, phenylephrine, serotonin, and histamine. Veins dilate in response to phenoxybenzamine, phentolamine, reserpine, guanethidine, barbiturates, and many anesthetic agents.[71] Therefore, circulating adrenergic and pharmacologic substances influence vein diameter. This may explain why central mechanisms may also be responsible for venous tone. In addition, local chemical changes produced through exercise also provide for the distribution of blood flow in accordance with local metabolic needs.

Evidence for a central sympathetic control of venoconstriction has been demonstrated by the failure of such venoconstriction to occur with tilting of sympathectomized patients.[72] Even the stress of mental arithmetic or unpleasant thoughts has been shown to activate adrenergic nerves connected to cutaneous veins.[64] Veins may become more distensible during sleep because of a change in either respiration or nerve stimulation.[73] This explains the need for continuous compression of sclerotherapy treated veins during the endosclerotic stages after treatment.

**REFERENCES**

1. Kosinski C: Observations on the superficial venous system of the lower extremity, J Anat 60:131, 1926.
2. Farber EM and Bates EE: Pathologic physiology of stasis dermatitis, Arch Dermatol 70:653, 1954.
3. Klein Ronweler BJF, Kuiper JP, and Brakkee HJM: Venous flow resistence and venous capacity in humans with primary varicosis of the long saphenous vein, Phlebology 5:31, 1990.
4. McPheeters HO and Rice CO: Varicose veins: the circulation and direction of venous flow, Surg Gynecol Obstet 49:29, 1929.
5. Kuster G, Lofgren EP, and Hollinshead WH: Anatomy of the veins of the foot, Surg Gynecol Obstet 127:817, 1968.
6. Jacobsen BJ: The venous drainage of the foot, Surg Gynecol Obstet 131:22, 1970.

7. Fox RH and Gardner AMN: Video-phlebography in the investigation of venous physiology and disease. In Negus D and Jantet G (editors): Phlebology 85, London, 1986, Libbey.
8. McMullin G et al: An assessment of the effect of the foot pump on venous emptying in chronic venous insufficiency. In Davy A and Stemmer R (editors): Phlebologie 89, Blanche, France 1989, John Libbey Eurotext Ltd.
9. Bouissou H et al: Vein morphology, Phlebology 3, Suppl 1:1, 1988.
10. Laufman H: Silvergirl's surgery: the veins, ed 1, Austin, Texas, 1986, Silvergirl Inc.
11. Myers TT: Varicose veins. In Allen EV, Barker NW, and Hines EA: Peripheral vascular diseases, ed 3, Philadelphia, 1962, WB Saunders Co.
12. Thurner J and Mar R: Probleme der Phlobopathologie mit besonderer Berucksichtigung der Phlebosklerose, Zentralblatt Fuer Phlebologie 6:404, 1967.
13. Reference deleted in proofs.
14. Villavicencio JL: Personal communication, 1989.
15. Cotton LT: Varicose veins: gross anatomy and development, Br J Surg 48:589, 1961.
16. Greenfield ADM: Physiology of the veins. In Luisada AA (editor): Cardiovascular functions, New York, 1962, McGraw-Hill Book Co.
17. Psaila JV et al: Do varicose veins have abnormal viscoelastic properties? In Davy A and Stemmer R (editors): Phlebologie 89, Blanche, France, 1989, John Libbey Eurotext Ltd.
18. Fegan G: Varicose veins: compression sclerotherapy, London, 1967, William Heinemann Medical Books Ltd.
19. Eger SA and Wagner FB Jr: Etiology of varicose veins, Postgrad Med 6:234, 1949.
20. Braverman IM and Keh-Yen A: Ultrastructure of the human dermal microcirculation. IV. Valve-containing collecting veins at the dermal-subcutaneous junction, J Invest Dermatol 81:438, 1983.
21. Thompson H: The surgical anatomy of the superficial and perforating veins of the lower limb, Ann R Col Surg Eng 61:198, 1979.
22. Browse NL, Burnand G, and Thomas ML: Diseases of the veins: pathology, diagnosis, and treatment, London, 1988, Edward Arnold.
23. Sherman RS: Varicose veins: anatomy re-evaluation of Trendelenburg tests and operating procedure, Surg Clin North Am 44:1369, 1964.
24. Dodd H and Cockett FB (editors): The pathology and surgery of the veins of the lower limb, ed 2, Edinburgh, 1976, Churchill Livingstone Inc.
25. Zimmerman LM and Rattner H: Infra-red photography of subcutaneous veins, Am J Surg 27:502, 1935.
26. Bjordal RI: Circulation patterns in incompetent perforating veins in the calf and in the saphenous system in primary varicose veins, Acta Chir Scand 136:251, 1972.
27. Limborgh J van: L'anatomie du systeme veineux de l'extremite inferieure en relatio avec la pathologie variqueuse, Folia Angiologica 8:3, 1961.
28. Stolic E: Terminology, division, and systematic anatomy of the communicating veins of the lower limb. In May R, Partsch H, and Straubesand J (editors): Perforating veins, Munich, 1981, Urban & Schwarzenberg Inc.
29. Sherman RS: Varicose veins: further findings based on anatomic and surgical disections, Ann Surg 130:218, 1949.
30. Arnoldi CC: Venous pressure in patients with valvular incompetence of the veins of the lower limb, Acta Chir Scand 132:628, 1966.
31. Linton R: Communicating veins of the lower leg and the operative technique for their ligation, Ann Surg 107:582, 1938.
32. Wupperman T, Mellimann J, and von Sclweder WJ: Morphometric characteristics of incompetent perforating veins in primary varicosis of the lower leg, Vasa 7:66, 1978.
33. Dodd H: The varicose tributaries of the superficial femoral vein passing into Hunter's canal, Postgrad Med J 35:18, 1959.
34. Sherman RS: Varicose veins: anatomic findings and an operative procedure based upon them, Ann Surg 120:772, 1944.
35. Cockett FB: The pathology and treatment of venous ulcers of the leg, Br J Surg 43:260, 1955.
36. Fischer R, Fullemann HJ, and Alder W: Zum phlebogischen Dogma der Pradilektionsstellen der Cockettschen Venae perforantes, Phlebo u Proktol 16:184, 1987.
37. Raivio EVL: Untersuchungen die Venen der unteren Extremitaten mit besonderer Bevuckgichtigunu der gegenseihgen Verbindungen zwischen den oberflachlichen und tiefen Venen, Ann Med Exp Fenn 26(suppl):1, 1948.
38. Kubik S: Anatomie der Beinvemen. In Wuppermann TW (editor): Varizen ulcus cruris und Thrombose Berlin, 1986, Springer-Verlag.
39. Miller SS: Investigation and management of varicose veins, Ann Col Surg Eng 55:245, 1974.
40. Foote RR: Varicose Veins, St Louis, 1949, The CV Mosby Co.

41. Wokalek H et al: Morphology and localization of sunburst varicosities: an electron microscopic and morphometric study, J Dermatol Surg Oncol 15:149, 1989.
42. Moreno AH et al: Mechanics of distension of dog veins and other very thin-walled tubular structures, Circ Res 29:1069, 1970.
43. Strandness DE Jr and Thiele BI: Selected topics in venous disorders: pathophysiology, diagnosis, and treatment, New York, 1981, Futura Publishing Co.
44. Rhodin Johannes AG: Histology: a text and atlas, New York, 1974, Oxford University Press.
45. Barrow DW: The clinical management of varicose veins, ed 2, 1957, Hoeber-Harper.
46. Vanhoutte PM: The role of systemic veins: an update, Phlebology 3 Suppl 1:13, 1988.
47. Ehinger B, Falck B, and Sporrong B: Adrenergic fibers to the heart and to peripheral vessels, Bibl Anat 8:35, 1966.
48. Edwards JE and Edwards AE: The saphenous valves in varicose veins, Am Heart J 19:338, 1940.
49. Kugelgen A: Uber des Verhaltnis von Ringmuskulatur und Innendruck in menschlichen grossen Venen, Z Zellforsch Mikrosk Anat 43:168, 1955.
50. Leu HJ, Vogt M, and Pfrunder H: Morphological alterations of nonvaricose and varicose veins, Basic Res Cardiol 74:435, 1979.
51. Braverman IM: Ultrastructure and organization of the cutaneous microvasculature in normal and pathologic states, J Invest Dermatol 93:28, 1989.
52. Miani A and Rubertsi U: Collecting venules, Minerva Cardioangiol 41:541, 1958.
53. Braverman IM and Keh-Yen A: Ultrastructure of the human dermal microcirculation. IV. Valve-containing collecting veins at the dermal-subcutaneous junction, J Invest Dermatol 81:438, 1983.
54. Benninghoff, quoted by Moretti G. In Jadassho J (editor): Handbuch der Haut- und Geschlechtskrangheiten, Berlin, 1968, Springer Verlag.
55. Bargmann W: Histologie und mikroskopische Anatomie des Meerschen, Stuttgart, 1956, Georg Thieme.
56. Goldman MP and Bennett RG: Treatment of telangiectasia: a review, J Am Acad Dermatol 17:167, 1987.
57. Bean WB: Vascular spiders and related lesions of the skin, Springfield, Ill, 1958, Charles C Thomas Publisher.
58. Bodian EL: Sclerotherapy, Sem Dermatol 6:238, 1987.
59. de Faria JL and Moraes IN: Histopathology of the telangiectasias associated with varicose veins, Dermatologia 127:321, 1963.
60. Wokalek H et al: Morphology and localization of sunburst varicosities: an electron microscopic and morphometric study, J Dermatol Surg Oncol 15:149, 1989.
61. Fried SZ and Lynfield L: Unilateral facial telangiectasia macularis eruptiva perstans, J Am Acad Dermatol 16:250, 1987.
62. Azizkhan RG et al: Mast cell heparin stimulates migration of capillary endothelial cells in vitro, J Exp Med 152:931, 1980.
63. Folkman J: Regulation of angiogenesis: a new function of heparin, Biochem Pharmacol 34:905, 1985.
64. Shepherd JT: Reflex control of the venous system. In Bergan JJ and Yao JST (editors): Venous Problems, Chicago, 1978, Year Book Medical Publishers.
65. Kaiser GA, Ross J Jr, and Braunwald E: Alpha and Beta adrenergic receptor mechanisms in the systemic venous bed, J Pharmacol Exp Ther 144:156, 1964.
66. Johansson B and Ljung B: Role of myogenic propagation in vascular smooth muscle response to vasomotor nerve stimulation, Acta Physiol Scand 73:501, 1968.
67. Speden RN: Excitation of vascular smooth muscle. In Bulbring E et al (editors): Smooth muscle, Baltimore, 1970, Williams & Wilkins.
68. Vanhoutte PM and Shepherd JT: Thermosensitivity and veins, J Physiol (Paris) 63:449, 1970.
69. Vanhoutte PM and Shepherd JT: Effect of temperature on reactivity of isolated cutaneous veins of the dog, Am J Physiol 218:187, 1970.
70. Wood JE and Eckstein JW: A tandem forearm plethysmograph for study of acute responses of the peripheral veins of man: the effect of environmental and local temperature change and the effect of pooling blood in the extremities, J Clin Invest 37:41, 1958.
71. Mellander S: Operative studies on the adrenergic neuro-hormonal control of resistance and capacitance blood vessels in the cat, Acta Phys Scand 50:5, 1960.
72. Peterson LH: Some characteristics of certain reflexes which modify the circulation in man, Circulation 2:351, 1950.
73. Watson WE: Distensibility of the capacity blood vessels of the human hand during sleep, J Physiol (Lond) 161:392, 1962.

# 2 | Adverse Sequelae and Complications of Venous Hypertension

## PATHOGENESIS

Venous insufficiency may be defined as relative impedance of venous flow back to the heart. When this occurs in the lower extremities, the normal reabsorption of perivascular fluids by osmotic and pressure gradients is impaired, resulting in accumulation of perivascular and lymphatic fluid. This leads to edema and impaired oxygenation of surrounding tissue (Figs. 2-1 and 2-2). This disruption of the normal vascular and lymphatic flow of the lower extremities may result in pain, cramping (especially at night), restless feelings, pigmentary changes, dermatitis, and ulceration (Fig. 2-3).[1-3] The association of abnormal venous flow with various signs and symptoms has been noted for centuries; it was first noted by Hippocrates in the fourth century BC[3] and was first reported by Wiseman in England in 1676.[4] It has been estimated that chronic venous insufficiency will develop in almost 50% of patients with major varicose veins.[5,6]

Several alterations of normal venous flow cause venous hypertension. Such hypertension in the lower extremities is usually caused by a loss or disruption of the normal one-way valvular system. This usually occurs because of deep vein thrombosis (DVT), thrombophlebitis, or a dilation of veins resulting from other causes.[7,8] When communicating vein valvular function becomes incompetent, there may be shunting of blood flow from the deep to the superficial venous system through incompetent communicating veins, with resultant adverse sequelae.[9-11] The superficial veins respond by dilating to accommodate the in-

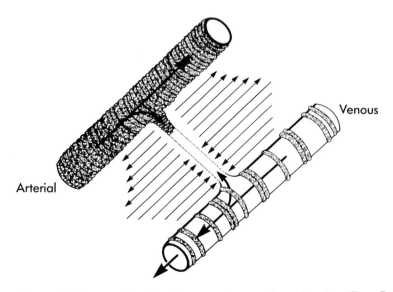

Venous

Arterial

**Fig. 2-1**  Schematic diagram showing the normal resorption of pericapillary fluid in response to precapillary and postcapillary pressure and interstitial pressures.

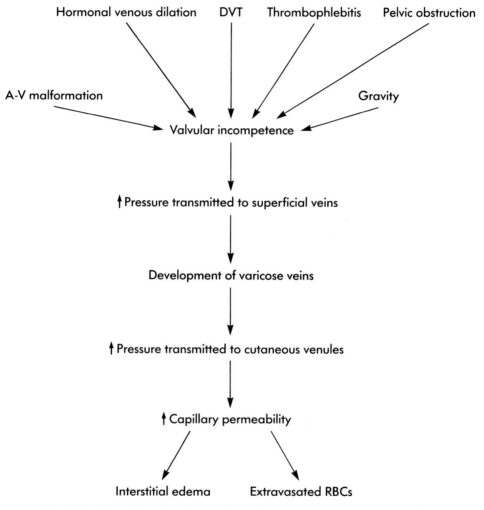

**Fig. 2-2**    Flowchart showing etiology of cutaneous venous hypertension.

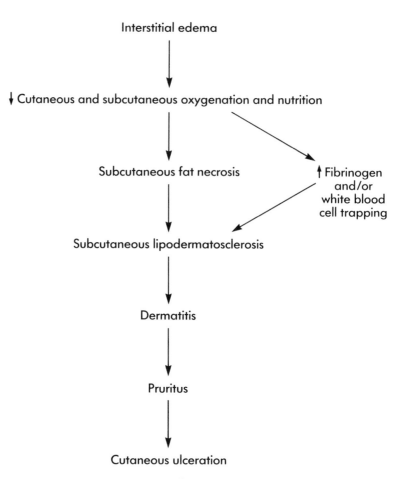

**Fig. 2-3** Flowchart showing etiology of cutaneous manifestations of venous hypertension.

creased blood flow, which produces superficial valvular incompetence leading to the development of varicosities.[12] In addition, with muscular movement in the lower limbs, the high venous pressure normally occurring within the calf is transmitted straight to the superficial veins and subcutaneous tissues.[13,14] Venous pressure in the cuticular venules may greatly exceed the normal 100 mm Hg in the erect position.[15] This causes venular dilation over the whole area resulting in capillary dilation, increased permeability,[16-19] and an increase in the subcutaneous capillary bed.[17,20] This is manifested as telangiectasia and venectasia (Fig. 2-4). Fortunately, both sclerotherapy and surgical treatment are capable of normalizing abnormal venous hypertension.

The lymphatic system also becomes overloaded because of interstitial edema.[21-23] Dilated lymphatics, resulting from venous obstruction, have been shown to fibrose.[21,24-26] Thus lymphatic stasis adds to venous stasis edema and may persist even after venous stasis has resolved. This may cause elephantiasis of the limb[12] or lymphostasis verrucosa cutis (Fig. 2-5).[27,28] Permanent disruption of the normal cutaneous and subcutaneous venous outflow ensues producing poor tissue nutrition and oxygenation.[2,29] Subcutaneous fat necrosis may develop with subsequent reorganization of the subcutaneous tissue forming a hard plate.[22,30] The combined effects of venous hypertension and lymphatic stasis re-

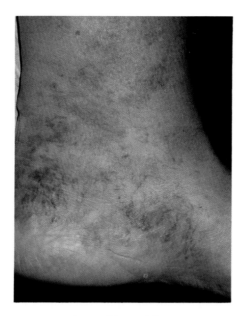

**Fig. 2-4**    Telangiectasia in the medial ankle/pedal area in a patient with chronic venous insufficiency referred to as *corona phlebectasia.*

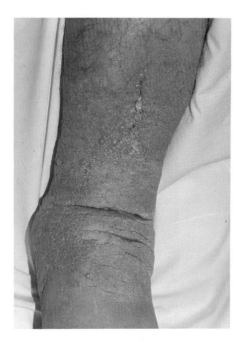

**Fig. 2-5**    Lymphostasis verrucosa cutis in a patient with long-standing venous hypertension resulting from deep venous thrombosis and thrombophlebitis.

sult in profound changes in the cutaneous and subcutaneous tissues. These changes are collectively referred to as *lipodermatosclerosis.*

The formation of subcutaneous lipodermatosclerosis is thought to be caused in part by an increase in the local and perivascular concentration of fibrinogen. Burnand et al.[17] have measured a high local concentration of fibrinogen and other macromolecules in the interstitial fluid after the production of increased venous pressure through an arteriovenous fistula in experimental animals. Hypercoagulability of the interstitial fluid then produces localized fibrin formation, which in turn may be responsible for the development of lipodermatosclerosis and subsequent cutaneous breakdown. Alternatively, perivascular fibrin cuffing (Fig. 2-6) may decrease diffusion of gases with resultant tissue hypoxia, which in turn may produce venous ulceration.[31,32] However, the fibrin cuff has not been proven to be a true barrier to oxygen diffusion,[33] thus casting some doubt on this theory.

A new hypothesis to explain the cause of venous ulceration and cutaneous disease has recently been proposed.[33] Bollinger et al.,[34] observed that patients with chronic venous insufficiency who demonstrated areas devoid of cutaneous blood flow had this flow restored with the use of graduated compression stockings. It has been proposed that the capillary occlusion is a result of white blood cells sticking to the endothelial surface of intradermal capillaries blocking blood flow.[33,35,36] It is thought that the trapped white blood cells release toxic oxygen metabolites and proteolytic enzymes that damage capillaries, increasing their per-

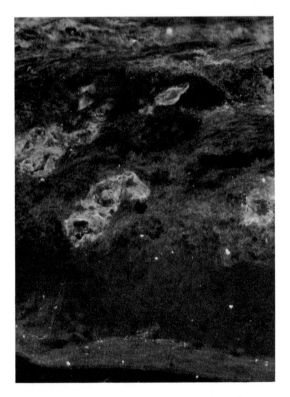

**Fig. 2-6** Skin biopsy specimen taken from the edge of a venous ulceration. The tissue was stained by direct immunofluorescence with a polyclonal antifibrinogen antibody. There is intense pericapillary staining for fibrinogen and fibrin (250×). (Courtesy Vincent Falanga, M.D., University of Miami School of Medicine.)

meability and resulting in leakage of fibrinogen and other plasma proteins. This could lead to the formation of the fibrin cuff. Trapped white blood cells may also prevent circulation in the subcutaneous capillary loops, which then increases tissue ischemia.

Histologic examination of skin over areas of venous stasis demonstrates an increase in the number of dermal capillaries. These also appear elongated and tortuous.[18] Unlike cutaneous capillaries in the normal leg, these remain dilated in the supine position and do not change in caliber when subjected to pressure.[37] These capillaries also have been demonstrated to be encased in a fibrin cuff[31] as described previously.

Venous hypertension is not a benign condition. The cutaneous chain of events following the onset of venous stasis is thought to occur in the following temporal order: localized edema, induration, pigmentation, dermatitis, atrophie blanche, and in untreated cases, eventual ulceration, infection, scarring, and further complications, including lymphatic obstruction, sensitization to applied medications, protein loss, and many other unwanted effects.

## INCIDENCE

Varicose veins have been estimated to occur in 7% to 60% of the adult United States population.[5,15,38-41] Varicose veins have been noted to increase in incidence with age. Varicose veins occur in 8% of women between ages 20 and 29, increasing to 41% in the fifth decade and 72% in the seventh decade of life.[39,42] A similar rate of increase in the incidence of varicose veins occurs in men. In men the incidence of varicose veins is 1% in the third decade, increasing to 24% in the fourth decade, and 43% in the seventh decade.[39,42] The Basle Study III[5] found that the greatest correlation between age and incidence of varicose veins occurred in those with varicose veins only and not in those with the presence of telangiectasias (hyphenwebs) or reticular veins (Fig. 2-7).

Varicosities in childhood are rare, occurring almost exclusively in association

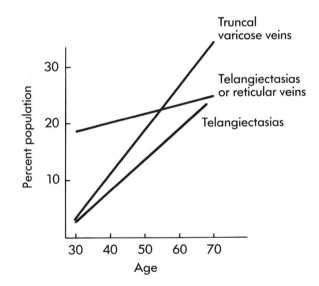

**Fig. 2-7**   Risk of varicosity by age. Increasing age best correlated with the development of varicose and/or reticular veins. (From Widmer L: Peripheral venous disorders: prevalence and socio-medical importance observations in 4529 apparently healthy persons. Basle Study III. Bern, Switzerland, 1978, Hans Huber Publishers.)

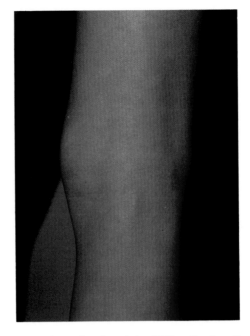

**Fig. 2-8**   Subtle, asymptomatic varicosity of the SSV at the junction in the popliteal fossa of an 11-year-old girl. There is no significant family history of varicose veins.

with congenital vascular malformations (see Chapter 3). When they do occur, they usually appear as a subtle physical finding such as a slight bulge over the popliteal fossa (Fig. 2-8). One estimation on the incidence of telangiectasias in children was performed by Oster and Nielsen in Denmark.[43] Of 2171 Danish schoolchildren examined, 46.2% of the girls and 35.1% of the boys had telangiectasias on the nape of the neck; 1% of whom had pronounced telangiectasias elsewhere, that is, on the shoulders, thorax, cheeks, and ears. No mention was made of the occurrence of telangiectasias on the legs. An examination of 403 children, aged 8 to 18, in East Germany disclosed a 50% incidence of "very discrete" venous abnormalities of leg veins. Of the children examined, 15% had clear symptoms (without visible varices) that could be assigned to a prospective varicose disease. Only between the ages of 17 and 18 could reticular varicose veins be identified. In these 403 children studied by venous Doppler, 2.3% had incompetent communicating veins and 3.2% had an incompetent saphenofemoral junction.[44] A more complete study of 518 children aged 10 to 12 years, using photoplethysmography in addition to venous Doppler, demonstrated a 10.2% incidence of reticular varicose veins without any other venous abnormalities.[45] When these children were examined 4 years later, the incidence of reticular veins was 30.3%; 2% of the children had developed varicose veins, and 4% had developed incompetent communicating veins. Therefore, although rare, venous disease can be demonstrated in a small number of children, and its progression can be documented.

## SYMPTOMS

Varicose veins may be symptomatic in addition to being large and unsightly (see box on p. 39). They may produce a dull aching of the legs, particularly after prolonged standing or during certain times of the menstrual cycle (especially during

**SYMPTOMS OF VARICOSE VEIN/VENOUS STASIS DISEASE
(CHRONIC VENOUS INSUFFICIENCY)**

Cosmetic                              Dermatitis
Aches and pains                       Ulceration
Night cramps                          Hemorrhage
Edema                                 Superficial thrombophlebitis
Cutaneous pigmentation

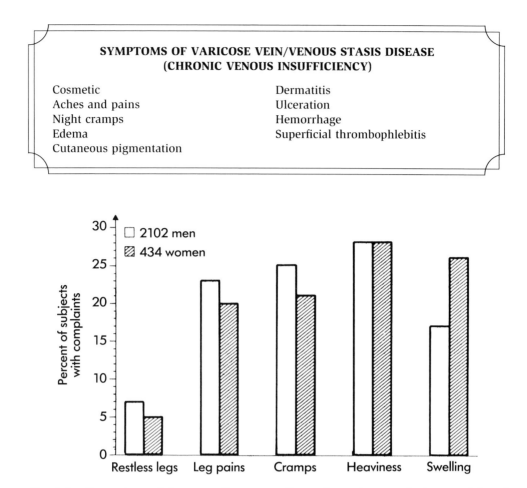

**Fig. 2-9**  Type of complaints according to sex. Except for an increase in the complaint of ankle swelling, men with varices have complaints similar to those of women. (From Widmer L: Peripheral venous disorders: prevalence and socio-medical importance observations in 4529 apparently healthy persons. Basle Study III. Bern, Switzerland, 1978, Hans Huber Publishers.)

menses).[46] A small number of women will also experience painful varicose veins after sexual intercourse.[47] It is proposed that the increase in venous pressure with distention of the varicose vein contributes to the heaviness and tightness of the lower legs.[4,48] The Basle Study III[5] found a similar range of complaints in both men and women (Fig. 2-9) and also found an increased incidence of complaints among women and older patients.

Symptoms in varicose veins are often disproportionate to the amount of actual pathologic change. Patients with small, early stage varices may complain more than those with large, long-standing varicosities.[49,50] A recent survey of 350 patients who presented for sclerotherapy treatment of veins less than 1 mm in diameter noted that 53% of these patients complained of swelling, burning, throbbing, and cramping of the legs in addition to a "tired feeling."[51] These symptoms are so insidious that most patients fail to realize how good their legs could feel until after treatment of these blood vessels by either compression sclerotherapy or the wearing of lightweight (<20 mm Hg) graduated compression stockings.[41]

---

**DIFFERENTIAL DIAGNOSIS OF LEG PAIN**

Varicose veins                     Achilles tendonitis or tear
Thrombophlebitis                   Intermittent (arterial) claudication
Osteoarthritis                     Venous claudication
Rheumatoid arthritis               Spinal claudication
Malignancy                         Myalgia
Osteomyelitis                      Peripheral neuropathy
Meniscial tears                    Lymphedema

---

From Browse NL, Burnand KG, and Thomas ML: Diseases of the veins: pathology, diagnosis, and treatment, London, 1988, Edward Arnold.

One American health survey found that nearly 50% of those with varicose veins were bothered by their symptoms once in a while, and 18% noted frequent to continuous symptoms.[52] The increased incidence of symptomatic varicose veins may have a hormonal etiology. It has been estimated that 27.7% of women with varicose veins have premenstrual pain in their varices.[53] Varicose veins during pregnancy appear to be more symptomatic than those unassociated with pregnancy. In a study of 150 pregnant women with varicose veins, 125 noted pain and 26 were unable to stand for more than 1 to 2 hours because of the pain.[54]

The differential diagnosis of leg pain is extensive and not necessarily attributable to a patient's varicosities (see box above). Symptoms derived from varicose veins can usually be distinguished from arterial symptoms. Pain associated with arterial diseases often disappears at rest and is exacerbated with walking. Pain associated with varicosities is dull, vague, and localized on the medial side of the legs. It is usually relieved with walking. In addition to the dull aching, varicose veins associated with venous hypertension may produce cramping or painful spasms of the legs and an increase in leg fatigue and restless legs, especially at night. Unfortunately, a patient's perception and reporting of pain is subjective in nature and difficult to document. Browse, Burnand, and Thomas[55] advocate the use of compression hosiery as a diagnostic test to determine if the pain is from venous origin.

## SIGNS

In addition to the direct symptoms of varicose and telangiectatic veins, varicose veins may also be a cutaneous marker for venous insufficiency (see box on p. 41).[24,56,57] It has been estimated that at least 50% of people with varicose veins have a cutaneous finding.[2] The cutaneous manifestation appears as edema, hyperpigmentation, dermatitis, or ulceration. Over 1 million Americans suffer from skin ulcers caused by abnormal circulation resulting from varicose veins, and nearly 100,000 Americans are totally disabled by this condition.[39] Thus varicose and telangiectatic leg veins are not merely of cosmetic concern, but represent a widespread and potentially serious medical problem.

## Edema

Ankle edema is usually the first manifestation of chronic venous insufficiency.[58] Ankle edema tends to be worse in warm weather[2] and toward the end of the day.[41] It is especially common in persons who stand a great deal.[41] True "pitting"

---

**VENOUS STASIS DISEASE SIGNS**

| | |
|---|---|
| Ankle edema | Pigmentation |
| Dilated veins and venules | Venous dermatitis |
| Telangiectasias | Atrophie blanche |
| Corona phlebectasia | Ulceration |

---

**DIFFERENTIAL DIAGNOSIS OF ANKLE EDEMA**

Cardiac failure
Renal failure
Deep vein thrombosis
Venous obstruction from other causes
Hypoalbuminemia
Fluid retention syndromes
Lymphedema
Lipodystrophy
Hemihypertrophy (Klippel-Trenaunay syndrome)
Venous valvular agenesis

---

edema is rare,[23] perhaps resulting from lipodermatosclerosis. The edema usually found is restricted to a limited area drained by capillaries that empty directly into the varicose veins and/or incompetent communicating veins.[59] This area has been termed the *gaiter area* and refers to the ankle and lower calf. (In the 1800s it was commonly covered by a cloth or leather material [gaiter] to protect the ankle and instep from the environmental elements. Such protection is still used today by cross-country skiers.) Ankle edema caused by venous hypertension and varicose veins must be differentiated from that caused by other conditions (see box above).

The protein-rich edema fluid stimulates fibroblastic activity, which entangles blood vessels and lymphatics into a fibrous mass.[60] The resulting lymphedema and hypertrophy of the skin and subcutaneous tissues disrupts the flow of cutaneous nutrition. In women with venous stasis and fat, hairless, erythrocyanoid-type ankles, the resulting decrease in nutrition for the sizeable fatty subcutaneous tissue and the decrease in local tissue oxygenation may result in sudden and massive fat necrosis of the subcutaneous tissue.[2,15] The affected area may then appear erythematous, indurated and tender to the touch.

Treatment of ankle edema caused by increased venous pressure with or without lipodermatosclerosis is primarily directed toward prevention of trauma and alleviation of superficial venous hypertension.[19] Temporizing treatments include leg elevation, systemic diuretics, and localized compression bandaging.[19] Recently, fibrinolytic enhancement has been reported to be successful in improving symptoms, induration, and cutaneous thickening in patients with lipodermatosclerosis.[61] The authors of that report used stanazol (5 mg by mouth, twice daily) in 14 patients with long-standing lipodermatosclerosis resulting from venous disease. Of these 14 patients, 11 noted improvement within 3 months. Long-term follow-up was not given nor has this treatment been accepted elsewhere.

## Pigmentation

Pigmentation (Fig. 2-10) is also a sign of venous stasis disease. The elongated vascular system underlying areas of stasis is more susceptible to trauma than normal. Even minor blunt injuries may cause rupture of the vascular wall with extravasation of erythrocytes into the cutis.[12,18,60] Histologically, cutaneous hyperpigmentation represents extravasated erythrocytes and hemosiderin-laden macrophages interspersed between dilated and tortuous capillaries.[12] Extravasated erythrocytes may also be found in the deep dermis around adnexal structures (Fig. 2-11). A more acute "eruptive" cutaneous pigmentation has also been noted as a "blow-out" of erythrocytes into the dermis as a result of tremendous back pressure within the cutaneous microvasculature.[62] This phenomenon has been ascribed as the cause of lichen aureus (Fig. 2-12) by Shelley et al.[63] The only treatment for this condition is correction of the underlying venous hypertension including graduated compression stockings and leg elevation. Eventually, some of the pigment darkening will fade with the passage of time.

## Venous (Stasis) Dermatitis

The next dermatologic manifestation to occur in the chain of events following venous hypertension/stasis is "stasis" dermatitis. This dermatitis has been given many names including stasis eczema, varicose eczema, stasis syndrome, hypostatic eczema, congestive eczema, and dermatitis hypostatica. Since there may not be a true "stasis" in the lower leg with venous insufficiency, but rather venous hypertension, this condition is best referred to as "venous" dermatitis.

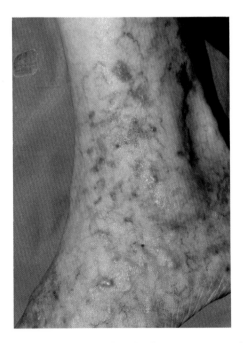

**Fig. 2-10** Hyperpigmentation around dilated telangiectasias and venules in a 70-year-old man. There has been no history of cutaneous trauma.

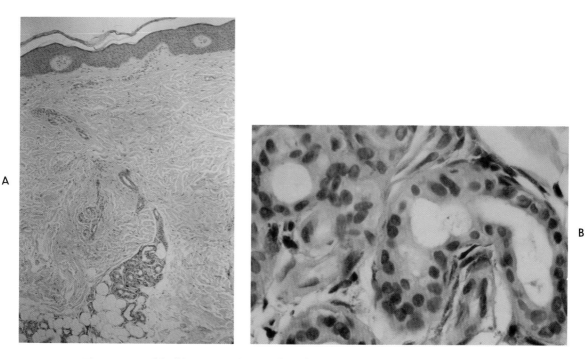

**Fig. 2-11**  Skin biopsy specimen taken from the medial malleolar area of a 38-year-old man with ankle/pedal telangiectasias and venulectases with associated hyperpigmentation. Note hemosiderin-laden macrophages interspersed among eccrine glands in the deep dermis. (Hematoxylin-eosin; **A,** 50×; **B,** 200×.)

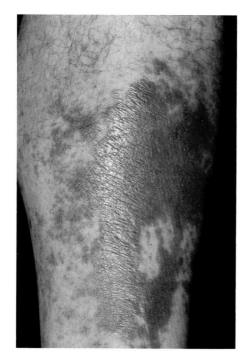

**Fig. 2-12**  Woman, 52 years old, with onset of cutaneous hyperpigmentation over 1 to 2 years of the anterior tibial and medial malleolar areas. Venous Doppler examination was diagnostic for an incompetent communicating vein.

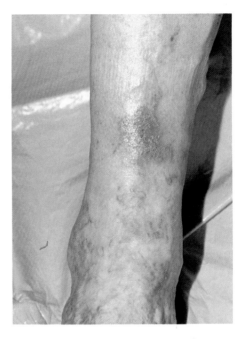

**Fig. 2-13**    Early venous eczema appearing as a nummular eczema overlying prominent dilated venules and reticular veins in a 58-year-old woman.

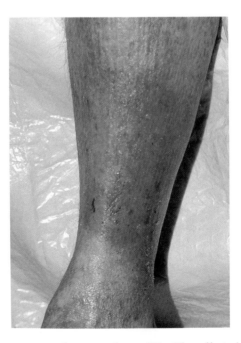

**Fig. 2-14**    Typical appearance of venous dermatitis. The affected area is erythematous, poorly marginated, and scaly with hyperpigmentation and excoriations.

Venous dermatitis occurs more frequently in women, obese people, middle-aged men and women, and in those with a history of deep venous thrombosis and thrombophlebitis.[3] Edema, which causes the change from the normal cutaneous venous circulation to a high pressure system with increased vascular permeability, is the precursor of this dermatitis.[3,64-66]

The dermatitis usually begins in the medial paramalleolar region. This region is particularly vulnerable because the vascular supply, skin nutrition, and subcutaneous tissue are less abundant here than in other areas of the lower extremity.[67] Venous dermatitis appears clinically as a sharply marginated, erythematous, crusted plaque (Fig. 2-13). With time and cutaneous trauma resulting from pruritus, overlying lichenification may occur[3] as well as exudation, depending on the extent of the inflammation and associated edema. However, an indolent venous flow may make the skin assume a much paler color with less moisture.[68] The color of the lesion darkens as a result of an increase in melanin and dermal hemosiderin (Fig. 2-14).[2,69] The dermatitis may also be complicated by a generalized systemic hypersensitivity or "ID" reaction.[2]

Histologic examination (Fig. 2-15) of the dermis demonstrates a diffuse homogenization of collagen, fragmentation or absence of elastic fibers, thickening and partial occlusion of arterioles, and atrophic changes of appendages.[12,70] There may also be an associated acanthosis and hyperkeratosis of the epidermis, which rarely results in pseudoepitheliomatous hyperplasia.[3] The lymphatic vessels are usually thickened and fibrotic, and there may be an associated dermal inflammatory infiltrate.[3] Since these changes are those of a nonspecific dermatitis, the histologic diagnosis of venous dermatitis can be certain only with clinical correlation.

## Atrophie Blanche

Atrophie blanche is the descriptive name given to the appearance of porcelain-white scars seen on the lower extremities as a result of infarctive lesions of the skin (Fig. 2-16). This condition was originally attributed to syphilis or tuberculosis in 1929.[71] The white plaques are bordered by hyperpigmentation and telangiectasias. The process usually occurs in middle-aged women with associated varicose veins and signs of venous insufficiency. However, this descriptive term represents the sequelae of many disease processes including venous dermatitis, arteriosclerosis, dysproteinemia, diabetes mellitus, hypertension, systemic lupus erythematosus, scleroderma, juvenile rheumatoid arthritis, and idiopathic segmental hyalinizing vasculitis. Therefore, this physical condition is best thought of as an intermediate stage between venous dermatitis and varicose ulceration; the term *atrophie blanche* is best reserved for the idiopathic vasculitic condition.

## Ulceration

Cutaneous ulceration represents the end-stage manifestation of venous stasis disease. This relationship has been noted for centuries. Hippocrates was the first to record the association.[72] Over 300 years ago, Wiseman noted that valvular incompetence caused by venous thrombosis could result in a circulatory defect leading to ulceration of the skin.[73]

Varicose or postthrombophlebitic ulcers (Fig. 2-17) occur in up to 600,000 adults in the United States and 250,000 adults in England. The prevalence has been estimated to be up to 1% of the United States population and 2% of the Swedish population.[3,74,75] Seventy-two different causes of leg ulcers have been recognized and grouped into three categories,[76] but 75% to 90% of all of these causes are of venous etiology,[3,77,78] 40% to 60% of which are associated with var-

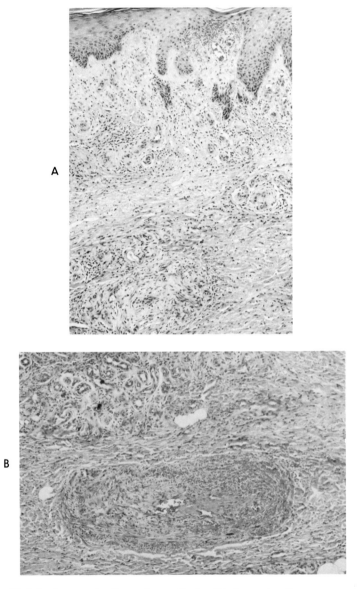

**Fig. 2-15**    Histologic examination of a patient with long-standing venous hypertension and overlying venous dermatitis. (For description see text.) (Hematoxylin-eosin; **A**, 50×; **B**, 200×.)

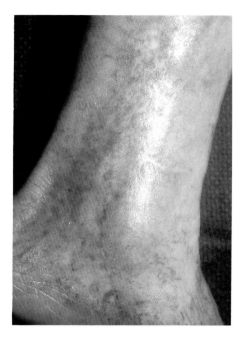

**Fig. 2-16** Middle-aged woman with venous insufficiency and atrophie blanche of the medial malleolar area. (Courtesy Kim Buterwick, M.D.)

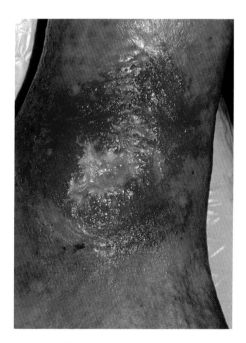

**Fig. 2-17** Chronic venous insufficiency with cutaneous ulceration in a 68-year-old man before treatment.

icose veins,[3,77-79] and 35% to 90% associated with a past history of DVT.[3,30,77-80] In one practice of over 20,000 lifetime patients, it was estimated that nearly 15% of patients with major varicose veins will develop ulcerations.[6] Nonvenous causes of leg ulceration include arterial disease (8%) and ulcers caused by trauma or that have bacteriologic, mycotic, hematologic, neoplastic, neurologic, or systemic origins (2%).[76]

Cutaneous ulceration usually occurs 10 to 35 years (mean 24 years) after the onset of varicose veins[81] and is specifically associated with incompetent calf perforating veins (see Chapter 9).[15,82,83] Dodd and Cockett[15] surgically explored 135 limbs with ankle ulceration and found that the most severe lesions always were associated with an incompetent perforating vein. Lawrence et al.[83] studied patients with varicosities, both with and without associated ulceration, with Doppler ultrasound. They found sustained retrograde flow in incompetent veins in eight of nine ulcer patients, but found it in only one of seven patients with varicose veins without ulceration. Thus any operative procedure on varicose ulcers must correct the underlying abnormal communicating or perforating veins. Interestingly, no evidence or history of DVT was reported in up to 24% of patients with chronic venous leg ulcers.[79,84] Therefore, the etiology may be multifactorial, with the majority of patients having a similar initiating event: superficial venous hypertension from incompetent communicating or perforating veins or an unrecognized deep venous thrombosis of the lower leg.

Stasis ulcerations, unlike most other causes of cutaneous ulcerations, appear in the gaiter area.[31,79] The ulcers appear cyanotic, edematous, and friable. The base usually is covered with thick granulation tissue that rarely penetrates the deep fascia. The skin edges are painless, thickened, and bleed easily. Adjacent skin is edematous and inflamed with associated dilated venules, eczematous changes, and pigmentation.[30,85] Calcification of the subcutaneous tissue, often not even adjacent to the ulceration, occurs in a significant number of patients,[64,86,87] up to 25% in one study.[88] The calcium, acting as a foreign body, may perpetuate the ulceration or may actually be an essential cause of the lesion. Calcification is probably caused by venous insufficiency and represents the last stage of the inflammatory response. It almost always precedes the ulceration.[64]

### Malignant degeneration

A potentially fatal, but fortunately rare, secondary change in venous ulcers is malignant degeneration (Fig. 2-18). There have been fewer than 75 case reports of malignant degeneration of a stasis ulcer in the world literature.[89-101] The incidence of malignant degeneration appears to be no greater than 0.4% of all varicose ulcers.[95] The average duration of the ulcer before tumor growth is 21 years, with a reported span of 10 to 40 years.[93] The onset of malignant change usually appears as a rapid growth of exuberant cauliflower-like masses, an increase in pain, or in a smaller number of cases, a rapid extension of the ulcer crater.[93] An increase in induration of the ulcer borders and surrounding tissue and a failure of the ulcer to respond to prolonged conservative treatment is also suspect.[99] The reason for the transition into a malignant growth is thought to be the result of chronic dermatitis, irritation, and/or infection.[92,99] Therefore, it seems only prudent to biopsy the base and border areas of ulcers with these characteristics or ulcers over 4 months in duration.

## Secondary Complications of Venous Hypertension/Stasis

In addition to the varicose ulcers and dermatologic abnormalities already discussed, external hemorrhage, superficial thrombophlebitis, and deep vein thrombosis (DVT) are the three most severe and acute complications of varicose veins.

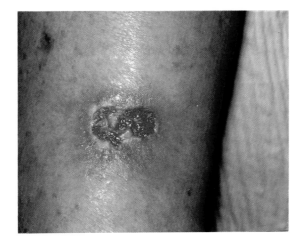

**Fig. 2-18**    Basal cell carcinoma (keratinizing type) arising in an ulcer in the setting of chronic venous insufficiency in a 77-year-old woman. The ulceration has been present for at least 6 years. An incompetent communicating vein was found at the base of the ulceration.

### Hemorrhage

Hemorrhage from varicose veins may not be a rare event. Tretbar[102] has reported treating 12 patients in 3 years for 18 episodes of hemorrhagic varicose veins. All but two of his patients had varicose veins for over 20 years. The bleeding area typically consisted of a mat of "blue blebs" 1 to 2 mm in diameter on the medial ankle. Doppler examination usually disclosed an underlying incompetent communicating vein. None of Tretbar's patients developed serious sequelae from the bleeding episodes, and all were treated successfully with compression sclerotherapy of the affected veins. However, bleeding can be profuse and, if unnoticed or treated improperly, can be fatal.[103-105] Hemorrhage is usually spontaneous but may also occur when the skin overlying a varicose vein becomes traumatized or eroded. Twenty-three fatal cases of hemorrhage were reported from England and Wales in 1971.[103] The patients most at risk are the solitary elderly patients with long-standing varicose veins. If the varicose vein is under high pressure from venous insufficiency, as it usually is, the acute hemorrhage may appear to be arterial in origin. This may result in the inappropriate application of a tourniquet, which will only serve to increase venous hypertension. Properly recognized, bleeding of venous origin is easily controlled by raising the affected area above the level of the heart and applying localized pressure to the bleeding vein.

### Superficial thrombophlebitis

Superficial thrombophlebitis (ST) is a painful condition that fortunately seldom results in serious embolic complications. In the absence of malignancy, thrombophlebitis of the leg is almost invariably associated with varicose veins.[4,106] It results from the development of a clot in a varicose vein caused by one or more of the following factors: trauma to the varicosity, stasis of blood flow, or occlusion of blood flow. Fifty percent of cases may occur spontaneously.[106,107] The greater saphenous system is the usual site of ascending ST. Clinically, one notes a painful, tender, hot, erythematous swelling along the course of the vein with a variable amount of perivascular edema. The pain associated with ST is often severe, probably resulting from inflammation of the dense network of somatic nerve fibers in the associated subcutaneous tissue.[4]

ST increases in incidence with increasing age and inactivity and with bed rest as the result of surgery, childbirth, or cardiac disease.[108,109] ST has been estimated to occur in 0.7% of women in their fourth decade of life, increasing to 2.6% of women in the seventh decade.[39] In men the incidence of ST has been estimated to be 0.4% in the fourth decade, increasing to 1.7% in the seventh decade.[39] A review of the lifetime work of one physician with over 20,000 patients notes an incidence of ST in up to 20% of patients with prominent major varicosities.[6] Older papers have estimated a 50% lifetime incidence of thrombophlebitis in patients with varicose veins.[110] Therefore, for both men and women the incidence of ST is estimated to occur in about 4% of those with varicose veins.[47] Coon et al.[39] estimated in 1973 that ST occurred in 123,000 persons in the United States yearly.

Although the condition is usually treated as a benign complication of varicose veins, the development of DVT, venous hypertension, and pulmonary emboli may occur in a significant percentage of patients.[106,107,111-113] A review of 340 cases of ST in a university hospital disclosed a 10% incidence of pulmonary emboli with 5 deaths.[107] This risk has been confirmed by others.[114] The development of pulmonary emboli may also be related in some cases to a coexistent DVT.[4]

DVT and pulmonary emboli, by definition, do not complicate ST unless the thrombus progresses into the deep venous system. This may occur because of either progression into a communicating vein or ascending involvement of the common femoral vein at the saphenofemoral junction (Fig. 2-19). When either of these events occurs, superficial or deep venous hypertension occurs as a result of valvular destruction.[109] Propagation of the thrombotic process into the deep system has been reported to occur in 6%[115] to 32%[111] of all cases of ST. In an 11-year retrospective series, 17% of 133 patients were noted to have extension of the clot into the deep system.[116] Surgical exploration of the saphenofemoral junction followed by ligation, thrombectomy, and limited vein stripping has been advocated particularly if clinical signs of thrombophlebitis reach the midthigh.* Alternatively, full anticoagulation is advocated by some.[125] Surgical removal of the thrombosed vein segments and associated varicosities shortens the convalescence and mitigates recurrences.[115,118] Unfortunately, this latter form of treatment usually results in extensive scarring. Finally, because DVT may manifest itself partly in the appearance of ST, patients should be carefully examined.

### Deep venous thrombosis

Varicose veins, by virtue of their low blood flow, are considered a risk factor for postoperative deep venous thrombosis (DVT).[123-129] This may be related to the increased incidence of thrombophlebitis in varicose veins in the postoperative period with an incidence estimated at 6% versus the normal 0.5% to 0.7% incidence.[130] Therefore, all patients with varicose veins who are about to undergo surgery or who are bedridden or pregnant should receive thrombosis prophylaxis, such as wearing a graduated support stocking, to prevent this potentially fatal, albeit rare, complication of varicose veins.

In summary, varicose veins are associated with a number of serious medical problems and are not just of cosmetic concern. Basle Study III[5] found that the incidence of the major complications of varicose veins — chronic venous insufficiency, phlebitis, and pulmonary embolism — increases with the severity of the varicosity (Fig. 2-20). Even patients with minor telangiectasias and reticular veins

---

*References 106, 109, 113-115, 117-124.

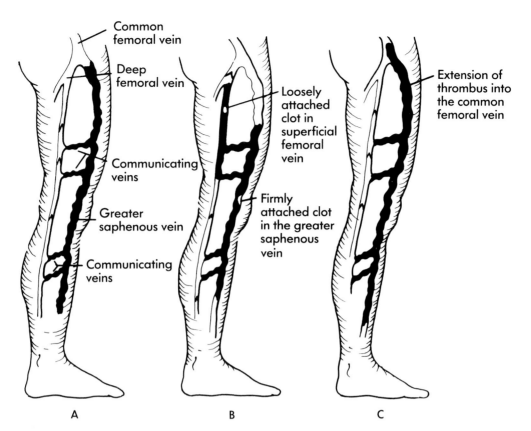

**Fig. 2-19** Diagrammatic representation of three methods of propagation of superficial thrombophlebitis. **A,** Thrombophlebitis limited to the superficial system with blockage by the communicating vein valves and at the saphenofemoral junction. **B,** Extension of the thrombus into the deep system via destruction and incompetence of communicating veins. **C,** Direct extension of the thrombus into the femoral vein at the saphenofemoral junction. (Redrawn from Totten HP: Angiology, The Journal of Vascular Diseases, Fig 2, vol 16:37, 1965. Reproduced with permission of the copyright owner; Westminster Publications, Inc, Roslyn, New York. All rights reserved.)

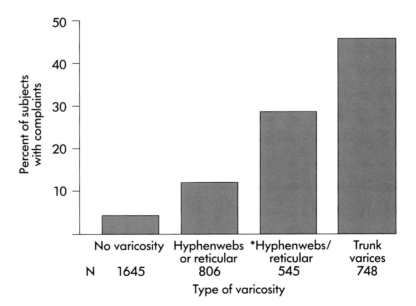

**Fig. 2-20** Complications according to the type of varicose vein; *N* represents the number of persons in the defined group; *hyphenweb* refers to telangiectatic veins; * refers to the group composed of both telangiectasia and reticular veins. (Redrawn from Widmer L: Peripheral venous disorders: prevalence and socio-medical importance observations in 4529 apparently healthy persons. Basle Study III. Bern, Switzerland, 1978, Hans Huber Publishers.)

**Table 2-1**   Classification of varicosities of the lower extremities

| Group | Varicosities | Saphenous system |
|:-----:|--------------|------------------|
| 1 | Spider bursts; telangiectatic veins | Competent |
| 2 | Mild or moderate varicosities | Competent |
| 3 | Mild, moderate, or marked varicosities | Incompetent |

From Heyerdale WW and Stalker LK: The management of varicose veins of the lower extremities, Ann Surg 114:1042, 1941.

---

**ADVANTAGES OF LIGATION OF INCOMPETENT GREAT SAPHENOUS VEIN**

1. Continuity of the vein is interrupted at the most proximal point
2. Possibility of cannulization is reduced to a minimum
3. Number of local injections necessary for obliteration is decreased
4. Period of treatment is shortened
5. Adequate complete thrombosis is obtained with greater ease
6. Pulmonary showers are less likely to occur

From Heyerdale WW and Stalker LK: The management of varicose veins of the lower extremities, Ann Surg 114:1042, 1941.

---

in combination demonstrated a significant increase of these serious medical complications when compared to patients without these types of veins.

## CLASSIFICATION

A classification of varicose veins should be based on anatomic and/or subsequent therapeutic considerations. The first anatomic classification was proposed by Heyerdale and Stalker[131] in 1941 (Table 2-1). This classification is useful in determining when surgical ligation of the great saphenous vein is advantageous before performing sclerotherapy. The list of advantages presented by Heyerdale and Stalker still holds true today (see box above). The Basle study[132] classified varicose veins into three groups:

1. Dilated saphenous veins (stem veins)
2. Dilated superficial branches (reticular veins)
3. Dilated venules (hyphenwebs)

Recently, Duffy[133] proposed a more complete classification of "unwanted leg veins." Since one purpose of a classification is to provide a mechanism for evaluating pathophysiology and treatment, a modification of the Duffy classification appears useful. It provides comprehensive clinical and therapeutic criteria in an effort to optimize treatment (see box on p. 56) (Figs. 2-21 to 2-26).

Varicose veins can also be classified into four developmental stages. The first stage appears as a somewhat dilated blue vein in association with a normal long and short saphenous vein. This stage usually occurs in teenagers with a family history of varicose veins. It is asymptomatic.

The second stage appears as a palpable, bulging, moderately dilated vein usually in association with a larger saphenous vein. Venous Doppler examination is normal. Duplex scanning may show a dilated but competent saphenofemoral and/or saphenopopliteal junction. These veins may be symptomatic after prolonged immobilization or standing.

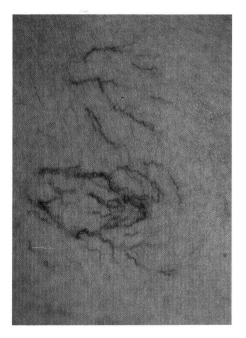

**Fig. 2-21**   Duffy type 1 (telangiectasia) on the inner thigh of a 58-year-old woman.

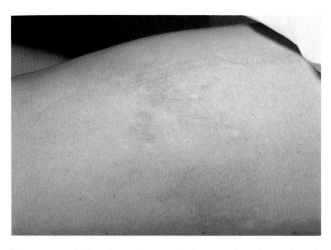

**Fig. 2-22**   Duffy type 1A (telangiectatic matting) 6 weeks after sclerotherapy treatment on the lateral calf. Note associated reticular veins, postsclerotherapy hyperpigmentation, and bruising.

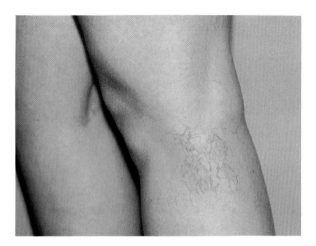

**Fig. 2-23**    Duffy type 1B (communicating telangiectasia) in a 20-year-old woman.

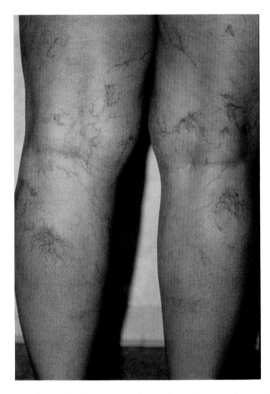

**Fig. 2-24**    Duffy type 2 (mixed telangiectasia and varicose veins with no direct communication with the saphenous system) in a 54-year-old woman. There was no evidence (venous Doppler) of incompetence of the saphenofemoral or saphenopopliteal junctions or of perforating veins.

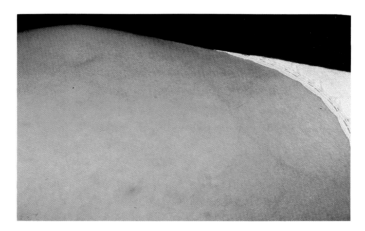

**Fig. 2-25**    Duffy type 3 (nonsaphenous varicose [reticular] veins) in a 24-year-old woman located over the proximal anterolateral thigh.

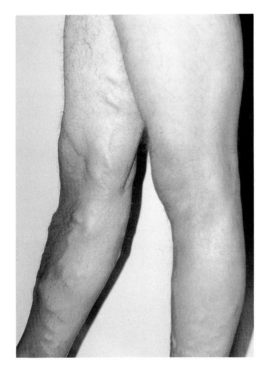

**Fig. 2-26**    Duffy type 4 (saphenous varicose veins). Varicose LSV with incompetent valvular function throughout its length and a grossly incompetent saphenofemoral junction in a 32-year-old man.

## VESSEL CLASSIFICATION

**TYPE 1-TELANGIECTASIA, "SPIDER VEINS"**
0.1-1.0 mm diameter
Red to cyanotic

**TYPE 1A-TELANGIECTATIC MATTING**
<0.2 mm diameter
Red

**TYPE 1B-COMMUNICATING TELANGIECTASIA**
Type 1 veins in direct communication with varicose veins of the saphenous system

**TYPE 2-MIXED TELANGIECTATIC/VARICOSE VEINS (NO DIRECT COMMUNICATION WITH THE SAPHENOUS SYSTEM)**
1.0-6.0 mm diameter
Cyanotic to blue

**TYPE 3-NONSAPHENOUS VARICOSE VEINS (RETICULAR VEINS)**
2-8 mm diameter
Blue to blue-green

**TYPE 4-SAPHENOUS VARICOSE VEINS**
Usually over 8 mm in diameter
Blue to blue-green

Modified from Duffy DM: Small vessel sclerotherapy: an overview. In Callen et al, editors: Advances in dermatology, vol 3, Chicago, 1988, Year Book Medical Publishers.

The third stage represents established varicose vein disease. The long and/or short saphenous veins are dilated over all or part of their length. There are associated varicose veins over the thigh and lower leg with accompanying venules and spider veins. The varicose veins themselves may or may not be incompetent, but gross incompetence is present at the saphenofemoral and/or saphenopopliteal junctions.

The final, or fourth, stage consists of complications arising from chronic venous insufficiency and varicose veins. Perforating vein incompetence is present along with cutaneous manifestations of venous stasis disease including ulcerations.

The development of varicose vein disease is generally progressive. Certain patients may experience spontaneous stabilization of the disease in the early stages. Treatment of early stage disease may prevent the progression and cause regression of the disease process. A complete understanding of the anatomy and pathophysiology of the venous system with regard to varicose veins allows the development of a rational treatment plan.

## REFERENCES

1. Baron HC: Varicose veins, Consultant, May:108, 1983.
2. Hobbs JT: The problem of the post-thrombotic syndrome, Postgrad Med J (Aug Supp):48, 1973.
3. Beninson J and Livingood CS: Stasis dermatitis in clinical dermatology. In Demis DJ, editor: Clinical dermatology, vol 2, Philadelphia, 1985, Harper and Row Publishers.
4. Strandness DE Jr and Thiele BL: Selected topics in venous disorders, Mt Kisco, NY, 1981, Futura Publishing Co.
5. Widmer LK: Peripheral venous disorders: prevalence and socio-medical importance observations in 4529 apparently healthy persons. Basle Study III. Bern, Switzerland, 1978, Hans Huber Publishers.
6. Gallagher PG: Major contributing role of sclerotherapy in the treatment of varicose veins, J Vasc Surg 20:139, 1986.
7. Homans J: The operative treatment of varicose veins and ulcers, based upon a classification of these lesions, Surg Gynecol Obstet 22:143, 1916.
8. Haeger KHM and Bergman L: Skin temperature of normal and varicose veins and some reflections on the etiology of varicose veins, Angiology 14:473, 1963.
9. Linton R: The post-thrombotic ulceration of the lower extremity: its etiology and surgical treatment, Ann Surg 138:415, 1953.
10. Burnand KG et al: The relative importance of incompetent communicating veins in the production of varicose veins and venous ulcers, Surgery 82:9, 1977.
11. Warren R, White EA, and Belcher CB: Venous pressure in the saphenous system in normal, varicose, and post-phlebitic extremities, Surgery 26:435, 1949.
12. Farber EM and Batts EE: Pathologic physiology of stasis dermatitis, Arch Dermatol 70:653, 1954.
13. Smith HG: Complicating factors in the surgical management of varicose veins, Surgery 17:590, 1945.
14. Cockett FB and Jones BE: The ankle blow-out syndrome: a new approach to the varicose ulcer problem, Lancet 1:17, 1953.
15. Dodd H and Cockett FB: The pathology and surgery of the veins of the lower limbs, ed 2, London, 1976, Churchill Livingstone Inc.
16. Landis EM: Factors controlling the movement of fluid through the human capillary wall, Yale J Biol Med 5:201, 1933.
17. Burnand KG et al: The effects of sustained venous hypertension of the skin capillaries of the canine hind limb, Br J Surg 69:41, 1982.
18. Ryan TJ and Wilkinson DS: Diseases of the veins: venous leg ulcers. In Rook A, Wilkinson DS, and Ebling FTG, editors: Textbook of dermatology, ed 3, London, 1979, Blackwell Scientific Publications.
19. Ryan TJ: Diseases of the skin: management of varicose ulcers and eczema, Br Med J 1:192, 1974.
20. Whimster I. Cited in Dodd H and Cockett FP: The pathology and surgery of the veins of the lower limb, Edinbugh & London, 1956, Churchill Livingstone Inc.
21. Calman JS et al: Venous obstruction in the aetiology of lymphoedema praecox, Br J Med 2:221, 1964.
22. Farber EM and Barnes VR: The stasis syndrome, Arch Dermatol Syph 73:277, 1956.
23. Lofgren KA: Varicose veins: their symptoms, complications, and management, Postgrad Med 65:131, 1979.
24. Veal JR and Hossey H: The pathologic physiology of the circulation in the post-thrombotic syndrome, Am Heart J 23:390, 1942.
25. Drinker CK, Field ME, and Homans J: Experimental production of edema and elephantiasis as a result of lymphatic obstruction, Am J Physiol 108:509, 1934.
26. Isenring G, Franzeck UK, and Bollinger A: Lymphatische Mikroangiopathie bei Chronisch-Venoeser Insuffizienz (CVI), Vasa 11:104, 1982.
27. McMaster PD: Changes in the cutaneous lymphatics of human beings and in the lymph flow under normal and pathological conditions, J Exp Med 65:345, 1937.
28. Campbell RT: Chronic varicose ulcer with pseudoepitheliomatous hyperplasia, Proc R Soc Med 44:923, 1951.
29. Nemeth AJ et al: Ulcerated edematous limbs: effect of edema removal on transcutaneous oxygen measurements, J Am Acad Dermatol 20:191, 1989.
30. Dodd H and Cockett FB: The pathology and surgery of the veins of the lower limbs, Edinburgh & London, 1956, ES Livingstone Ltd.
31. Falanga V et al: Dermal pericapillary fibrin in venous disease and venous ulceration, Arch Dermatol 123:620, 1987.

32. Browse NL and Burnand KG: The cause of venous ulceration, Lancet 2:243, 1982.
33. Coleridge Smith PD et al: Causes of venous ulceration: a new hypothesis, Br Med J 296:1726, 1988.
34. Bollinger A et al: Fluorescence microlymphography in chronic venous incompetence, Int Angiol 8:23, 1989.
35. Thomas PRS, Nash GB, and Dormandy JA: White cell accumulation in dependent legs of patients with venous hypertension: a possible mechanism for trophic changes in the skin, Br Med J 296:1693, 1988.
36. Nash GB, Thomas PRS, and Dormandy JA: Abnormal flow properties of white blood cells in patients with severe ischemia of the leg, Br Med J 296:1699, 1988.
37. Allen JC: The micro-circulation of the skin of the normal leg in varicose veins and in the post-thrombotic syndrome, S Afr J Surg 10:29, 1972.
38. Strandness DE Jr: Varicose veins. In Demis DJ, editor: Clinical dermatology, Philadelphia, 1985, Harper and Row Publishers.
39. Coon WW, Willis PW III, and Keller JB: Venous thromboembolism and other venous disease in the Tecumseh community health study, Circulation 48:839, 1973.
40. Engel A, Johnson ML, and Haynes SG: Health effects of sunlight exposure in the United States: results from the first national health and nutrition examination survey, 1971-1974, Arch Dermatol 124:72, 1988.
41. Dinn A and Henry M: Value of lightweight elastic tights in standing occupations, Phlebology 4:45, 1989.
42. Lake M, Pratt GH, and Wright IS: Arteriosclerosis and varicose veins: occupational activities and other factors, JAMA 119:696, 1942.
43. Oster J and Nielsen A: Nuchal naevi and intrascapular telangiectasies, Acta Paediat Scand 59:416, 1970.
44. Heede G: Prevaricose epidemiological symptoms in 8 to 18 aged pupils. In Davy A and Stemmer R, editors: Phlebologie '89, Montrouge, France, 1989, John Libbey Eurotext Ltd.
45. Schultz-Ehrenburg U et al: Prospective epidemiological investigations on early and preclinical stages of varicosis. In Davy A and Stemmer R, editors: Phlebologie '89, Montrouge, France, John Libbey Eurotext Ltd.
46. McPheeters HO: The value of estrogen therapy in the treatment of varicose veins complicating pregnancy, Lancet 69:2, 1949.
47. Fegan G: Varicose veins, London, 1967, William Heinemann Medical Books, Ltd.
48. Summer DS: Hemodynamics and pathophysiology of venous disease. In Rutherford RB, editor: Vascular surgery, Philadelphia, 1984, WB Saunders Co.
49. Sumner DS: Venous dynamics-varicosities, Clin Obstet Gynecol 24:743, 1981.
50. Burnand KG: Management of varicose veins of the legs, Nursing Mirror 144:45, 1977.
51. Weiss R and Weiss M: Resolution of pain associated with varicose and telangiectatic leg veins after compression sclerotherapy, J Dermatol Surg Oncol, 16:333, 1990.
52. Wilder CS: Prevalence of selected chronic circulatory conditions, Vital Health Stat 94:1, 1974.
53. Fegan WG, Lambe R, and Henry M: Steroid hormones and varicose veins, Lancet 1:1070, 1967.
54. MacCausland AM: Varicose veins in pregnancy, Ca West Med 50:258, 1939.
55. Browse NL, Burnand KG, and Thomas ML: Diseases of the veins: pathology, diagnosis, and treatment, London, 1988, Edward Arnold.
56. Gay J: On varicose disease of the lower extremities, London, 1868, J Churchill & Sons.
57. Pleuss J: Contribution a letude etiopathogenique des ulceres de jambe, Bull Soc Franc Phlebologie 4:137, 1952.
58. Allen EV, Barker NW, and Hines EA Jr: Peripheral vascular diseases, Philadelphia, 1946, WB Saunders Co.
59. Hojensgard IC and Sturup H: On the function of the venous pump and the venous return from the lower limbs, Acta Derm Venerol Stockn 29(suppl):169, 1952.
60. Ryan TJ: Microvascular injury: vasculitis, stasis, and ischemia, London, 1976, WB Saunders Co.
61. Browse NL et al: The treatment of liposclerosis of the leg by fibrinolytic enhancement: a preliminary report, Br Med J 2:434, 1977.
62. Hobbs JT: The post-thrombotic syndrome. In Hobbs JT, editor: The treatment of venous disorders, Philadelphia, 1977, JB Lippincott Co.
63. Shelley WB, Swaminathan R, and Shelley ED: Lichen aureus: a hemosiderin tattoo associated with perforator vein incompetence, J Am Acad Dermatol 11:260, 1984.
64. Gravatational eczema. In Rook A et al, editors: Textbook of dermatology, ed 4, Melbourne, 1986, Blackwell Scientific Publications.
65. McPheeters HO and Anderson JK: Injection treatment of varicose veins and hemorrhoids, Philadelphia, 1943, FA Davis Co.

66. Zimmerman LM and Rattner H: Infra-red photography of subcutaneous veins, Am J Surg 27:502, 1935.
67. Larsen WG and Maibach HI: Dermatitis and eczema. In Mosschella SL and Hurley HJ, editors: Dermatology, ed 2, Philadelphia, 1985, WB Saunders Co.
68. Biegeleisen HI: Varicose veins, related diseases, and sclerotherapy: a guide for practitioners, London, 1984, Eden Press.
69. Jeghers H and Edelstein L: Skin color in health and disease. In MacBryde CM and Blackslow RS, editors: Signs and symptoms, ed 6, Philadelphia, 1983, JB Lippincott Co.
70. Kulwin MH and Hines EA Jr: Blood vessels of the skin in chronic venous insufficiency: clinical pathologic studies, Arch Dermatol Syph 62:293, 1950.
71. Milian G: Les atrophies cutanees syphilitiques, Bull Soc Franc Dermatol Syph 36:865, 1929.
72. Anning ST: Leg ulcers: their causes and treatment, London, 1954, J & A Churchill, Ltd.
73. Wiseman R: Severall chirurgical treatises, London, 1676, Royston and Took.
74. Dale WA and Foster J: Leg ulcers: comprehensive plan of diagnosis and management, Med Sci 15:56, 1964.
75. Callam MJ et al: Chronic ulceration of the leg: extent of the problem and provision of care, Br Med J 290:1855, 1985.
76. Haeger K, editor: Venous and lymphatic disorders of the leg, Lund, Sweden, 1966, Bokforlaget Universitet och Skola.
77. Sicard JA, Forestier J, and Gaugier L: Treatment of varicose ulcers, Proc R Soc Med 21:1837, 1929.
78. Sigg K: Varizen, ulcus cruris, und Thrombose, Berlin, 1958, Springer-Verlag.
79. Ruckley CV et al: Causes of chronic leg ulcer, Lancet 2:615, 1982.
80. Bauer G: Heparin as a therapeutic against thrombosis: results of a one-year treatment at Mariestal Hospital, Acta Chir Scand 86:217, 1942.
81. Hoare MC et al: The role of primary varicose veins in venous ulceration, Surgery 92:450, 1982.
82. Editorial: Venous ulcers, Lancet 1:522, 1977.
83. Lawrence D, Fish PJ, and Kakkar VV: Blood-flow in incompetent perforating veins, Lancet 1:117, 1977.
84. Burnand K et al: Relationship between postphlebitic changes in the deep veins and results of surgical treatment of venous ulcers, Lancet 1:936, 1976.
85. Lofgren EP: Leg ulcers: symptoms of an underlying disorder, Postgrad Med 76:51, 1984.
86. Lippman HI: Subcutaneous ossification in chronic venous insufficiency, presentation of 23 cases: preliminary report, Angiology 8:378, 1957.
87. Ward WH: Leg ulcers, Australas J Dermatol 5:145, 1960.
88. Lippman HI and Goldin RR: Subcutaneous ossification of the legs in chronic venous insufficiency, Radiology 74:279, 1960.
89. Michael: Uber der primaren Krebs der Extremitaten, Tübingen, Germany, 1890, Inaug Diss.
90. Druckenmuller: Beitrag zur Kasuistik der Carcinom entwicklung auf Unterschenkel Geschwuren, Greifswald, Germany, 1895, Inaug Diss.
91. Gottheil WS: Cancerous degeneration in chronic leg ulcers, JAMA 59:14, 1912.
92. Grusser M: Cancer of leg, Arch f Klin f Klin Chir 127:529, 1923; abstr JAMA 81:2156, 1923.
93. Knox LC: Epithelioma and the chronic varicose ulcer, JAMA 85:1046, 1925.
94. Von Volkmann R: Samml Klin Vortr 1886-1890, Chir 335:235, 1925. In Bang: le Cancer des Cicatrices Etude Clinque et Expérimentale, Assoc Franc Pour l'Etude du Cancer 14:203, 1925.
95. Tenopyr J and Silverman I: The relation of chronic varicose ulcer to epithelioma, Ann Surg 95:754, 1932.
96. Glasser ST: Sarcomatous degeneration on a varicose ulcer, Am J Surg 43:776, 1939.
97. Black W: Neoplastic disease in varicose ulcers or eczema: a report on six cases, Br J Cancer 5:120, 1952.
98. Levine MR and Fung FL: Malignant degeneration in varicose ulcers of the lower extremities, Can Med Assoc J 76:961, 1957.
99. Pannell TC and Hightower F: Malignant changes in post-phlebitic ulcers, S Med J 58:779, 1965.
100. Dawson EK and McIntosh D: Granulation tissue sarcoma following longstanding varicose ulceration, J R Coll Surg Edinb 16:88, 1971.
101. Balestrino E et al: Malignant degeneration of chronic venous ulcer (Marjolin's ulcer), Min Chir 38:211, 1983.
102. Tretbar LI: Bleeding from varicose veins, treatment with injection sclerotherapy. In Davy A and Stemmer R, editors: Phlebologie '89, Montrouge, France, 1989, John Libby Eurotext Ltd.
103. Evans GA et al: Spontaneous fatal hemorrhage caused by varicose veins, Lancet 2:1359, 1973.
104. Harman RRM: Haemorrhage from varicose veins, Lancet 1:363, 1974.
105. Du Toit DF, Knott-Craig C, and Laker L: Bleeding from varicose veins — still potentially fatal, S Afr Med J 67:303, 1985.

106. Husni EA and Williams WA: Superficial thrombophlebitis of the lower limbs, Surgery 91:70, 1982.

107. Zollinger RW, Williams RD, and Briggs DO: Problems in the diagnosis and treatment of thrombophlebitis, Arch Surg 85:18, 1962.

108. Raso AM et al: Studio su 357 casi di flebite degli arti inferiori su due campioni interregionali, Minerva Chir 34:553, 1979.

109. Totten HP: Superficial thrombophlebitis: observations on diagnosis and treatment, Geriatrics 22:151, 1967.

110. Edwards EA: Thrombophlebitis of varicose veins, Gynecol Obstet 60:236, 1938.

111. Gjores JE: Surgical therapy of ascending thrombophlebitis in the saphenous system, Angiology 13:241, 1962.

112. Husni EA, Pena LI, and Lenhert AE: Thrombophlebitis in pregnancy, Am J Obstet Gynecol 97:901, 1967.

113. Osius EA: Discussion of Hermann's paper, AMA Arch Surg 64:685, 1952.

114. Guilmot J-L, Wolman F, and Lasfargues G: Thromboses veineuses superficielles, Rev Prat 38:2062, 1988.

115. Zollinger RW: Superficial thrombophlebitis, Surg Gynecol Obstet 124:1077, 1967.

116. Hafner CD et al: A method of managing superficial thrombophelbitis, Surgery 55:201, 1964.

117. Martin P et al: Peripheral vascular disorders, Edinburgh and London, 1956, E & S Livingstone Ltd.

118. Lofgren EP and Lofgren KA: The surgical treatment of superficial thrombophlebitis, Surgery 90:49, 1981.

119. Totten HP: The surgical treatment of acute ascending superficial thrombophlebitis, Angiology 16:37, 1965.

120. Lilly GD: Discussion of paper by Sawyer et al, Surgery 55:121, 1964.

121. Glover WJ et al: Venous thrombectomy in the management of acute venous thrombosis of the saphenous system, Am J Surg 93:798, 1957.

122. Lowenberg EL: Significance and management of acute spontaneous thrombophlebitis in the superficial veins of the lower extremities, J Internat Col Surg 18:422, 1952.

123. Barrow DW: The clinical management of varicose veins, ed 2, New York, 1957, Paul H. Hoeber, Inc.

124. Foote RR: Varicose veins, St Louis, 1949, The CV Mosby Co.

125. Bergan J: Personal communication, 1989.

126. Clayton JK, Anderson JA, and McNicol GP: Preoperative prediction of post-operative deep vein thrombosis, Br Med J 2:910, 1976.

127. Crandon AJ et al: Post-operative deep vein thrombosis: identifying high-risk patients, Br Med J 281:343, 1980.

128. Lowe GD et al: Prediction and selective prophylaxis of venous thrombosis in elective gastrointestinal surgery, Lancet 1:409, 1982.

129. Rakoczi I et al: Prediction of post-operative leg-vein thrombosis in gynecological patients, Lancet 1:509, 1978.

130. Matyas M: The clinical management of varicose veins, ed 2, New York, 1957, Paul H Hoeber, Inc.

131. Heyerdale WW and Stalker LK: The management of varicose veins of the lower extremities, Ann Surg 114:1042, 1941.

132. Widmer LK: Peripheral venous disorders: prevalence and socio-medical importance observations in 4529 apparently healthy persons. Basle Study III, Bern, Switzerland, 1978, Hans Huber.

133. Duffy DM: Small vessel sclerotherapy: an overview. In Callen et al, editors: Advances in dermatology, vol 3, Chicago, 1988, Year Book Medical Publishers Inc.

# 3 | Pathophysiology of Varicose Veins

There are essentially three components of the venous system of the leg that act in concert: deep veins, superficial veins, and perforating/communicating veins. Dysfunction in any of these three systems results in dysfunction of the other two. When the superficial veins are placed under high pressure, they dilate and elongate to accommodate the increased blood volume. The tortuous appearance thus produced is termed *varicose,* derived from the Greek term for "grape-like." This term applies to both the large protruding veins within the superficial subcutaneous fascia and the smaller venectasia "spider veins" that occur just beneath the epidermis.

The World Health Organization[1] defines varicose veins as "Saccular dilatation of the veins which are often tortuous." Further, this definition specifically excludes any tortuous veins associated with previous thrombophlebitis or an arteriovenous fistula or with venectasia.

## HISTOCHEMICAL PHYSIOLOGY OF VARICOSE VEINS

Varicose veins may differ from nonvaricose veins in physiologic function. Endothelial damage has been noted to occur in parts of a varicose vein.[2] Also varicose veins have been noted to have a considerable degree of smooth muscle hypertrophy and a 15% increase in muscle content compared with normal veins.[3] This is thought to be a secondary response to venous hypertension. Other investigators have found that smooth muscle cells are capable of phagocytosis and decomposition of collagen fibers.[4] Thus these cells may be part of the cellular basis for collagen breakdown. Some investigators have found that varicose veins have an extremely dense and compact fibrosis between the intima and adventitia, with a diminished and atrophied elastic network and a disorganized muscular layer (Fig. 3-1).[5-7] Thickening and fibrillation of individual collagen fibers has also been noted.[2,6,8]

The loss of tonicity of varicose veins is primarily the result of this loss of coordinated communication between vein wall smooth muscle cells as previously described. Electron microscopic studies of nonvaricose veins demonstrate the close approximation of smooth muscle cells. When veins become varicose, smooth muscle cells become vacuolated and are separated by collagen.[5,6] With increasing varicose changes, intercellular collagen deposition accumulates and separates the smooth muscle cells that atrophy (Fig. 3-2). It is suggested that the resulting separation of smooth muscle cell hemidesmosomes results in inefficient smooth muscle contraction and increased venous distensibility.[6,9] However, at least some varicose veins are capable of constricting in response to an infusion of dihydroergotamine. This venoconstriction is even more pronounced than that which occurs in normal veins.[10] The reason for this paradoxical effect is unknown. Therefore, the varicose vein appears to be a dysplastic vein characterized by malformations. Whether this is the result of continual high venous pressure or is the primary etiologic event in the development of valvular incompetence is unknown.

Although collagen accumulation is thought to separate smooth muscle cells

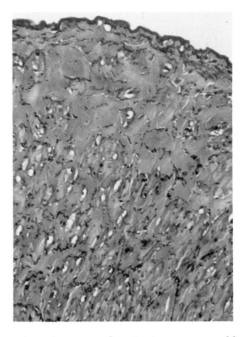

**Fig. 3-1** Cross section of a tributary to the LSV in a 46-year-old man, stained with Verhoeff-van Gieson (×150). Note extensive fragmentation of elastin fibers interspersed between irregularly oriented muscle bundles with marked hypertrophy of collagen fibers. Elastic fibers stain *black;* collagen: *red;* muscle: *brown-yellow.*

within the varicose vein wall, the collagen content of varicose veins is less than that in normal tissues.[3] The bulk of the varicose vein wall is made up of mucopolysaccharides and other ground substances. Varicose veins contain 67% more hexosamine (which composes about 0.3% of normal vein dry material) as compared with normal veins.

Dysplasticity of the varicose vein wall may explain why varicose veins have an even greater susceptibility to pressure-induced distention than nonvaricose veins. This anatomico-pathophysiologic correlation has been demonstrated by pharmacologic studies that show reduced maximal contraction of varicose veins as compared with control veins.[2,9] However, some investigations have failed to disclose a significant difference in the degree of intimal fibrosis between varicose and nonvaricose veins.[11] Therefore, fibrosis of the vein wall alone is not totally responsible for development of varicose veins.

Finally, a decrease in tocopherol concentration has been noted in varicose veins.[12] There also appears to be a significant correlation between the inhibition of vessel wall tissues on lipoperoxidation and their tocopherol concentration, independent of serum concentrations. This may be the result of the protective effect of blocking peroxidation of membrane-associated fatty acids by tocopherol and other antioxidants to prevent vein wall damage.[13] It is clear that the dysplasticity of varicose veins correlates with the changes in their pharmacodynamics and histochemistry. Varicose veins have a demonstrated loss of contractility.[14] In addition, histochemical examination discloses a marked increase in the activity of lysosomal enzymes,[15] acid phosphatase, β-glucuronidase, and anaerobic isoenzymes (lactodehydrogenase) in primary varicose veins.[16-18] These enzyme patterns suggest a decline in energy metabolism and an increase in cellular damage in the varicose veins. Also, varicose veins accumulate and metabolize norepi-

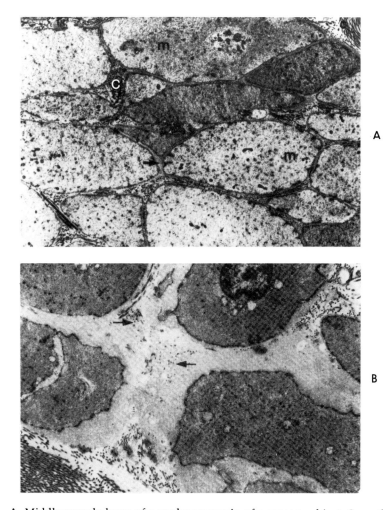

**Fig. 3-2** **A,** Middle muscle layer of a saphenous vein of a young subject. Smooth muscle cells, *(m);* narrow perimyocytic spaces containing collagen fibers, *(c).* The basilar membrane of smooth muscle is clearly visable, *(arrow).* (Uranyl acetate–lead citrate; ×4000.) **B,** Muscle fibers in an aged subject showing the wide separation of dystrophic muscle cells. A few collagen fibers are visible, *(arrows).* (Uranyl acetate–lead citrate; ×5000.) (From Bouissou H et al: Phlebologie 3(suppl 1):1, 1988.

nephrine less efficiently than normal veins.[19] Therefore, both an anatomic and a biochemical breakdown in the varicose vein undoubtedly contribute to its easy distensibility.

## PATHOPHYSIOLOGY

Approximately 75% of the body's total blood volume is contained within the peripheral venous system.[20] The quantity of blood within the legs is a function of body position. When erect, 300 to 800 ml of extracellular and vascular fluids (the quantity varies as to the experimental method and the size of the subject measured) collect in the legs.[21-23] This includes a 15% increase of blood volume.[21] Thus the venous system, especially in the legs, is an important component of the cardiovascular system's circulatory reservoir. However, the arterial system plays an equally important role in cardiovascular adaptation to postural changes by virtue of changes in arterial resistance. In fact, studies have demonstrated that reflex changes in venous tone are not essential for this fluid shift.[24]

Venous blood pressure is determined by several factors. Among these are pressure generated by the heart, the energy lost in the peripheral resistance of arterioles, hydrostatic gravitational forces, blood volume, anatomic composition of the venous wall, efficiency of one-way valves, vein wall distensibility (determined by hormonal, systemic alcohol, and other factors), and the contraction of venous smooth muscle as influenced by ambient temperature and sympathetic and parasympathetic nerve tone (Fig. 3-3).

Although arterial pressure does comprise one factor in the development of venous pressure, arterial hypertension has been noted to be associated with the development of varicose veins in some epidemiologic studies[25] but not others.[26] At rest, in the erect position, pressure in the saphenous vein is determined primarily by the height of the column of blood from the right atrium to the site of measurement (90 to 120 mm Hg at the ankle) (Fig. 3-4).[27,28] Contraction of calf muscles generates pressures between 200 and 300 mm Hg.[29-31]

Pressure generated deep to the fascia, outside of muscles, is between 100 and 150 mm Hg.[31,32] However, with muscular activity, pressure in the normal saphenous vein at the level of the malleoli falls 45 to 68 mm Hg below the resting level.[33] It is reduced from 80 to 40 mm Hg in the posterior tibial vein.[34] Because of the one-way valves, blood flow is directed from the superficial venous system to the deep venous system via communicating or perforating vessels. This has been visually demonstrated by serial phlebography of the normal lower leg (see Fig. 1-6).[35] The venous blood then flows towards the heart.

Respiration produces alterations in intraabdominal venous pressure. This "abdominal venous pump" contributes to the flow of blood even when an individual is erect.[23,36] Inspiration produces a rise in venous pressure in the external iliac vein, common iliac vein, and inferior vena cava when measured in both the horizontal and erect positions, 6.3 mm Hg and 8.7 mm Hg respectively.[36]

In the supine position, blood flows evenly along all superficial and deep vessels toward the heart. It is propelled by the relatively small vis-à-tergo from the capillaries[34] and the respiration-induced aspiration of blood into the abdominal and thoracic veins. In contrast to deep veins, superficial veins have smooth muscle in their walls. This allows contraction of these vessels in response to cold and to drugs such as dihydroergotamine[37,38] and allows dilation in response to topical and systemic alcohol, estrogen, and light physical trauma.[34] As previously described, part of the pathophysiology of varicose veins may be a diminished response of such smooth muscle contraction.

Regardless of its cause, chronic venous hypertension in the lower extremities causes an increase in venous diameter. This may lead to valvular insufficiency, which usually causes a reversal of blood flow from the deep veins into the superficial veins through incompetent communicating veins. This "private circulation" may account for up to 20% to 25% of the total femoral flow to be involved in a circular retrograde flow (Fig. 3-5).[39]

Direction of venous flow in varicose veins has been examined by McPheeters and Rice[40] by fluoroscopy. Reversal of flow caused by incompetent perforator valves is beneficial during sclerotherapy. When a superficial varicosity is injected, its venous flow is forced distally to the smaller branching veins where it is arrested (see Chapter 8).[40] Thromboembolic disease is thereby prevented.

Superficial veins respond to increased pressure by dilating. Valvular incompetence occurs and varicosities appear.[41] In addition, in muscular contraction, high compartmental pressure that normally occurs within the calf muscle pump

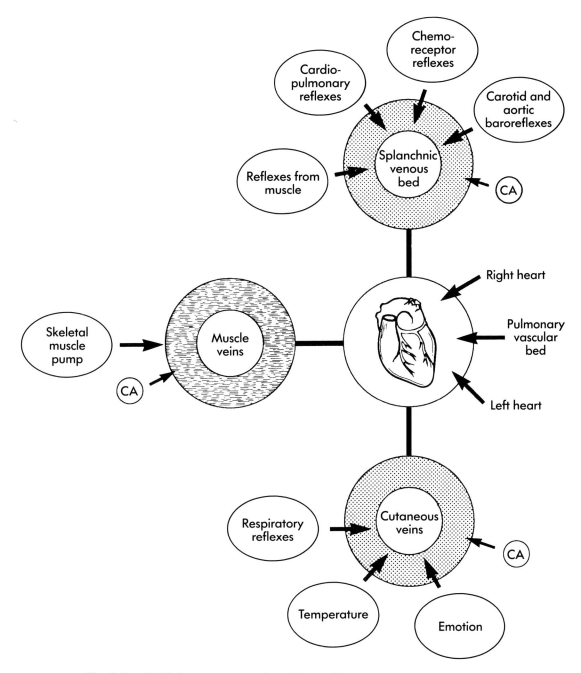

**Fig. 3-3** Multiple environmental and internal factors act on the venous system to influence its dilation and constriction. (*CA* = catecholamines.)

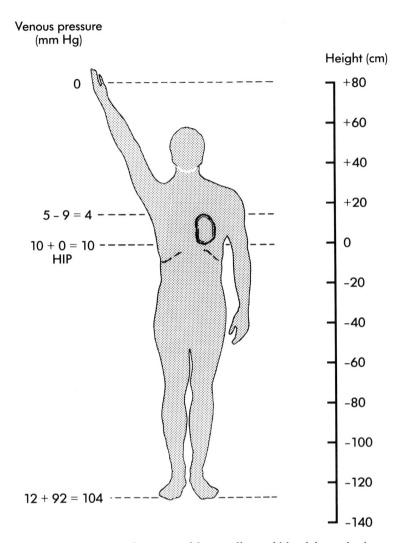

**Fig. 3-4** Venous pressure is that exerted by a collum of blood from the heart to the location of measurement.

is transmitted directly to the superficial veins and subcutaneous tissues drained by communicating veins.[42,43] When this occurs, venous pressure in the cuticular venules may reach 100 mm Hg in the erect position.[34] This causes venular dilation over a broad area and may cause capillary dilation, increased permeability,[44-47] and an increase in the subcutaneous capillary bed.[45,48] This is expressed clinically in venous blemishes. Histologically, cutaneous and subcutaneous hemosiderin deposition may also occur. This, in time, results in cutaneous pigmentation (see Chapter 2).

A special situation develops in the area of the medial malleolus. In this area perforating veins are not surrounded by deep or superficial fascia. Therefore, any increased deep venous pressure is transmitted directly through perforating veins to superficial connecting veins. This causes high cutaneous venous pressures and a transudation of extracellular fluid. This, in turn, leads to perivascular fibrin deposition, which may play a role in decreased oxygenation of cutaneous

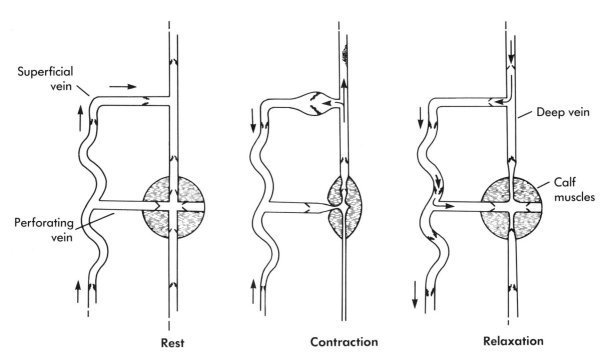

**Fig. 3-5**    Private circulation of blood flow in primary varicose veins demonstrating a retrograde circuitous blood flow with muscle contraction and relaxation.

and supporting tissues, which contributes to cutaneous ulceration (see Chapter 2).[45,49,50]

The effect of temperature variations on the venous system is well studied.[51,52] The cutaneous vasculature is intimately involved in thermoregulation. An increase in body core temperature results in cutaneous vasodilation. This occurs not as a result of relaxation of venous smooth muscle, but because of reduction in the vasoconstrictor impulses to the vein wall. Such vasodilation also occurs in varicose veins. Recently strain gauge venous occlusion plethysmography has shown an increase in venous distensibility associated with temperature elevation.[53] Similarly, alcohol ingestion may influence the development of varicose veins. Alcohol intake, like increased environmental temperature, causes cutaneous vasodilation. In an examination of 136 men with primary varicose veins greater than 4 mm in diameter, it was found that a significantly increased incidence of varicose veins occurs among men who consume 4 oz of alcohol a day.[54] Unfortunately, further experimental evaluations of this association have not been performed.

In summary, pathologic development of varicose veins can be divided into four broad categories. These may overlap. Increased deep venous pressure, primary valvular incompetence, secondary valvular incompetence, and hereditary factors such as vein wall weakness all coexist and are influenced by temperature, alcohol, and hormonal and other vasodilatory stimuli (see box, p. 68).

## Increased Deep Venous Pressure

An increase in the deep venous pressure may be of proximal or distal origin. Proximal causes include pelvic obstruction (resulting in indirect venous obstruction); increased intraabdominal pressure caused by straining during defecation or

## PATHOPHYSIOLOGY OF VARICOSE VEINS

**INCREASED DEEP VENOUS PRESSURE**
*Proximal*
Pelvic obstruction (indirect venous obstruction)
Intraabdominal pressure caused by straining at defecation or micturition, wearing constrictive clothing, standing, chair sitting, leg crossing, squatting, obesity, or running
Saphenofemoral incompetence
Venous obstruction

*Distal*
Communicating or perforating vein valvular incompetence
Venous obstruction
Arteriovenous anastomosis

**PRIMARY VALVULAR INCOMPETENCE**
Venous obstruction (thrombosis)
Thrombophlebitis with destruction of venous valves
Congenital absence of venous valves (agenesis)
Decreased number of venous valves

**SECONDARY VALVULAR INCOMPETENCE**
Deep venous obstruction
Increased venous distensibility
   Hormonal (pregnancy; estrogens, progesterone, and their relative concentrations)

**HEREDITY**
Vein wall weakness
   Inherited deficiency of vein wall collagen
Primary valvular dysfunction/agenesis
ABO blood group

Modified from Goldman MP and Fronek A: Anatomy and pathophysiology of varicose veins, J Dermatol Oncol 15:138, 1989.

micturition, wearing constrictive clothing, sitting in chairs, obesity, and running; saphenofemoral incompetence; and intraluminal venous obstruction. Distal causes include communicating vein valvular incompetence, arteriovenous anastomoses, and intraluminal venous obstruction.

### Proximal

*Pelvic obstruction.* Pelvic obstruction is an uncommon cause of varicose veins. Extravascular abdominal tumors such as ovarian and uterine carcinoma or teratoma may be causes of obstruction, but more commonly, it is relative pelvic obstruction that provides a mechanism for impedance of return blood flow. Relative obstruction may occur in the third trimester of pregnancy, particularly during recumbency when the gravid uterus compresses the inferior vena cava against the lumbar spine and/or psoas muscles. Phlebographic studies have shown complete obstruction of the inferior vena cava at the confluence of the iliac veins in third-trimester pregnancies.[55] Partial obstruction has been shown in earlier months of pregnancy. Some degree of compression is evident using phlebography even in the left lateral decubitus position.

*Increased intraabdominal pressure.* One popular hypothesis for the development of varicose veins is Western dietary and defecation habits that cause an increase in intraabdominal pressure. A distended cecum or sigmoid colon resulting from constipation may drag on the iliac veins, obstructing venous return from the legs.[56] Population studies have demonstrated that a high-fiber diet is evacuated within an average of 35 hours.[57] In contrast, a low-fiber diet has an average transit time of 77 hours. An intermediate diet has a stool transit time of 47 hours. When a diet intermediate between Western low-fiber and high-fiber diets is consumed, the prevalence of varicose veins is also found to be in an intermediate range.[58]

It is possible that the small increase in abdominal intravenous pressure caused by less than optimal bowel habits, when transmitted intravenously distally, gradually breaks down venous valves of leg veins.[59,60] Evidence in support of this hypothesis is seen in populations who eat unprocessed high-fiber food. These persons are free from constipation and varicose veins.[61,62] However, if this population's diet is changed to low fiber, the incidence of varicose veins increases.[56,63-65]

Also, defecatory straining induced by Western-style toilet seats has been cited as a cause of varicose veins in contrast to the African custom of squatting during defecation.[64] However, venous pressures of subjects measured while in both the sitting and squatting positions during defecation have not shown a significant difference.[66] Venous flow has not been accurately examined in constipated and nonconstipated populations.

Finally, there are other dietary factors besides fiber content that may explain the differences in prevalence of varicose veins. An increased incidence of varicose veins is found in populations who consume diets high in long-chain fatty acids as opposed to a diet high in short-chain fatty acids.[67] Long-chain fatty acids have been shown in experimental systems to enhance blood coagulation and stimulate the development of blood clots.[68-70] And clot lysis times were lower in the population group that consumed long-chain fatty acids.[67] Accordingly, the *type* of dietary fatty acids consumed may also predispose one to the development of varicose veins. In addition, the Western diet has also been found to be relatively deficient in vitamin E.[71] It is hypothesized that the slight vitamin E deficiency, when aggravated by pregnancy, may predispose the vein wall to coagulation and fibrinolysis, thus causing the veins to become more sensitive to venous stasis and venous hypertension. Therefore, although it would seem prudent to recommend a high-fiber diet for several medical reasons, it remains an unproven treatment for the prevention of varicose veins.

An association between prostatic hypertrophy, inguinal hernia, and varicose veins may also be caused by straining at micturition with a resultant increase in intraabdominal pressure.[72]

Another mechanism for increasing distal venous pressure by proximal obstruction is the practice of wearing girdles or tight-fitting clothing. A statistically significant excess of varicose veins is noted in women who wear corsets compared with women who wear less constrictive garments.[73] A similar increased incidence was noted in women who stand at work compared with those whose jobs entail more walking and sitting.[26,27,73,74]

Leg crossing and chair sitting are two other potential mechanisms for producing a relative impedance in venous return. Habitual leg crossing is commonly thought to result in extravenous compression, but this has never been scientifically verified. A decreased incidence of varicose veins has also been noted in population groups that do not sit in chairs.[75,76] It is thought that sitting may produce some compression on the posterior thigh that produces a relative impedance to blood flow. Wright and Osborn[77] have shown that the linear velocity of venous flow in the lower limbs in the recumbent position is reduced by half in the standing position and by two thirds when sitting. Alexander[76] found that the circumferential stress on the saphenous vein at the ankle was 2.54 times greater with chair sitting than with ground sitting. This may explain the increased incidence of varicose veins in men versus women in population groups where only men sit on chairs and women sit on the floor. In this population study,[75] varicose veins were present in 5.1% of men and only 0.1% of women. Finally, the practical implications regarding chair sitting concerns those who travel for long periods in airplanes. Pulmonary thromboembolism has occurred in multiple people after prolonged air travel and has been termed *economy class syndrome.*[78] Although preexisting venous disease, dehydration, and immobility are all contributing factors, chair sitting adds another insult to the venous system.

Some,[25,26,79-81] but not all,[82] studies have found obesity to be associated with the development of varicose veins. Obesity was especially correlated with the development of varicose veins in women when the varicosities occurred in unison with cutaneous changes indicative of venous stasis (see Chapter 2).[83,84]

Running has also been demonstrated to raise the intraabdominal pressure by 22 mm Hg.[85] This increase in abdominal pressure occurs because of a reflex tightening of abdominal muscles during running, which prevents the pelvis from tipping forward during thigh flexion induced by contraction of the iliopsoas muscle group.[86] Therefore, during strenuous leg exercise, elevated abdominal pressures may impede venous return. By way of comparison, a Valsalva maneuver was shown to elevate the intraabdominal pressure by 50 mm Hg or more.[85] Strenuous exercise, particularly long-distance running, is often associated with prolonged increases in limb blood flow, which could theoretically overload the venous system and lead to progressive dilation.[41] Usually, dilated veins that occur in this situation are normal and do not require treatment.

*Saphenofemoral incompetence..* Saphenofemoral impedance rarely occurs because of anatomic abnormalities in the saphenofemoral triangle. When it does, pelvic tributary veins or accessory saphenous veins may converge in such a manner that flow to the femoral vein is impeded.[87] Likewise, iliac venous incompetence caused by congenital absence of or acquired damage to venous valves via thrombosis may cause distal venous hypertension.

### Distal

*Valvular incompetence.* Unlike the foregoing, clearly, incompetence of the saphenofemoral junction does produce distal retrograde flow into the LSV and thus produces distal venous hypertension. The LSV then dilates producing further distal valvular incompetence sequentially. Retrograde flow thus produced is channeled via the perforator veins back into the deep venous system. This produces a private circuit of blood flow from the femoral vein to the saphenous vein back to the femoral vein via perforating veins.[39] This paradoxical circulation can be maintained for a long time, but eventually the quantity of blood channeled by the perforator veins increases. As this happens, they hypertrophy and dilate. This produces valvular incompetence and localized varicose veins.

Perforator incompetence in the lower part of the leg may occur from localized thrombosis in the vein following trauma. It is believed that the localized thrombosis is usually masked by the local tissue injury. The valve cusps become involved by the thrombus and after recanalization remain functionless.[88] Dodd and Cockett[34] found on examination of 54 legs with perforator incompetence that the lower leg incompetent perforators were in communication with the soleal plexus of veins and, as such, were the channels most likely to be damaged as a result of thrombotic episodes in this region. In support of this concept, Fegan,[89] Hobbs,[90] Lofgren,[91] and Beninson and Livingood[92] have all pointed out that the treatment of varicosities may have no effect on superficial venous pressure. They hold that treatment of communicating or perforating veins draining the ankle and lower calf area is important.[42,90,93-95] These vessels may be either surgically ligated[42,93-95] or sclerosed (see Chapter 9).[90] Only then will retrograde flow under high pressure via the calf muscle pump be diverted upstream away from the skin. When this is done, a lowering of cuticular venous pressure and a decrease in dermal capillary pressure is accomplished. The excess transudation of fluid producing edema and the associated decrease in tissue oxygenation and nutrition is halted. Quill and Fegan[96] have clearly demonstrated the narrowing of the proximal LSV after obliteration of incompetent distal perforating veins in 9 of 11 cases. This suggests that dilation and incompetence of the saphenous vein may be caused by distal reflux as well as primary or irreversible abnormalities of the proximal venous wall. Diagnosis and treatment of incompetent communicating veins will be discussed in subsequent chapters.

*Venous obstruction.* Venous obstruction may occur proximal or distal to varicose veins. An obstruction is typically produced by thrombus that may extend proximally and distally from its origin. The thrombus may also extend into communicating or perforating veins. Depending on the extent of thrombus, venous blood may be forced into the superficial veins in either a retrograde or lateral direction (see Fig. 1-11).

Finally, it is interesting to speculate that the wearing of high-heeled shoes may lead to distal compression of the vein walls by leg muscles that are strained as a result of these shoes. This secondary, logical factor has been proposed previously but awaits experimental confirmation.[97]

*Arteriovenous anastomosis.* Another important factor that may lead to increased venous pressure in cutaneous veins is the opening of arteriovenous communications. Arteriovenous anastomoses (AVAs) were suggested as being a component in the pathogenesis of varicose veins in 1949 by Pratt[98] and by Piulachs, Vidal-Barraquer, and Biel[99] in 1952. Pratt hypothesized that they represented the failure of closure of femoral artery branches to the saphenous system.

A clue to the presence of AVAs is often provided by the presence of varicosities in an unusual anatomic location in the absence of detectable abnormalities of the deep venous system.[41] Physical examination often shows lack of complete emptying of the varicose veins when the limb is elevated, very rapid refilling of the varicose vein or venules with diascopy, warmth over affected varicose veins, and the rare presence of a bruit or thrill over these vessels.[98] Often arterial Doppler sounds are demonstrated over varices, especially when they are associated with bright red venectasia.

AVAs have also been demonstrated by direct operative microscopic dissection by Schalin[100] and Gius.[101] In addition, Schroth[102] and Haeger and Bergman[103] have indirectly supported these findings by evaluations of oxygen content of varicose blood and skin temperature over varicose veins. They estimate that

AVAs occur in up to 64% of patients with varicose veins. Pratt[98] estimated that AVAs occur in 24% of varicose veins and in 50% of patients with recurrent varicose veins after surgical ligation and stripping.

Schalin has demonstrated AVAs with thermography (Fig. 3-6). Schalin[104] has recently reviewed the role of arteriovenous shunting in the development of varicose veins and has concluded that the recurrent and varying flow of arterial flow transmitted to veins over years causes the venous wall to distend. He has observed this to occur by operative microscopy demonstrating that AVAs connect to varicose veins at the convex curves. Although AVAs are difficult to detect ra-

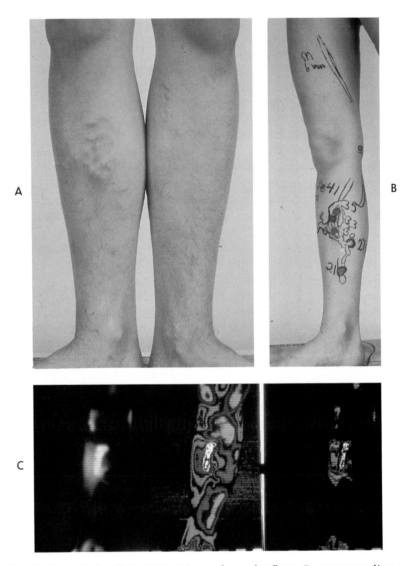

**Fig. 3-6**   At the medial calf, **A**, 33 to 35 cm above the floor, **B**, corresponding to a thermographically hot (35° centigrade) varicosity, **C**, of a woman 27 years of age, two small pulsating vessels were identified at cautious dissection using an operation microscope, **D**. These arteries joined the meandering (tortuous) vein at the convex bends. No alternative arterial run off was identified. The drawing, **E**, illustrates the connection of the arteries with the varicose vein. (Courtesy Lars Schalin, M.D.)

diographically in association with varicose veins,[105] rapid venous filling is commonly seen in arteriograms of limbs with severe venous stasis.

Opening of the AVA may occur through developmental or functional abnormalities of vasa vasorum of the venous wall. In one scenario, an association of excessive alcohol consumption in male patients with varicose veins has been proposed to cause arteriolar dilation and new capillary formation, which may act like multiple AVAs.[54] Alternatively, opening of the AVA may be caused by proximal venous hypertension that breaks down the capillary barrier.[105] Once dysfunction of the AVA is established, shunting of arterial blood directly into the

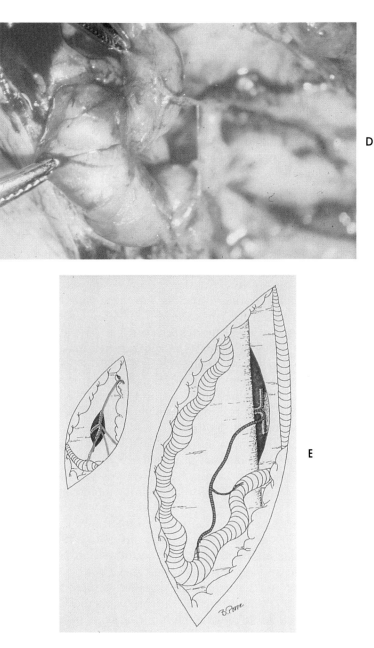

**Fig 3-6, cont'd.**  For legend see opposite page.

venous system further increases venous dilation. It is still uncertain whether AVAs are the cause or the result of varicosities. Despite this, there are common observations that tend to support the concept of AVA-induced varicosities. Varicose veins may recur after anatomically correct sclerotherapy that obliterates all perforating veins. This may result from an AVA distal to the point of injection. Also, the bright red color of some leg telangiectasias may be caused by underlying AVA. Finally, cutaneous ulceration after sclerotherapy treatment may also be related to injection of venules and their associated AVAs (see Chapter 8). Therefore, the AVA is important either as an etiologic or as an associated factor in the cause of and treatment of varicose veins.

## Primary Valvular Incompetence

Primary valvular incompetence is a serious precursor of varicose veins because, by definition, such valves are permanently damaged, absent, or incompetent. Thus, as originally suggested by William Harvey,[106] an incompetent valve causes distention of the distal vein by gravitational back pressure and may produce a varicosity. Many things may be responsible for the development of valvular incompetence including developmental abnormalities and destruction of the venous valves.

Congenital valvular agenesis is a very rare cause of varicose veins.[107-111] Multiple case reports and a series of 14 patients have been described.[107,112] Such patients have partial or complete absence of deep vein valves in the lower extremities. Familial occurrence in two pedigrees suggested a simple dominant mode of inheritance. Clinically, such patients are detected by development of venous insufficiency at an early age. Interestingly, signs and symptoms invariably occurred only after puberty. The most serious physical finding was cutaneous ulceration in the typical medial malleolar area. The most notable physical finding was ankle edema occurring during the day with complete resolution at night or during rest. Another common sign was marked orthostatic hypotension from venous pooling in the legs. In these patients, wide variations in the number of valves was seen. This ranged from complete agenesis in both lower extremities to agenesis in only one leg or even partial agenesis. Therefore, although rarely reported, valvular agenesis in some degree may be found on careful examination of some patients. Its diagnosis is critical before performing injection sclerotherapy because a major complication of injecting veins without valves is a possible progression of venous fibrosis and thrombosis to the deep venous system. This could cause a worsening of venous insufficiency, even to the extent of jeopardizing the viability of the limb.

Scientific evaluation of the relative significance of valvular deficiency in relation to the development of varicose veins is not as clear. A recent autopsy study showing decrease in number of venous valves in the left internal iliac vein as compared with the right iliac vein is emblematic. This could explain the relative increased incidence in left-sided varicose veins; the relative obstruction caused by the right iliac artery may be unimportant.[113] Anatomic studies do not define functional significance of venous valves. In a radiographic functional study of external iliac and femoral valves performed on 12 male volunteers with and without varicose veins, it was found that subjects with a family history of varicose veins did not have femoral or external iliac valves.[114] Conversely, those men without a family history of varicose veins did have such valves. Another study of 54 normal adults and 19 children of patients with varicose veins also confirmed these findings. Using venous Doppler examination, incompetent iliofemoral valves were present in 16% of the normal adults and 32% of the children of patients with varicose veins.[115] These studies lend support to the theory of descending sequential valvular incompetence as a pathogenic mechanism for the development of varicose veins.

Unfortunately, other studies have failed to show a convincing association between the absence of iliofemoral valves and the presence of LSV incompetence.[116] In addition, veins that have been reversed, rendering their valves incompetent, and used as arterial grafts fail to elongate or dilate. They certainly do not develop into varicose veins.[117] Therefore, primary valvular deficiency with or without increased transmural pressure may not be important as an etiologic factor in all patients with varicose veins.

Common mechanisms for the destruction of these valves is deep venous thrombosis (DVT) and thrombophlebitis. DVT is estimated to precede the development of varicose veins in as many as 25% of patients.[118] Incompetence of the veins may also occur because of destruction of the valves by the inflammatory process of thrombophlebitis.[119-121] In addition to spontaneous DVT, thrombophlebitis may occur as a result of chemical or mechanical trauma or inflammatory bowel disease. Also, it may occur postsurgically in association with various malignancies or as a result of hormonal elevations in conjunction with birth control pills or postpartum or even as a result of smoking.[121]

Finally, chronic venous dilation may in itself result in valvular fibrosis. Venous dilation increases tension on the cusps of the valves, which causes them to project into the lumen of the vein as rigid flanges (Fig. 3-7). The resultant turbulence of blood flow is thought to cause sclerosis and contraction of the valve and its eventual disappearance. This has been noted on histologic examination of varicose veins removed at surgery or postmortem.[122]

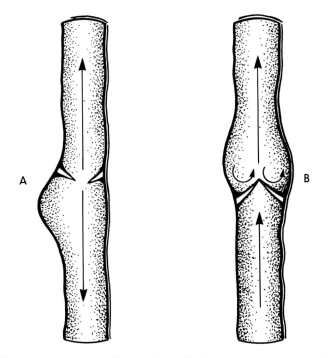

**Fig. 3-7**    A, Diagram of eccentric dilation beneath the valve cusps in a varicose vein. B, A normal valve is shown for comparison. (From Cotton L: Br J Surg 48:589, 1961.)

## Secondary Valvular Incompetence

Secondary valvular incompetence is a common cause of varicose veins. In this situation the valves are normal but become incompetent because of dilation of the vein wall. Secondary valvular incompetence may occur as a result of destruction of the valvular system after DVT or because of the expansion in the diameter of the vein. This later process may occur via an increase in venous volume, obstruction in venous return, or a hormonally induced increase in venous distensibility. Thrombotic destruction of venous valves usually begins in the venous sinuses, such as in the soleal sinuses. Here the thrombus may spread to the posterior tibial vein and then subsequently into the ankle communicating veins.[34] Organization and recanalization of the thrombus destroys the valves.[34] An even more dangerous event occurs when the thrombus spreads proximally as a precursor to development of pulmonary embolism.

Pregnancy is typically associated with secondary valvular incompetence. Varices are often first noted during pregnancy and are exceedingly rare before puberty.[123] Indeed, population studies have found that only 12% of women with varicose veins have never been pregnant.[124] It has been suggested that increased total blood flow in the iliac veins from the uterine and ovarian veins may explain the occurrence of varicose veins in early pregnancy.[125] Blood flow through the uterine veins is increased 4 to 16 times in the first 2 months of pregnancy and doubles again during the third month.[126] Although uterine obstruction to venous flow and an increase in iliac blood volume and flow are measurable physiologic factors in pregnancy, it is obvious that factors other than venous congestion are important in the development of varicose veins.

Femoral vein obstruction by the gravid uterus also may lead to secondary valvular incompetence through an increase in proximal venous pressures. The obstructive effects of the uterus do not develop during pregnancy until the second and third trimesters.[127] A sequential study of 50 gravid women through the first, second, and third trimesters using Doppler ultrasound demonstrated that femoral venous flow was obstructed in 72% of erect patients in the second trimester and 86% of patients in the third trimester.[128] An additional study of femoral blood flow in 61 pregnant patients demonstrated that the most significant decrease in femoral blood flow occurred when the head of the fetus became engaged during the latter part of the third trimester.[129] The effect of the gravid uterus on the impedance of femoral blood flow may be influenced by hereditary factors. Although some investigators have not found a consistent relationship between the presence or absence of varicose veins and the obstruction to venous flow,[128] others[130] have measured venous pressure in the popliteal vein in pregnant patients in the third trimester and found a marked increase in venous pressure only in those women with varicose veins. Therefore, both an increase in blood volume and an obstruction of venous return are responsible for the development of varicose veins in pregnancy. However, these two factors do not account for the development of smaller telangiectasias and venectasias. They also do not account for the development of varicose veins in the first trimester.

In pregnancy, hormonal factors are primarily responsible for venous dilation. As many as 70% to 80% of patients develop varicose veins during the first trimester when the uterus is only slightly enlarged (Fig. 3-8). In the second trimester, 20% to 25% of patients develop varicose veins, and 1% to 5% of patients develop them in the third trimester.[131-133]

Varicose veins of the legs are first apparent as early as 6 weeks into gestation, a time when the uterus is not yet large enough to impede venous return from the leg veins significantly. In contrast, vulvar varices usually develop in the

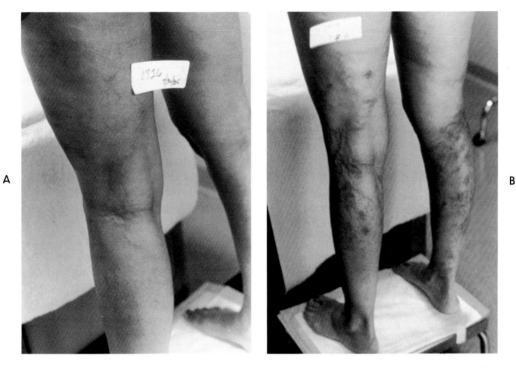

**Fig. 3-8**   Woman, 33 years old. **A,** Before pregnancy. **B,** 20 weeks into pregnancy with a 15-lb weight gain. Note the dramatic increase in the size and number of varicose veins. (Courtesy Anton Butie, M.D.)

third trimester but may appear in the late first trimester.[125,134] Furthermore, Mullane[133] notes that symptoms of varicose veins may be the first sign of pregnancy and can occur even before the first missed menstrual period. This confirms observations of many multiparous women and argues for a profound influence of progesterone on venous dilation and valvular insufficiency. Siegler[135] states that 40% of all pregnant patients are affected and maintains that all women will develop varicosities if they have a sufficient number of pregnancies. In support of this theory is Mullane's patient who developed varicose veins for the first time in her eleventh pregnancy.[133] However, some epidemiological studies have failed to confirm this association when the effect of age is controlled.[26]

Venous distensibility has been found to increase in both forearm and calf veins with the progression of pregnancy, particularly after the thirteenth week of pregnancy.[136] The increase in distensibility was greater in the calf than in the forearm and returned to normal by the eighth postpartum week.[136]

Incompetence of the saphenous veins may occur because of excessive dilation of the vein when there is sufficient separation of the valve cusps.[120] Interestingly, retrospective studies have shown that 40% to 78% of patients note the development of varicosities during the second pregnancy rather than the first.[6,132,133] Rose and Ahmed[6] postulate that veins that become subclinically varicose after the first pregnancy become clinically obvious after the second.

The pregnant state is associated with elevations of multiple hormones. Estrogen produces a relaxation of smooth muscle and softening of collagen fibers in general, which may explain the increased distensibility of veins.[137,138] The increased distensibility of vein walls has been reported to occur as a result of estrogen therapy.[139,140] McCausland[132] believes that the progesterone level, and, more importantly, the estrogen/progesterone ratio is primarily responsible for increased venous distensibility. Supporting this theory is the marked venous distensibility demonstrated in women given a synthetic progesterone.[141] Furthermore, a study reported in 1946 found that the administration of an estrogenic substance, diovocylin (CIBA Pharmaceutical Company), to 27 pregnant patients with either varicose or telangiectatic veins in weekly doses throughout pregnancy actually produced an amelioration of the smaller and larger types of veins and a reduction of peripheral edema and subjective complaints in a majority of patients.[142] This was confirmed in a subsequent study of 34 patients treated with oral ethinyl estradiol 0.05 mg two to four times daily.[143] Presumably, administration of this substance altered the progesterone/estrogen ratio. (No mention was made of feminization of male babies on follow-up examination.) An additional study has also demonstrated a complete relief of symptoms in 13 of 15 patients with angiectids (small intradermal, raised; bluish mats of blood vessels) in pregnancy with diethylstilbestrol (E. R. Squibb & Sons, Inc.) in doses ranging from 50 to 150 mg daily.[144] In this regard, the degree of pain and disability caused by the angiectid was frequently related to the level of subnormal estrogen. Symptomless angiectids were correlated with low normal amounts of estrogen and progesterone. Therefore, the hormonal factor responsible for the development or exacerbation of varicosities in pregnancy may very well be related to estrogen-progesterone balance.

In pregnancy two factors operate to dilate leg veins: increased venous distensibility from hormonal stimulation and increased venous pressure from obstruction by the gravid uterus and an increased blood volume. Sumner[145] has estimated that 80% to 90% of varicose veins tend to regress during the puerperium. He advises physicians to wait 6 to 12 weeks postpartum before performing surgery or sclerotherapy to allow time for the varices to regress. This will not only enhance treatment efficacy, but also allow the physician to make a more accurate assessment of the true extent and severity of the disease.

The hormonal influence on the venous system also extends beyond pregnancy. Studies have also demonstrated that the increase in venous distensibility is different for different oral contraceptive agents. Oral contraceptives with a high progestogen component appear to increase venous capacitance and may induce venous stasis, whereas coagulability is partially enhanced by estrogen-dominant contraceptives.[146] Finally, it has been noted by Gallagher[147] in his practice of 20,000 patients that the incidence of minor asymptomatic varices decreases after menopause. This is correlated with a fall in estradiol production and plasma concentration. Therefore, estrogen or progesterone alone do not seem to be an independent factor influencing venous capacitance; their proportional concentrations may be more important.

A change in venous distensibility also occurs during the menstrual cycle.[141,146] Venous distensibility is higher during the luteal phase than during the follicular phase of the menstrual cycle.[146] This increase in distensibility correlates most closely with progesterone levels.[141] However, studies on vein distensibility do not distinguish between relaxation of smooth muscle and alteration in the visoelastic properties of the venous wall. Also, these studies do not exclude the possibility that the increased distensibility may also result from the release of vasoconstrictor tone. Therefore, it is difficult to make recommendations regarding the timing of sclerotherapy with the menstrual cycle or on the necessity to discontinue oral contraceptives during sclerotherapy.

Of more clinical concern is postpartum thrombophlebitis and its attendant dangers of pulmonary embolism and eventual development of the postphlebitic syndrome.[148] The reported incidence of thrombophlebitis in pregnancy may be as high as 0.35% with a 0.085% incidence in the antepartum group as compared with 0.27% in the postpartum group.[149] There are multiple factors responsible for the increased incidence of thrombophlebitis in this group of patients. In late pregnancy the blood volume is increased, the uterus impedes venous return, and elevated hormonal levels produce an increased distensibility of veins with resulting valvular incompetence. In addition, multiple factors are present at childbirth, including increased clotting factors and a hormonal environment conducive to clotting, which appear to predispose this physiologic milieu to the development of thrombophlebitis.[150,151] Therefore, graduated elastic support hosiery should be worn before, during, and immediately after delivery.[148]

## Heredity

Although development of varicose veins can usually be ascribed to one of the above-mentioned pathologic states, postmortem examination may not disclose the apparent source of the high-pressure leak from the deep to the superficial system.[152] Therefore, other inherent factors such as vein wall weakness, increased primary valvular dysfunction or agenesis, and other genetic factors may enhance the development of varicose veins.

A familial tendency towards the development of varicose veins has previously been described.[153,154] A limited study of 50 patients with varicose veins in Great Britain disclosed a simple dominant type of inheritance.[155] Only 28% of patients had no family history of varicose veins. In Scandinavia questionnaires completed by 124 women with varicose veins disclosed a 72% prevalence of varicose veins in the women's siblings of an autosomal type.[154] Of these cases, 28% were of a recessive pattern. Troisier and LeBayon[156] examined 154 families with 514 descendants. They found if both parents had varicose veins, 85% of children had evidence of varicose veins, whereas 27% of children were affected if neither parent had varicose veins, and 41% of children were affected if one parent had varicosities. These authors conclude that the inheritance of varicose disease is of a recessive type.

A single study on unselected twins found that 75% of 12 monozygotic pairs were concordant with regard to varicose veins. Of 25 dizygotic, same-sexed pairs, 52% had varicose veins.[157]

Other studies have found more of a multifactorial inheritance. In a detailed study from Sweden of 250 probands of patients with varicose veins presenting for treatment, the overall frequency of varicose veins in female relatives was 43% as compared with 19% in male relatives.[158]

The absence of venous valves in the external iliac and femoral veins has been shown to be a marker of varicose veins in a limited radiographic study of 12 male volunteers, some with and some without varicose veins,[114] and in a venous Doppler study of 54 patients with varicose veins.[159] In addition, a simple dominant mode of inheritance has been reported in 14 patients with congenital partial or total absence of venous valves of the leg.[107] Thus this genetic predisposition may be the result of multiple factors, and the subsequent development of varicose veins may depend on one or more occupational or hormonal factors.

Congenitally weak or nonfunctioning venous valves may be an initiating factor in the altered venous hemodynamics that lead to the formation of varicose veins.[160] The argument against this theory is that valvular cusps consist of a fibrous tissue core covered by endothelium. This structure has been demonstrated to be extremely strong in experimental models.[161] In fact, it has been estimated that experimentally valves will not rupture at the physiologic pressures to which a valve might be subjected during life. Therefore, it is most likely alterations in the vein wall, and not valve strength, that are responsible for the development of incompetence.

Rose and Ahmed[6] have postulated that an inherited alteration in vein wall collagen and/or elastin, or an increase in vein wall collagen deposition with separation of smooth muscle cells (as previously described) is a major etiologic precursor to the development of varicose veins. They reason that increased venous pressure should lead to hypertrophy of the vein wall as demonstrated in arterialized venous bypass coronary grafts[161-165] and not the dilation associated with varicose veins. Accordingly, dilation of varicose veins, at times only in certain areas of the vein, must be caused by a vein wall defect — not caused merely by the presence of high venous pressure. A generalized increase in venous distensibility was found in superficial forearm and hand veins in patients with a saphenous varicosity as compared with patients without varicosities.[166,167] Abnormal distensibility curves were found to be similar regardless of the age and sex of the patient. This may be related to a reported decrease in collagen content in the saphenous veins of patients with varicosities, which occurs even in vein segments that are not varicose.[17] However, this theory does not explain why correction of proximal valvular dysfunction with a tourniquet can correct abnormal venous pressures distally if, indeed, it is the vein wall that is abnormally distensible.[168]

Another interesting relationship is the recently described association of varicose veins with the ABO blood group system. Numerous studies have demonstrated a relationship between blood groups of the ABO system and DVT of the lower limbs.[169-171] A study of 569 French men and women has shown the risk of varicose veins in patients with type A blood to be double that for patients with all other blood groups.[172] Varicose veins were defined as the presence in the standing position of a permanent dilation of at least one leg vein with a diameter of 3 mm or more with reflux. The risk of varicose veins persisted after adjustment for age, sex, paternal or maternal history, or personal history of DVT. No association was found between rhesus factor and varicose veins. Therefore, the authors conclude that a patient's blood group should be taken into account when assessing the need for prophylactic treatment of varicose veins or assessing the risk of postoperative venous thrombosis.

In conclusion, multiple studies of population groups have documented a significant relationship between heredity and the development of varicose veins.[173-175] In addition, there appears to be a significant difference in the incidence of varicose veins among different cultures with a rarity of varicose veins in non-Westernized populations.[176] Therefore, multiple factors — pathologic, intrinsic, and extrinsic — all contribute to the development of varicose veins.

## REFERENCES

1. Prerovsky I: Disease of the veins, internal communication, MHO-PA 10964, World Health Organization.
2. Thulesius O et al: The varicose saphenous vein: functional and ultrastructural studies with special reference to smooth muscle, Phlebology 3:89, 1988.
3. Svjcar J et al: Biochemical differences in the composition of primary varicose veins, Am Heart J 67:572, 1964.
4. Jurukova Z and Milenkov C: Ultrastructural evidence for collagen degradation in the walls of varicose veins, Exp Mol Path 37:37, 1982.
5. Bouissou H et al: Vein morphology, Phlebology 3(suppl 1):1, 1988.
6. Rose SS and Ahmed A: Some thoughts on the aetiology of varicose veins, Cardiovasc Surg 27:534, 1986.

7. Acsady G and Lengyel I: Modifications between histomorphological and pathobiochemical changes leading to primary varicosis. In Davy A and Stemmer R, editors: Phlebologie 89, Montrouge, France, 1989, John Libbey Eurotext Ltd.

8. Zwillenberg LO, Laszt L, and Willenberg H: Die Feinstruktur der Venenwand bei Varikose, Angiologica 8:318, 1971.

9. Merlen JF et al: Le devenir histologique d'une veine sclerosee, Phlebologie 31:17, 1978.

10. Partsch H and Mostbeck A: Constriction of varicose veins and improvement of venous pumping by dihydroergotamine, Vasa 14:74, 1985.

11. Leu HJ, Vogt M, and Pfrunder H: Morphological alterations of nonvaricose and varicose veins, Basic Res Cardiol 74:435, 1979.

12. Deby C et al: Decreased tocopherol concentration of varicose vein associated with a decrease in antilipoperoxidant activity without similar changes in plasma, Phlebology 4:113, 1989.

13. Kontos HA and Hess ML: Oxygen radicals and vascular damage, Adv Exp Med Biol 161:365, 1983.

14. Felix W: Pharmakologische BeeinfluBbarkeit kapazitativer Venen. In Schneider KW, editor: Die venose Insuffizienz, Wittstock, East Germany, 1972, Baden-Baden.

15. Kreysel HW, Nissen HP, and Enghofer E: A possible role of lysosomal enzymes in the pathogenesis of varicosis and the reduction in their serum activity by venostasis, Vasa 12:377, 1983.

16. Haardt B: Histological comparison of the enzyme profiles of healthy veins and varicose veins, Phlebology 39:921, 1986.

17. Svejcar J et al: Content of collagen, elastine, and hexosamine in primary varicose veins, Clin Sci 24:325, 1963.

18. Niebes P: Biochemical studies of varicosis, Monogr Stand Cardioangeiological Methods 4:233, 1977.

19. Branco D and Osswald W: The influence of Ruscus extract on the uptake and metabolism of noradrenaline in the normal and varicose vein, Phlebology 3(suppl 1):33, 1988.

20. Mellander S: Operative studies on the adrenergic neuro-hormonal control of resistance and capacitance blood vessels in the cat, Acta Physiol Scand 50:5, 1960.

21. Waterfield RL: The effect of posture on the volume of the leg, J Physiol 72:121, 1931.

22. Ludbrook J and Loughlin J: Regulation of volume in postarteriolar vessels of the lower limb, Am Heart J 67:493, 1964.

23. Rushmer RF: Effects of posture. In Rushmer RF: Cardiovascular dynamics, ed 4, Philadelphia, 1976, WB Saunders Co.

24. Samueloff SL, Browse NL, and Shepherd JT: Response of capacity vessels in human limbs to head-up tilt and suction on lower body, J Appl Physiol 21:47, 1966.

25. Reinis Z et al: Incidence of diseases of veins of the lower extremities in the population, Vnitr Lek 29:105, 1983.

26. Abramson JH, Hopp C, and Epstein LM: The epidemiology of varicose veins: a survey in Western Jerusalem, J Epidemiol Community Health 35:213, 1981.

27. Pollack AA et al: The effect of exercise and body position on the venous pressure at the ankle in patients having venous valvular defects, J Clin Invest 28:559, 1949.

28. Pollack AA and Wood EH: Venous pressure in the saphenous vein at the ankle in man during exercise and changes in posture, J Appl Physiol 1:649, 1949.

29. Barcroft H and Dornhorst AC: The blood flow through the human calf during rythmic exercise, J Physiol (Lond) 107:402, 1949.

30. Wells HS, Youmans JB, and Miller DG: Tissue pressure, intracutaneous, subcutaneous, and intramuscular, as related to venous pressure, capillary filtration, and other factors. J Clin Invest 17:489, 1938.

31. Ludbrook J: The musculo-venous pumps of the human lower limb, Am Heart J 71:635, 1966.

32. Hojensgard IC and Sturup H: Static and dynamic pressures in superficial and deep veins of the lower extremity in man, Acta Physiol Scand 27:49, 1953.

33. Arnoldi CC: Venous pressure in the leg of healthy human subjects at rest and during muscular exercise in the nearly erect position, Acta Chir Scand 130:570, 1965.

34. Dodd H and Cockett FB, editors: The pathology and surgery of the veins of the lower limb, ed 2, Edinburgh, 1976, Churchill Livingstone.

35. Almen T and Nylander G: Serial phlebography of the normal lower leg during muscular contraction and relaxation, Acta Radiol 57:264, 1962.

36. Fegan WG, Milliken JC, and Fitzgerald DE: Abdominal venous pump, Arch Surg 92:44, 1966.

37. Lange L and Echt M: Comparative studies on drugs which increase venous tone using noradrenaline, ethyl-andrianol, dihydroergotamine, and horsechestnut extract, Fortschr Med 90:1161, 1972.

38. Mellander S and Nordenfelt L: Comparative effects of dihydroergotamine and noradrenaline on resistance, exchange, and capacitance functions in the peripheral circulation, Clin Sci 39:183, 1970.

39. Bjordal R: Simultaneous pressure and flow recordings in varicose veins of the lower extremities, Acta Chir Scand 136:309, 1970.

40. McPheeters HO and Rice CO: Varicose veins: the circulation and direction of venous flow, Surg Gynecol Obstet 49:29, 1929.

41. Farber EM and Bates EE: Pathologic physiology of stasis dermatitis, Arch Dermatol 70:653, 1954.

42. Negus D and Friedgood A: The effective management of venous ulceration, Br J Surg 70:623, 1983.

43. Cockett FB and Jones BE: The ankle blow-out syndrome: a new approach to the varicose ulcer problem, Lancet 1:17, 1953.

44. Landis EM: Factors controlling the movement of fluid through the human capillary wall, Yale J Biol Med 5:201, 1933.

45. Burnand KG et al: The effect of sustained venous hypertension on the skin capillaries of the canine hind limb, Br J Surg 69:41, 1982.

46. Ryan TJ and Wilkinson DS: Diseases of the veins: venous ulcers. In Rook A, Wilkinson DS, and Ebling FJG, editors: Textbook of dermatology, ed 3, London, 1979, Blackwell Scientific Publications.

47. Ryan TJ: Diseases of the skin: management of varicose ulcers and eczema, Br Med J 1:192, 1974.

48. Whimster I. Cited in Dodd H and Cockett FB, editors: The pathology and surgery of the veins of the lower limb, ed 2, Edinburgh, 1976, Churchill Livingstone.

49. Falanga V et al: Dermal pericapillary fibrin in venous disease and venous ulceration, Arch Dermatol 123:620, 1987.

50. Lotti T, Fabbri P, and Panconesi E: The pathogenesis of venous ulcers, J Am Acad Dermatol 16:877, 1987.

51. Ludbrook J and Loughlin J: Regulation of volume in postarteriolar vessels of the lower limb, Am Heart J 67:493, 1964.

52. Shepherd JT and Vanhoutte PM: Role of the venous system in circulatory control, Mayo Clin Proc 53:247, 1978.

53. Boccalon H and Ginestet MC: Influence of temperature variations on venous return: clinical observations, Phlebology 3(suppl 1):47, 1988.

54. Tanyol H and Menduke H: Alcohol as a possible etiologic agent in varicose veins: a study of drinking habits in 136 patients with varicose veins and in 70 control patients, Angiology 12:382, 1961.

55. Kerr MG, Scott DB, and Samuel E: Studies of the inferior vena cava in late pregnancy, Br Med J 1:532, 1964.

56. Cleave TL: On the causation of varicose veins and their prevention and arrest by natural means, Bristol, 1960, Wright & Sons.

57. Cambell GC and Cleave TL: Diverticular disease of colon, Br Med J 3:741, 1968.

58. Richardson JB and Dixon M: Varicose veins in tropical Africa, Lancet 1:791, 1977.

59. Beaglehole R: Epidemiology of varicose veins, World J Surg 10:898, 1986.

60. Burkitt DP: Varicose veins: facts and fantasy, Arch Surg 111:1327, 1976.

61. Foote RR: Varicose veins, St Louis, 1949, The CV Mosby Co.

62. Pirner F: Der varikose Symptomen-komplex mit seien Folgen und Nachkrakheiten un ter besonerer Bereichsichtigung der Fehlerquellen. In Diagnostik und Therapie, Stuttgart, 1957, ENKE.

63. Dodd H: The cause, prevention, and arrest of varicose veins, Lancet 2:809, 1964.

64. Burkitt DP: Varicose veins, deep vein thrombosis, and haemorrhoids: epidemiology and suggested etiology, Br Med J 2:556, 1972.

65. Stamler J: Epidemiology as an investigative method for study of human arteriosclerosis, J Natl Med Assoc, Tuskegee, Ala, 50:161, 1958.

66. Martin A and Odling-Smee A: Pressure changes in varicose veins, Lancet 1:768, 1976.

67. Malhotra SL: An epidemiological study of varicose veins in Indian railroad workers from the south and north of India, with special reference to the causation and prevention of varicose veins, Int J Epidemiol 1:117, 1982.

68. Connor WE, Hoak JG, and Warner EA: Massive thrombosis produced by fatty acid infusion, J Clin Invest 42:860, 1963.

69. Connor WE and Poole JCF: The effect of fatty acids on the formation of thrombi, Q J Exp Physiol 46:1, 1961.

70. Poole JCF: Effective diet and lipidemia on coagulation and thrombosis, Fed Proc 21(4), pt 2:20, 1962.

71. Melet JJ: La place de l'alimentation parmi les facteurs de rísque des maladies veineuses, Phlebologie 34:469, 1981.
72. Abramson JH et al: The epidemiology of inguinal hernia: a survey in Western Jerusalem, J Epidemiol Community Health 32:59, 1978.
73. Schilling RSF and Walford J: Varicose veins in women cotton workers: an epidemiological study in England and Egypt, Br Med J 2:591, 1969.
74. Askar O and Emara A: Varicose veins and occupation, J Egypt Med Assoc 53:341, 1970.
75. Stanhope JM: Varicose veins in a population of lowland New Guinea, Int J Epidemiol 4:221, 1975.
76. Alexander CJ: Chair-sitting and varicose veins, Lancet 1:822, 1972.
77. Wright HP and Osborn SB: Effect of posture on venous velocity, Br Heart J 14:325, 1952.
78. Symington IS and Stack BH: Pulmonary thromboembolism after travel, Br J Dis Chest 71:138, 1977.
79. Myers TT: Varicose veins. In Barker and Hines, editors: Barker and Hines's peripheral vascular diseases, ed 3, Philadelphia, 1962, WB Saunders Co.
80. Leipnitz G et al: Prevalence of venous disease in the population: first results from a prospective study carried out in greater Aachen. In Davy A and Stemmer R, editors: Phlebologie '89, Montrouge, France, 1989, John Libby Eurotext Ltd.
81. Beaglehole R, Almond CE, and Prior IAM: Varicose veins in New Zealand: prevalence and severity, NZ Med J 84:396, 1976.
82. Widmer LK: Peripheral venous disorders: prevalence and socio-medical importance: observations in 4529 apparently healthy persons, Basle Study III, Berne, Switzerland, 1978, Huber.
83. Ludbrook J: Obesity and varicose veins, Surg Gynecol Obstet 118:843, 1964.
84. Seidell JC et al: Fat distribution of overweight persons in relation to morbidity and subjective health, Int J Obesity 9:363, 1985.
85. Stegall HF: Muscle pumping in the dependent leg, Circ Res 19:180, 1966.
86. Floyd WF and Silver PHS: Electromyographic study of patterns of activity of the anterior abdominal muscles in man, J Anat 84:132, 1950.
87. Kriessmann A: Klinische Pathophysiologie des venosen Ruckstroms. In Ay RE and Kriessmann A, editors: Periphere Venendruckmessung, Stuttgart, 1978, Thieme Medical Publishers Inc.
88. Fegan G: Varicose veins: compression sclerotherapy, London, 1967, William Heinemann Medical Books Ltd.
89. Fegan WG: Continuous uninterrupted compression technique of injecting varicose veins, Proc R Soc Med 53:837, 1960.
90. Hobbs JT: The problem of the post-thrombotic syndrome, Postgrad Med J (Aug supp):48, 1973.
91. Lofgren EP: Leg ulcers: symptoms of an underlying disorder, Postgrad Med 76:51, 1984.
92. Beninson J and Livingood CS: Stasis dermatitis. In Demis DJ, editor: Clinical dermatology, vol 2, Philadelphia, 1985, Harper & Row, Publishers Inc.
93. Cockett FB and Thomas ML: The iliac compression syndrome, Br J Surg 52:816, 1965.
94. Kwaan JHM, Jones RN, and Connolly JE: Simplified technique for the management of refractory varicose ulcers, Surgery 80:743, 1976.
95. Lim LT, Michoda M, and Bergan JJ: Therapy of peripheral vascular ulcers: surgical management, Angiology 29:654, 1978.
96. Quill RD and Fegan WG: Reversibility of femorosaphenous reflux, Br J Surg 55:389, 1971.
97. Lake M, Pratt GH, and Wright IS: Arteriosclerosis and varicose veins: occupational activities and other factors, JAMA 119:696, 1942.
98. Pratt GH: Arterial varices: a syndrome, Am J Surg 77:456, 1949.
99. Piulachs P, Vidal-Barraquer F, and Biel JM: Considerations pathogeniques sur les varices de la grossesse, Lyon Chir 47:263, 1952.
100. Schalin L: Revaluation of incompetent perforating veins: a review of all the facts and observations interpreted on account of a controversial opinion and our own results. In Tese M and Dormandy JA: Superficial and deep venous diseases of the lower limbs, Torino, Italy, 1984, Edizioni Panminerva Medica.
101. Gius JA: Arteriovenous anastomoses and varicose veins, Arch Surg 81:299, 1960.
102. Schroth R: Venose Sauerstoffsattigung bei varicen, Arch Klin Chir 300:419, 1962.
103. Haeger KHM and Bergman L: Skin temperature of normal and varicose legs and some reflections on the etiology of varicose veins, Angiology 14:473, 1963.
104. Schalin L: Role of arteriovenous shunting in the development of varicose veins. In Etilof B et al, editors: Controversies in the management of venous disorders, England, 1989, Butterworth Publishers.
105. Haimovici H, Steinman C, and Caplan LH: Role of arteriovenous anastomoses in vascular diseases of the lower extremity, Ann Surg 164:990, 1966.
106. Bylebyl JJ: Harvey on the valves in the veins, Bull Hist Med 3:351, 1983.

107. Lindvall N and Lodin A: Congenital absence of venous valves, Acta Chir Scand 124:310, 1962.
108. Luke JC: The diagnosis of chronic enlargement of the leg: with description of a new syndrome, Surg Gynecol Obstet 73:472, 1941.
109. Norman AG: The significance of a venous cough impulse in the short saphenous vein, Angiology 7:523, 1956.
110. Ludin A: Congenital absence of valves in the veins. In Molen HR van der, editor: Progres clinques et Therapeutiques dans le domaine de la Phlebologie, Apeldoorn, Netherlands, 1970, Stenvert.
111. Lodin A: Congenital absence of valves in the deep veins of the leg: a factor in venous insufficiency, Acta Derm Venerol 62(41):1, 1961.
112. Lodin A, Lindvall N, and Gentele H: Congenital absence of venous valves as a cause of leg ulcers, Acta Chir Scand 116:256, 1958-1959.
113. Villavicencio JL: Personal communication, 1989.
114. Ludbrook J and Beale G: Femoral vein valves in relation to varicose veins, Lancet 1:79, 1962.
115. Reagan B and Folse R: Lower limb venous dynamics in normal persons and children of patients with varicose veins, Surg Gynecol Obstet 132:15, 1971.
116. Basmajian JV: The distribution of valves in the femoral, external iliac, and common iliac veins and their relationship to varicose veins, Surg Gynecol Obstet 95:537, 1952.
117. LiCalzi LK and Stansel HC Jr: Failure of autogenous reversed vein femoropopliteal grafting: pathophysiology, Surgery 91:352, 1982.
118. Gjores JE: The incidence of venous thrombosis and its sequellae in certain districts of Sweden, Acta Chir Scand [suppl] 206:11, 1956.
119. Miller RP and Sparrow TD: The pathogenesis diagnosis and treatment of varicose veins and varicose ulcers, NC Med J 9:574, 1948.
120. Lofgren KA: Varicose veins: their symptoms, complications, and management, Postgrad Med 65:131, 1979.
121. Beninson J: Thrombophlebitis. In Demis DJ, editor: Clinical dermatology, Philadelphia, 1986, Harper and Row Publishers.
122. Cotton LT: Varicose veins: gross anatomy and development, Br J Surg 48:589, 1961.
123. Tolins SH: Treatment of varicose veins, an update, Am J Surg 145:248, 1983.
124. Henry M and Corless C: The incidence of varicose veins in Ireland, Phlebology 4:133, 1989.
125. Nabatoff RA: Varicose veins of pregnancy, JAMA 174:1712, 1960.
126. Barrow DW: Clinical management of varicose veins, ed 2, New York, 1957, Paul B. Hoeber Inc.
127. McLennan CE: Antecubital and femoral venous pressures in normal and toxemic pregnancy, Am J Obstet Gynecol 45:568, 1943.
128. Ikard RW, Ueland K, and Folse R: Lower limb venous dynamics in pregnant women, Surg Gynecol Obstet 132:483, 1971.
129. Wright HP, Osborn SB, and Edmonds DG: Changes in the rate of flow of venous blood in the leg during pregnancy, measured with radioactive sodium, Surg Gynecol Obstet 90:481, 1950.
130. Veal JR and Hussey HH: Venous circulation in lower extremities during pregnancy, Surg Gynecol Obstet 72:841, 1941.
131. Tournay R and Wallois P: Les varices de la grossesse et leur traitment principalement par les injections sclerosantes, expansion, Paris, 1948, Scient Franc.
132. McCausland AM: Varicose veins in pregnancy, Cal West Med 50:258, 1939.
133. Mullane DJ: Varicose veins in pregnancy, Am J Obstet Gynecol 63:620, 1952.
134. Dodd H and Wright HP: Vulval varicose veins in pregnancy, Br Med J 1:831, 1959.
135. Siegler J: The treatment of varicose veins in pregnancy, Am J Surg 44:403, 1939.
136. Barwin BN and Roddie IC: Venous distensibility during pregnancy determined by graded venous congestion, Am J Obstet Gynecol 125:921, 1976.
137. Wahl LM: Hormonal regulation of macrophage collagenase activity, Biochem Biophys Res Commun 74:838, 1977.
138. Woolley DE: On the sequential changes in levels of oestradiol and progesterone during pregnancy and parturition and collagenolytic activity. In Piez KA and Eddi AH, editors: Extracellular matrix biochemistry, New York, 1984, Elsevier Science Publishing Co.
139. Reynolds RM and Foster I: Peripheral vascular action of estrogen, observed in the ear of the rabbit, J Pharmacol Exp Ther 68:173, 1940.
140. Goodrich SM and Wood JE: Peripheral venous distensibility and velocity of venous blood flow during pregnancy or during oral contraceptive therapy, Am J Obstet Gynecol 90:740, 1964.
141. McCausland AM, Holmes F, and Trotter AD Jr: Venous distensibility during the menstrual cycle, Am J Obstet Gynecol 86:640, 1963.

142. Marazita AJD: The action of hormones on varicose veins in pregnancy, Med Rec 159:422, 1946.
143. McPheeters HO: The value of estrogen therapy in the treatment of varicose veins complicating pregnancy, Lancet 69:2, 1949.
144. Fried PH, Perilstein PK, and Wagner FB: Saphenous varicosities vs angiectids consideration of so-called varicose veins of the lower extremities complicating pregnancy, Obstet Gynecol 2:418, 1953.
145. Sumner DS: Venous dynamics — varicosities, Clin Obstet Gynecol 24:743, 1981.
146. Fawer R et al: Effect of menstrual cycle, oral contraception, and pregnancy on forearm blood flow, venous distensibility, and clotting factors, Eur J Clin Pharmacol 13:251, 1978.
147. Gallagher PG: Major contributing role of sclerotherapy in the treatment of varicose veins, Vasc Surg 20:139, 1986.
148. Harridge WH: The treatment of primary varicose veins, Surg Clin North Am 40:191, 1960.
149. Husni EA, Pena LI, and Lenhert AE: Thrombophlebitis in pregnancy, Am J Obstet Gynecol 97:901, 1967.
150. Pechet L and Alexander B: Increased clotting factors in pregnancy, New Engl J Med 265:1093, 1961.
151. Wood JE: Oral contraceptives, pregnancy, and the veins, Circulation 38:627, 1968.
152. Thompson H: The surgical anatomy of the superficial and perforating veins of the lower limb, Ann R Coll Surg Engl 61:198, 1979.
153. von Curtius F: Untersuchungen uber das menschliche Venensystem, Deutsches Arch Klin Med 162:194, 1928.
154. Arnoldi C: The heredity of venous insufficiency, Dan Med Bull 5:169, 1958.
155. Ottley C: Hereditary and varicose veins, Br Med J 1:528, 1934.
156. Troisier J and Le Bayon: Etude génétique des varices, Ann de Med (Fr) 41:30, 1937.
157. Niermann H: Zwillingsdermatologie, Berlin, 1964, Springer-Verlag.
158. Gundersen J and Hauge M: Hereditary factors in venous insufficiency, Angiology 20:346, 1969.
159. Folse R: The influence of femoral vein dynamics on the development of varicose veins, Surgery 68:974, 1970.
160. Baron HC: Varicose veins, Consultant, p 108, May 1983.
161. Ackroyd JS, Pattison M, and Browse NL: A study of the mechanical properties of fresh and preserved human femoral vein wall and valve cusps, Br J Surg 72:117, 1985.
162. Campbell PA, McGeachie JK, and Prendergast FJ: Vein grafts for arterial repair: their success and reasons for failure, Ann R Coll Surg Engl 4:257, 1981.
163. Szilagyi DE et al: Biological fate of autologous vein implants as arterial substitutes, Ann Surg 178:232, 1973.
164. Fuchs JCA, Michener JS, and Hagen PO: Postoperative changes in autologous vein grafts, Ann Surg 188:1, 1978.
165. Brody WR, Kosek JC, and Angell WW: Changes in vein grafts following aorto-coronary bypass induced by pressure and ischaemia, J Thorac Cardiovasc Surg 64:847, 1972.
166. Zsoter T and Cronin RFP: Venous distensibility in patients with varicose veins, Can Med Assoc J 4:1293, 1966.
167. Eiriksson E and Dahn I: Plethysmographic studies of venous distensibility in patients with varicose veins, Acta Chir Scand Suppl 398:19, 1968.
168. Ludbrook J: Valvular defect in primary varicose veins: cause or effect? Lancet 2:1289, 1963.
169. Jick H and Porter J: Thrombophlebitis of the lower extremities and the ABO type, Arch Intern Med 138:1566, 1978.
170. Robinson WN and Roisenberg I: Venous thromboembolism and the ABO blood groups in a Brazilian population, Hum Genet 55:129, 1980.
171. Talbot S et al: ABO blood groups and venous thromboembolic disease, Lancet 1:1257, 1970.
172. Cornu-Thenard A et al: Relationship between blood groups (ABO) and varicose veins of the lower limbs: a case-control study, Phlebology 4:37, 1989.
173. Cepelak V et al: Genetic backgrounds of varicosity. In Molen HR van der, Limborgh J van, and Boersma W, editors: Progres cliniques et therapeutiques dans le domanie de la phlebologie, Apeldoorn, Netherlands, 1970, Stenvert.
174. Niermann H: Genetische Problematik des varikosen Symptomenkomplexes, Ergebn Angiol 4:25, 1970.
175. Gundersen J: Hereditare Faktoren bei der Entstehung der Varikosis. In Schneider KW, editor: Die venose Insuffizienz, Wittstock, East Germany, 1972, Baden-Baden.
176. Alexander CJ: The epidemiology of varicose veins, Med J Aust 1:215, 1972.

# 4 | Pathophysiology of Telangiectasias

The term *telangiectasia* was first coined in 1807 by Von Graf to describe a superficial vessel of the skin visible to the human eye.[1] Individually, they measure 0.1 to 1 mm in diameter and represent either an expanded venule, capillary, or arteriole. Telangiectasias that originate from arterioles on the arterial side of a capillary loop tend to be small, bright red, and do not protrude above the skin surface. Telangiectasias that originate from venules on the venous side of a capillary loop are blue, wider, and often protrude above the skin surface. Sometimes telangiectasias, especially those arising at the capillary loop, are at first red, but with time become blue, probably because of an increasing hydrostatic pressure and backflow from the venous side.[2]

## CLASSIFICATION

Redisch and Pelzer[3] classified telangiectasias into 4 types based on clinical appearance: (1) sinus or simple (linear), (2) arborizing, (3) spider or star, and (4) puntiform (papular) (Fig. 4-1). Papular telangiectasias are frequently present in patients with collagen vascular disease. Spider telangiectasias are red and arise from a central filling vessel of arteriolar origin. Red linear telangiectasias occur on the face (especially the nose) or legs. Blue linear or anastomosing telangiectasias are found most often on the legs. Patients most commonly seek treatment for the latter. This chapter discusses the pathophysiology and anatomy of telangiectasias that occur on the lower extremities.

## PATTERNS

Two common patterns of telangiectasias on the legs of women, besides red or blue streaks, are the parallel linear pattern, usually found on the medial thigh (Fig. 4-2), and the arborizing or radiating cartwheel pattern, seen most often on the lateral thigh (Fig. 4-3).[4] These two subsets of telangiectasias seem to run in families and may form anastomosing complexes that may be as large as 15 cm in diameter. They may appear with or without "feeding" reticular veins. These complexes have been termed *venous stars, sunburst venous blemishes,* and *spider leg veins* by various authors.

## PATHOGENESIS

The pathogenesis of each of the various types of telangiectasias is somewhat different. Many factors may play a role in the development of new blood vessels or the dilation of existing blood vessels (see Chapters 2 and 8). Also, acquired telangiectasias are thought to occur as a result of the release or activation of vasoactive substances such as hormones and chemicals under a multitude of conditions including anoxia, infection, and the presence of certain physical factors, which results in capillary or venular neogenesis.[3,5,6] The box on p. 89 (which is an extension of the observations of Shelley[7] and Anderson and Smith[8]) lists the major causes and diseases associated with telangiectasias that may appear on the lower extremities.

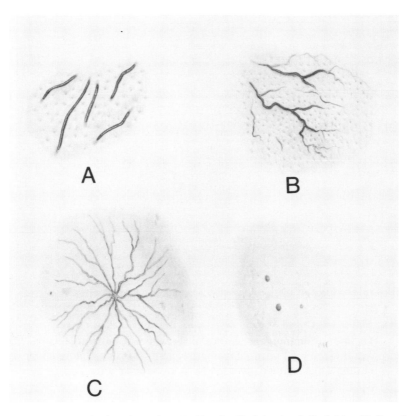

**Fig. 4-1**  Four types of telangiectasias. **A,** Simple. **B,** Arborized. **C,** Spider. **D,** Papular. (After Reddish W and Peltzer RH: Am Heart J 37:106, 1949.)

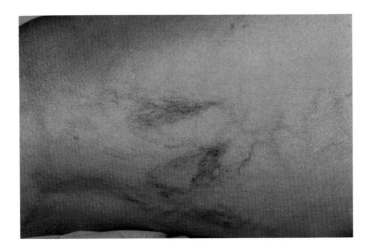

**Fig. 4-2**  Typical appearance of telangiectasia located at the medial thigh in a 54-year-old woman. Note the feeding reticular vein proximal to the telangiectasia.

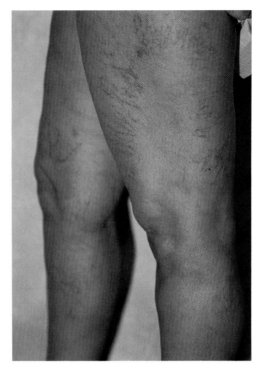

**Fig. 4-3**    Common appearance of cartwheel or radiating telangiectasia pattern on the lateral thigh of a 42-year-old woman. Note the feeding blue reticular vein at the distal aspect of the telangiectatic pattern.

## INCIDENCE

The incidence of varicose and telangiectatic leg veins in the general population is presented in Chapter 2. And since the relationship between varicose veins and spider leg veins (telangiectasias) is intimate, much of the anatomy and pathophysiology of telangiectasia is presented in Chapters 1 and 3. Two recent surveys have detailed the characteristics of patients seeking treatment of these unwanted spider leg veins. Duffy[9] in a nonrandomized survey of his patients reported a 90% family history of varicose or telangiectatic leg veins. The patients included three sets of identical twins with similar appearances of leg telangiectasia. Sadick[10] in a nonrandomized survey of 100 patients seeking treatment found a 43% family history of varicose or telangiectatic leg veins. Both surveys found that one third of the patients first noted the development of these veins during pregnancy. Duffy notes that the veins became most severe after the third pregnancy. Between 20% and 30% of patients developed these veins before pregnancy, and 18% of women noted the onset of the veins while ingesting progestational agents. Both authors conclude that the development of spider veins is probably a partially sex-linked, autosomal, dominant condition with incomplete penetrance and variable expressivity.

## PATHOPHYSIOLOGY

Many conditions — inherited, acquired, and iatrogenic — are known to be involved in the formation of telangiectasias.

## CAUSES OF CUTANEOUS TELANGIECTASIA OF THE LOWER EXTREMITIES

**GENETIC/CONGENITAL FACTORS**
Vascular nevi
  Nevus flammeus
    Klippel-Trenaunay syndrome
  Nevus araneus
  Angioma serpiginosum
Congenital neuroangiopathies
  Maffucci's syndrome
Congenital poikiloderma
  (Rothmund-Thomson syndrome)
Essential progressive telangiectasia
Cutis marmorata telangiectatica congenita
Diffuse neonatal hemangiomatosis

**ACQUIRED DISEASE WITH A SECONDARY CUTANEOUS COMPONENT**
Collagen vascular diseases
  Lupus erythematosus
  Dermatomyositis
  Progressive systemic sclerosis
Other
  Telangiectasia macularis eruptiva perstans (mastocytosis)
  Human immunodeficiency virus (HTLV-III)

**COMPONENT OF A PRIMARY CUTANEOUS DISEASE**
Varicose veins
Keratosis lichenoides chronica
Other acquired/primary cutaneous diseases
  Necrobiosis lipoidica diabeticorum
  Capillaritis (purpura annularis telangiectodes)
  Malignant atrophic papulosis (Degos' disease)

**HORMONAL FACTORS**
Pregnancy
Estrogen therapy
Topical corticosteroid preparations

**PHYSICAL FACTORS**
Actinic neovascularization and/or vascular dilation
Trauma
  Contusion
  Surgical incision/laceration
Infection
  Generalized essential telangiectasia
  Progressive ascending telangiectasia
  Human immunodeficiency virus (HTLV-III)
Radiodermatitis
Erythema ab igne (heat/infrared radiation)

Modified from Goldman MP and Bennett RG: Treatment of telangiectasia: a review, J Am Acad Dermatol 17:167, 1987.

## Genetic/Congenital Factors

Numerous genetic or congenital conditions (listed in the box on p. 89) display cutaneous telangiectasia. The pathogenesis for the development of telangiectasia in these syndromes is unknown. Genetic syndromes that may produce telangiectasias on the legs include nevus flammeus (either alone or as a component of Klippel-Trenaunay syndrome), nevus araneus, angioma serpiginosum, congenital neuroangiopathies (especially Maffucci syndrome), congenital poikiloderma, essential progressive or generalized telangiectasia, cutis marmorata telangiectatica congenita, and diffuse neonatal hemangiomatosis.

### Nevus flammeus

Nevus flammeus (port-wine stain) affects 0.3% to 1% of the population.[11,12] Women are affected twice as often as men.[13,14] The occurrence is usually sporadic, but a 10% familial incidence,[13] and an autosomal dominant inheritance have been described.[15-18] The lesions occur in various shapes and sizes on any part of the body. They most commonly occur on the face but may cover large areas of the skin including an entire arm, leg, or trunk (Fig. 4-4). Lesions often overlay the distribution of peripheral nerves. Nevus flammeus is usually macular and varies in color depending on the extent and depth of vascular involvement. Lesions become progressively nodular and darker with time and may ulcerate and bleed from minor trauma.

Histologic examination shows a collection of thin-walled capillary and cavernous vessels arranged in a loose fashion throughout the superficial and deep dermis (Fig. 4-5). These vessels represent dilations of the postcapillary venules of the superficial dermis with a mean vessel depth of 0.46 mm.[19] In infancy, histopathologic changes of the cutaneous vasculature are minimal. With advancing age, these lesions usually undergo a progressive ectasia and erythrocyte stasis.[19] Rarely, cavernous hemangiomas arising from arteriovenous malformations may occur within the lesions.[20] There may also be evidence of neovascularization or other vascular malformation.[19] Further, some lesions may be associated with prominent telangiectasias and reticular varicose veins when present over the lower limbs.

Nevus flammeus can also be a component of other congenital vascular diseases. The most commonly associated disease involving the leg is the Klippel-Trenaunay syndrome (KTS) (Fig. 4-6). With this latter entity, the cutaneous vascular abnormality is associated with underlying varicose and telangiectatic veins with or without significant abnormalities of the deep and superficial system or arteriovenous anastomoses. In addition, hypertrophy of soft tissue and bone may occur with overgrowth of the involved extremity (Figs. 4-7 and 4-8).

The cause of KTS is unknown. There is no apparent hereditary factor.[21] Some authors speculate that an atresia, agenesis, or compression of the deep venous system by fibrous tissue is the cause.[22] Other authors suggest that a congenital weakness of the venous wall in combination with vascular hypertension from an abnormal venous system leads to the development of KTS.[23]

When associated with KTS, cutaneous telangiectasias, venulectases, and varicose veins occur in the distribution of the underlying vascular malformation of the soft tissue and bone. Some patients may have a persistence of an embryologic lateral limb bud vein. The large drainage capacity of this vein may limit venous hypertension. In this instance microcirculatory, rather than large vessel, change may account for limb hypertrophy.[24]

Therefore, because KTS can be composed of a variable venous system, sclerotherapy treatment must only be performed after a thorough vascular evalua-

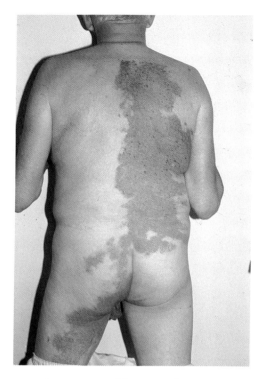

**Fig. 4-4** Nevus flammeus in a 68-year-old man without any associated soft tissue abnormalities. Note the lesion extends down the posterior thigh.

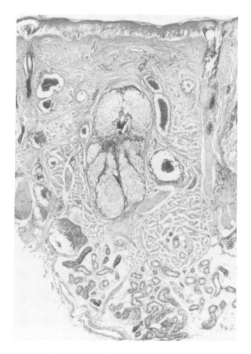

**Fig. 4-5** Histologic section of a nevus flammeus taken from the forehead of a 66-year-old man immediately after treatment with the argon laser. Note the location of the enlarged blood vessels within the middle and deep dermis. Since this lesion has just been treated, the overlying epidermis demonstrates thermal changes, and the vessels are thrombosed. (Hematoxylin-eosin, ×80) (Courtesy Richard Fitzpatrick, M.D.)

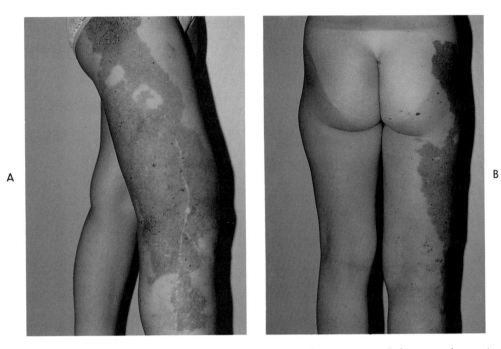

**Fig. 4-6**  **A** and **B,** Woman, 16 years old, with Klippel-Trenaunay syndrome and associated varicose veins and nevus flammeus of the right lower extremity from the toes to buttock.

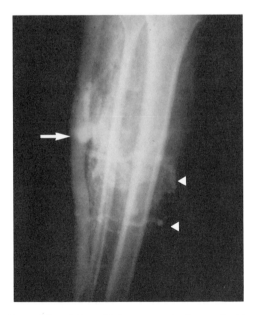

**Fig. 4-7**  Venogram film of the right calf (anteroposterior projection) of patient shown in Fig. 4-6. There are multiple dilated collateral dermal venules *(arrowheads)* and a grossly enlarged lateral accessory saphenous vein along the posterolateral aspect of the calf *(arrow),* which is avalvular. The deep venous system is absent. (Courtesy Christopher Sebrechts, M.D.)

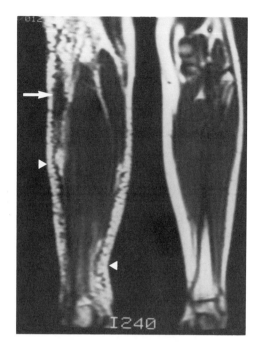

**Fig. 4-8**   Magnetic resonance image, coronal T1-weighted, of the calves (TR500, TE 20) of patient in Fig. 4-6. There are multiple small collateral vessels in the subcutaneous fat of the right calf seen as a spaghetti-like accumulation of dermal venulectases *(arrowheads)*. Note the enlarged lateral accessory vein present along the posterolateral aspect of the right calf *(arrow)*.

tion. In some patients it is possible to improve venous return and treat the cutaneous venectasia and nevus flammeus with a combination of sclerotherapy and pulsed-dye laser (Fig. 4-9) (see Chapter 12).

### Nevus araneus

Nevus araneus (spider telangiectasia) may occur as a component of a number of congenital and acquired diseases. They are found in up to 15% of the normal population and increase in number during pregnancy, liver disease, and many other conditions.[25] Ninety-nine percent occur above the umbilicus.[26] These lesions appear as bright red macules composed of a central red dot with fine blood vessels radiating out of the center (Fig. 4-10). The central vessel may pulsate indicating its arteriolar origin. Point compression of the central dot blanches the radiating vessels. One genetic disease with this form of telangiectasia distributed on the lower extremities is ataxia telangiectasia, which may have lesions in the popliteal fossae.[27]

Vascular spiders arise from a terminal arteriole (see Fig. 4-10).[3] The vessels arise within the deep dermis and push their way up into the superficial dermis as a space-occupying lesion. The central arteriole connects to dilated venous saccules with radiating venous legs in the papillary dermis.[25] Detailed histologic studies have provided little understanding of the factors responsible for the initial growth.[28]

Because the spider telangiectasia is composed of a central arteriole, sclerotherapy of these lesions usually produces cutaneous ulcerations (see Chapter 8). Therefore, treatment with the pulsed-dye laser, argon laser, or electrodesiccation to fibrose the central feeding arteriole is recommended (see Chapter 12).

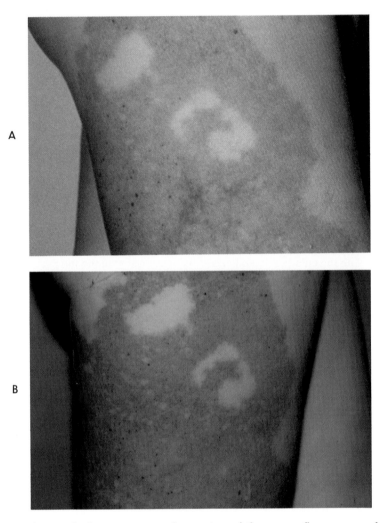

**Fig. 4-9**   Before and after treatment of a section of the nevus flammeus and associated superficial varicosity of patient shown in Fig. 4-6. The reticular veins were treated with Polidocanol 0.75% (6 ml total) followed by multiple impacts with the Candela SPTL-I pulsed dye laser at 8J/cm$^2$.

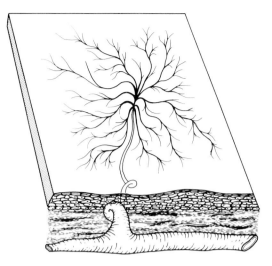

**Fig. 4-10** Schematic diagram of a nevus araneus (arteriolar spider) showing the origin at a dermal arteriole with coiled extension to the superficial dermis and branching horizontal "arms."

### Angioma serpiginosum

Angioma serpiginosum is a rare nevoid disorder of the upper dermal vasculature. The disease usually occurs in women on the lower extremities and has its onset in childhood. Although occurrence of most cases is sporadic, one family study suggests an autosomal dominant inheritance.[29] Lesions appear as small erythematous puncta occurring in groups that enlarge by forming new puncta at the periphery while those at the center fade. This results in a reticular or serpiginous pattern. A dilation of the subpapillary venous plexus may lead to telangiectasia. Histologic examination shows a number of ectatic capillaries in the superficial dermis. Endothelial cells appear hyperplastic and have an increased number of interendothelial junctions and vacuolization. Capillary walls are thickened with multiple basal laminae and a "heavy" precipitation of fine fibrillar material. The deeper dermis is unremarkable.[30] Therefore, angioma serpiginosum may represent a type of capillary nevus.

### Maffucci's syndrome

Maffucci's syndrome is a congenital dysplasia consisting of a constellation of vascular malformation and dyschondroplasia. Patients have single or multiple hemangiomas, varicosities, and telangiectasia of the legs. Dyschondroplasia and endochondromas occur as bony nodules on the fingers, toes, and extremities, and patients have unequal bone growth and slow union of easily sustained fractures. The distribution of vascular lesions often does not correspond to that of the skeletal lesions. In addition to the hemangioma, lymphangiomas and lymphectasis may be present.

The syndrome affects all races and equally affects men and women with no evidence of a familial tendency.[31] Twenty-five percent of patients have symptoms within the first year of life, and 78% manifest symptoms before puberty.[31] From 25% to 30% of patients will develop malignancies including chondrosarcoma, angiosarcoma, lymphangiosarcoma, glioma, fibrosarcoma, pancreatic carcinoma, and ovarian teratoma.[31-34]

### Congenital poikiloderma

Congenital poikiloderma (Rothmund-Thomson syndrome) is a rare neurocutaneous syndrome that has its onset in the first year of life. There appears to be a female predominance, and 70% of cases show a familial recessive inheritance.[35] A fine telangiectatic network first appears on the cheeks and progresses within a year to the head, arms, buttocks, and legs. There may be associated scaling of the skin and lichenoid papules. The hair is often sparse, and skin is soft and translucent. Dwarfism, cataracts, dental abnormalities, mental retardation, hypogenitalism, and diabetes mellitus may occur.[35]

### Essential progressive telangiectasia

Essential progressive telangiectasia (EPT) is a rare entity that has been reported in association with bronchogenic carcinoma,[36] angiokeratomas,[37] chronic sinusitis,[38] and an autoimmune setting.[39] It most commonly is essential in nature. EPT has been reported to be associated with small varicose veins that occur many years after disease onset.[40] Histochemical examination establishes the vessels in EPT to be venular in origin.[41] Lesions appear as blue to bright red telangioectasias 0.1 to 0.4 mm in diameter. There may be an associated peritelangiectatic atrophy of the subcutaneous tissues. Lesions most commonly appear on the feet and distal leg but rarely can involve the entire leg.

The treatment of these lesions is often fraught with complications because many of the telangiectasias are intimately associated with arterioles. This also leads to frequent recurrence of previously treated vessels. However, cautious treatment with either sclerotherapy or the pulsed-dye laser may be successful.[40]

### Cutis marmorata telangiectatica congenita

Cutis marmorata telangiectatica congenita is a rare congenital cutaneous vascular anomaly consisting of a sharply demarcated, reticulated vascular network of blue-violet venules associated with telangiectasias and dilated venules, with or without varicose veins. The cutis marmorata component is neither transient nor related to temperature. Telangiectasias may not appear in the first 2 years.[42-44] Lesions are most prominent on the lower extremities but may involve any cutaneous surface. Involvement may be unilateral or bilateral. Atrophy and ulcerations of the overlying skin may occur over time.[45] There may be an associated nevus flammeus. Lesions have also been reported to spontaneously improve in up to three fourths of patients within the first 2 years.[44]

Most cases of this disease occur sporadically, and two thirds of the approximately 80 reported cases occurred in women.[42-44,46] The pathogenesis is most likely multifactorial; genetic (autosomal dominant inheritance[47,48]) and teratogenic factors are most commonly cited.

Histologic examination demonstrates an abnormal dilation of capillaries and veins.[49] Associated congenital abnormalities have been reported in up to 50% of patients. These include structural defects of the musculoskeletal system, ocular and dental malformations, and arteriovenous malformations.[50]

### Diffuse neonatal hemangiomatosis

Diffuse neonatal hemangiomatosis is a rare congenital disorder of vascular development, occurring in infancy with multiple visceral hemangiomas. The combination of hepatic and cutaneous hemangiomas occurs twice as often in girls as in boys.[51] Hemangiomas are usually present on the skin and may be associated with large areas involved with telangiectasias and venulectases (Fig. 4-11).

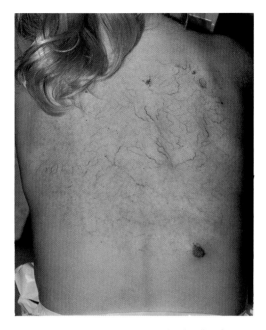

**Fig. 4-11**   Diffuse neonatal hemangiomatosis on the back of a 2½-year-old girl. The telangiectatic component was present at birth. Within the first few months cutaneous hemangiomas began to appear. A large mediastinal hemangioma was also noted surrounding the esophagus. Systemic treatment with corticosteroids did not result in any notable decrease in the size of the internal or cutaneous hemangiomas. The patient remains well now at age 9.

Infants with this disorder often die of high-output cardiac failure as a result of arteriovenous shunting of blood flow through the hemangiomas. Recognition of the cutaneous component, which may be minimal in some infants, will help prevent confusion of the cardiac failure with a congenital heart disease.[52] Therapy consists of systemic steroids, selective embolization, and/or surgical excision.[31] Selective sclerotherapy of the telangiectasias may be performed for cosmetic improvement.

## Acquired Disease with a Secondary Cutaneous Component

Telangiectasias occurring as a component of an acquired or primary cutaneous disease evolve because of a multitude of factors. When associated with collagen vascular diseases, relative tissue anoxia may result in the appearance of telangiectasias, especially in connection with an acral distribution. Alternatively, circulating cryoglobulins may lead to acral telangiectasia. Periungual telangiectasia is particularly common in lupus erythematosus and progressive systemic sclerosis. In addition, various vasculitic factors or other immunologic factors associated with these diseases may lead to the appearance of telangiectasias, particularly in areas where other physical factors (such as actinic damage) are prominent.

In some conditions (for example, mastocytosis), a component of the disease itself, such as the release of various mast cell vasoactive factors, especially histamine or heparin, may lead to the development of telangiectasias.[53,54] Recently histologic studies in a patient with unilateral facial telangiectasia macularis eruptiva perstans demonstrated an accumulation of mast cells.[55]

## Component of a Primary Cutaneous Disease
### Varicose veins

Varicose veins lead most likely to the development of telangiectasia either through associated venous hypertension with resulting angiogenesis or vascular dilation[25] or through an associated increased distensibility of the telangiectatic vein wall (see Chapter 3). Although telangiectasias associated with varicose veins may appear at first as erythematous streaks, with time they turn blue. Often they are directly associated with underlying varicose veins, so the distinction between telangiectasias and varicose veins becomes blurred.[25] (This concept is discussed on pp. 25-29.) In one study, telangiectasias were shown to be associated with underlying reticular veins. Tretbar[56] studied 100 patients with telangiectasias (<1 mm diameter) with the venous Doppler and found that they are connected with associated "feeding" reticular veins. These veins were separate from any truncal varicosities that may have been present. All blue reticular veins demonstrated reflux that did not appear to originate from the long or short saphenous veins. Of patients with blue reticular veins, 50% demonstrated reflux from incompetent calf perforating veins. In this situation, treatment of the feeding varicosity results in treatment of the distal telangiectasia (see Chapters 9 and 11). If no apparent connection exists between deep collecting or reticular vessels, the telangiectasia may arise from a terminal arteriole or arteriovenous anastomosis.[57]

Telangiectasias may be associated with underlying venous disease even when there are no clinical abnormalities. Thibault and Bray[58] have evaluated 83 patients with spider leg veins with duplex and Doppler examination. They found that 23% of these patients without clinically apparent varicose veins had incompetence of the superficial venous system. In addition, 1.2% had incompetence of a perforator vein. Nineteen patients, each with one clinically abnormal leg and one clinically normal leg, were also evaluated. Interestingly, 37% of clinically normal legs demonstrated incompetence of the superficial system. The abnormal legs in this group had a 74% incidence of incompetence of the superficial system, and 21% had saphenofemoral incompetence. This study demonstrates the need for both a clinical and noninvasive diagnostic work-up in patients who have spider veins and also reinforces the view that spider veins arise from underlying varicose veins via venous hypertension.

A proposed mechanism for the development of leg telangiectasia associated with underlying venous disease is that preexisting vascular anastomotic channels open in response to venous stasis.[59] And venous stasis with resulting venous hypertension leads to a reversal of flow from venules back to capillaries. The resulting capillary hypertension leads to opening and dilation of normally closed vessels. Consequently, relative anoxia as a result of reversed venous flow leads to angiogenesis. Merlen[57] states that capillaries and venules have an enhanced neogenic potential and a remarkable tendency towards neogenesis in a hypoxic atmosphere.

### Keratosis lichenoides chronica

Prominent telangiectasia of the feet and legs has been described in patients with keratosis lichenoides chronica.[60] This condition is usually not associated with telangiectasia.[61] However, severe pruritus was also present in these patients, and although the authors ascribed the development of the telangiectasia and lichenoid papules to the same process, it appears equally likely that both physical manifestations could be caused by chronic rubbing and scratching. Thus it is difficult to separate the development of telangiectasia into primary and secondary processes.

### Other acquired primary cutaneous disease

As with telangiectasia of acquired cutaneous disease, telangiectasia of primary cutaneous disease rarely affects the legs, with the obvious exception of varicose veins. Other cutaneous diseases with associated telangiectasia are necrobiosis lipoidica diabeticorum, capillaritis (purpura annularis telangiectodes), and malignant atrophic papulosis (Degos' disease).

Treatment of telangiectasias caused by an acquired or primary cutaneous disease usually is best accomplished by treatment of the acquired disease itself. The telangiectatic component of these lesions is usually asymptomatic and requires no treatment except for cosmesis. And in that case, electrodesiccation or the argon tunable continuous dye or pulsed dye laser may be the treatment of choice (see Chapter 12).

## Hormonal Factors
### Pregnancy and estrogen therapy

The hormonal influence in the development of telangiectasia is well known. Perhaps the most common physiologic condition that leads to the development of telangiectasia is pregnancy. Bean[25] has estimated that almost 70% of women develop telangiectasias during pregnancy, the majority of which disappear between 3 and 6 weeks postpartum (Fig. 4-12). Pregnant women often develop telangiectasias on the legs within a few weeks of conception, even before the uterus has enlarged to compress venous return to the pelvis.[62,63] Also, pregnant women and those taking birth control pills have been shown to have an increase in the distensibility of vein walls.[64] This increase in distensibility has also been noted to fluctuate with the normal menstrual cycle.[65] It was found that leg volume was greatest just before ovulation and during menses. The increased distensibility did not fully correlate with one specific hormone but was related to both estrogen

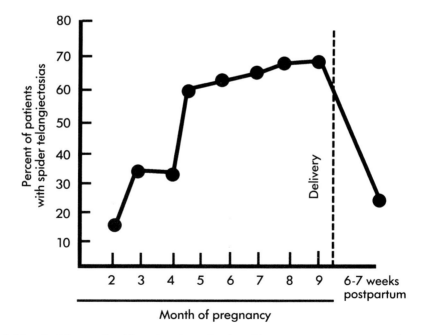

**Fig. 4-12** Incidence of spider telangiectasias in white pregnant women as a function of the duration of pregnancy. (From Bean WB: Vascular spiders and related lesions of the skin, Springfield, Ill, 1958, Charles C Thomas Publisher.)

and progesterone levels or ratios. Hormonal stimulation may also lead to the development of telangiectasia independent of the effect on venous distensibility. Paradoxically, estrogen has been found to be beneficial in controlling symptoms of venous distensibility during pregnancy (see Chapter 3).[66] Thus some hormonal influence is involved in the development of varicose veins and their associated telangiectasias in women (see Chapter 2), but the exact hormonal mechanism for telangiectasia development is unknown.

Davis and Duffy[67] have recently reported an apparent association of estrogen excess states with the development of telangiectatic matting after sclerotherapy of spider leg veins. In their selected patient population of 160, 29% of women who developed "new" telangiectasia were taking systemic estrogens or became pregnant as compared with 19% of patients on hormones who did not develop telangiectatic matting. One additional patient noted the disappearance of both spider veins and telangiectatic matting after taking the antiestrogen tamoxifen citrate (Nolvadex). Biopsies of these patients were not performed.

Estrogen acts by entering its target cell and associating with an extranuclear receptor protein. This complex then enters the nucleus and modulates ribonucleic acid (RNA) synthesis.[68] Since endothelial cells have been found to possess estrogen receptors, they may be potential target cells.[69] Sadick and Neidt[70] assayed 20 patients with leg telangiectasias for estrogen receptors. Interestingly, they failed to find any evidence of such receptors in their patient population. They postulated that either estrogen receptors are not present in increased numbers in leg telangiectasia or estrogen acts on endothelium through an indirect pathway. This pathway may be a stimulation of angiogenic factors (see Chapter 8) or an increase in vascular distensibility.

The hormonal influence in telangiectasia neogenesis has been noted in 10 of 15 reported cases of unilateral nevoid telangiectasia syndrome. In these female patients, the telangiectasias did not occur until triggered by pregnancy or puberty and correlated with high serum estrogen levels. Four of the remaining five cases were associated with alcoholic cirrhosis and one was congenital. There was no association with the development of varicose veins.[71]

### Topical corticosteroid preparations

The development of telangiectatic blood vessels may also occur from self-induced hormonal manipulation. A common form of iatrogenic telangiectasia may occur from the use of high potency topical steroid preparations. Leyden[72] first reported the development of rosacea associated with telangiectasia in 10 patients who regularly used topical fluorinated steroids on the face. Katz and Prawer[73] have demonstrated clinical cutaneous vascular dilation and network development within 2 weeks of treatment with superpotent topical steroids (betamethasone dipropionate in an optimized vehicle and clobetasol ointment). This type of steroid-induced telangiectasia probably reflects the loss of perivascular ground substance, allowing distention of existing vessels, or the capillary elongation and distortion generated to meet the requirement of the hyperplastic epidermis.[74] In support of this theory, covert vascular visualization has been shown to represent the early changes of cutaneous atrophy that occur as a result of steroid use.[75] Facial telangiectasia has also been reported to develop in association with long-term application of a topical corticosteroid to the scalp.[76] In this report the long-term use of betamethasone valerate lotion allowed percutaneous absorption of a sufficient amount to spread locally from the scalp to the face via the dermal vasculature. Therefore, topical application of corticosteroid preparations can induce the development or appearance of telangiectasia.

# Physical Factors

## Actinic neovascularization and vascular dilation

Physical factors are commonly responsible for acquired telangiectasia. Telangiectasias are noted to appear after many types of physical trauma. The most common form of physical damage to the skin is that caused from sun exposure.[77,78] Telangiectasia of the face is probably a manifestation of persistent active arteriolar vasodilation caused by weakness in the vessel wall resulting from degenerative elastic changes or weakness in the surrounding connective tissue caused by chronic sun exposure. These telangiectasias mostly arise from arterioles and are seen frequently in individuals with fair complexions, often on the nose, especially the ala and nasolabial crease. A similar mechanism of the pathogenesis of type I telangiectasias may also apply to their occurrence on the legs. Recently an examination of over 20,000 Americans[79] demonstrated the presence of fine telangiectasias in 17.3% of men and 11.6% of women with low sun exposure as compared with 30.1% of men and 26.2% of women who report high sun exposure. More significantly, 15.5% of men and 40.9% of women with actinic skin damage were shown to have spider leg veins as compared with 6% of men and 28.9% of women without actinic skin damage. Sun exposure with resulting damage to subcutaneous and cutaneous tissues is a significant etiologic factor in the appearance of telangiectasias.

## Trauma

*Contusion.* Various forms of physical trauma may lead to the development of new blood vessel growth. Contusion injuries are a common mechanism for the development of a localized growth of telangiectasias (Fig. 4-13). Neovascularization in this case is probably the result of epidermal and endothelial damage with the release of angiogenic factors including fibrin.[80] Trauma also causes a rapid change in the permeability of cutaneous blood vessels through the release of various mediators.[54] The increased permeability of endothelium may lead to angiogenesis through multiple mechanisms.[81]

Recently a solitary giant spider angioma with an overlying pyogenic granuloma was described.[82] This spider angioma was associated with alcoholic liver cirrhosis. The authors postulated that local mechanical irritation led to a reactive proliferation of the endothelial cells. When the central pyogenic granuloma was removed, the surrounding spider telangiectasia disappeared.

*Surgical incision/lacerations.* Surgical incision or cutaneous laceration are common events that require physiologic neovascularization. Here angiogenesis is a prerequisite for the development of wound healing.[80] Fibrin deposition appears to play a prominent role in wound healing by stimulating new blood vessel growth.[80,83] The resulting formation of blood vessels has been demonstrated to represent a dilation and extension of existing blood vessels.[54] Unfortunately, some postsurgical patients develop an exaggerated angiogenic response with resulting cutaneous telangiectasia. Although this may occur at sites of ligation for vein stripping (Fig. 4-14), the most common surgical event that leads to the development of telangiectasia is the skin flap procedure. When a skin flap is under excessive tension, telangiectasias may develop at the edge of the flap. This excessive blood vessel growth may result from the influence of mechanical forces on the wound. Histologic examination demonstrates the orientation of vascular fiber networks along lines of tension. This orientation may be related to the activation of cell growth through stretching.[84] Thus the vascularization of skin flaps and grafts supports the concept of an epidermal stimulus for vasculogenesis.[85,86]

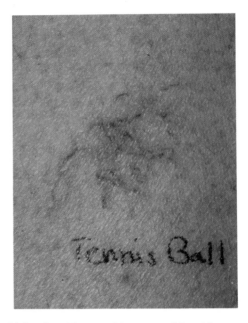

**Fig. 4-13**   Posterior thigh of a 35-year-old woman hit with a tennis ball 1 year previously. The resulting telangiectatic mass developed shortly after resolution of the bruise.

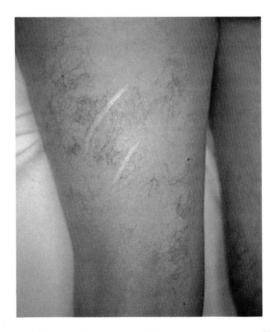

**Fig. 4-14**   At 18 years of age this woman underwent an extensive ligation and stripping of her varicose veins. She developed extensive telangiectasia around all of the surgical sites within weeks of the surgical procedure. This photograph was taken 22 years after the surgical procedure. (Courtesy John Bergan, M.D.)

## Infection

*Generalized essential telangiectasia.* Generalized essential telangiectasia is a benign form of telangiectasia of unknown etiology. It often begins in late childhood as extensive linear telangiectasia of the legs. It is more common in girls, but estrogen and progesterone receptors in the vascular lesions have not been found to be elevated.

Various infections have been associated with the development of this form of telangiectasia. Bacterium may stimulate endothelial proliferation in vitro.[87] Becker[88] in 1926 first noted the association of generalized telangiectasia with syphilitic infection in a review of patients with generalized telangiectasia. Of those patients, 16 had evidence of syphilis, and 4% had evidence of a focal infection. Ayres Jr., Burrows, and Anderson[89] later described a patient with generalized telangiectasia and sinus infection. Resolution of the sinusitis with antibiotic treatment resulted in the disappearance of the telangiectasia.

*Progressive ascending telangiectasia.* Finally, Shelley[90] and Shelley and Fierer[91] described two cases of essential progressive telangiectasia that resolved after empiric treatment with tetracycline and ketoconazole respectively. Electron microscopic studies in one patient[91] demonstrated focal fibrin clots in some of the dilated vessels, which disappeared within a month of ketoconazole therapy. They postulated a microbial-induced focal intravascular coagulation as the etiologic factor in the pathogenesis of this rare form of acquired telangiectasia.

*Human immunodeficiency virus.* Most recently, a HIV-positive hemophiliac man was seen with numerous telangiectasias on the shins, which resolved after treatment with tetracycline.[92] The specific infection involved is difficult to identify because a myriad of infections occur in this immunosuppressed population. Also, a recent survey of homosexual men with and without lymphadenopathy demonstrated that 47% had focal telangiectasias in a broad distribution across the anterior chest.[93] The presence of telangiectasias was significantly, although not exclusively, associated with HIV seropositivity. Telangiectasias in this group did not appear to be related to underlying bacterial or fungal infection or to sun exposure. The authors postulated that this clinical finding may be a direct manifestation of HIV infectivity.

Although not telangiectatic, bacillary angiomatosis (also called epitheliod angiomatosis) is a newly recognized disease most often characterized by multiple cutaneous reddish papules. Tissue sections of these lesions have demonstrated a weakly reactive gram-negative bacillus. The cutaneous lesions resolve with antibiotic therapy. Thus this new entity confirms an infectious etilogy for the stimulation of vascular proliferation.[94]

In summary, circumstantial evidence exists that indicates a systemic or localized infection promotes the development of neovascularization. Because this association is so rare, when one considers the ubiquitous occurrence of infections in man, the pathophysiology of this clinical association is obscure.

### Radiodermatitis

Therapeutic radiation therapy may also lead to the development of telangiectasia (Fig. 4-15). Chronic radiodermatitis has been noticeably decreased with the advent of mega-voltage equipment and better technique. Mega-voltage radiation beams are more penetrating than the older lower-energy beams, which minimizes the radiation dose to the skin. However, at least 5% of patients irradiated during therapeutic radiation therapy will develop cutaneous telangiectasia.[95] The

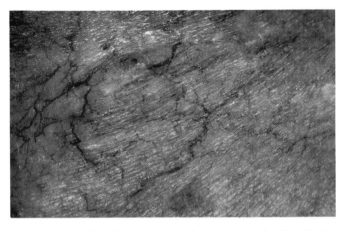

**Fig. 4-15**   Appearance of telangiectasia occurring as a result of radiation treatment on the lateral neck for laryngeal carcinoma 20 years previously.

fundamental pathology of chronic radiodermatitis is fibrosis of the vessels with occlusion and varying degrees of homogenization of the connective tissue. Residual superficial blood vessels are usually dilated.[96]

### Erythema ab igne

Infrared radiation/heat exposure can also lead to the appearance of telangiectasia. Erythema ab igne is a localized dermatosis that occurs as reticular pigmentation and telangiectasia produced by repeated exposures to heat. It is commonly seen on the legs of women who sit close to heating units in countries without central heating. Histologic findings include epidermal atrophy, vasodilation, a dermal mixed-cellular infiltrate, and an increase in melanophages and free-lying melanin granules.[97]

**REFERENCES**

1. Merlen JF: Red telangiectasia, blue telangiectasias, Soc Franc Phlebol 22:167, 1970.
2. Goldman MP and Bennett RG: Treatment of telangiectasia: a review, J Am Acad Dermatol 17:167, 1987.
3. Redisch W and Pelzer RH: Localized vascular dilatations of the human skin: capillary microscopy and related studies, Am Heart J 37:106, 1949.
4. Kaplan I and Peled I: The carbon dioxide laser in the treatment of superficial telangiectasias, Br J Plast Surg 28:214, 1975.
5. Ayres S Jr, Burrows LA, and Anderson NP: Generalized telangiectasias and sinus infection: report of a case with cure by treatment of chronic sinusitis, Arch Derm Syph 26:56, 1931.
6. Noe JM et al: Post rhinoplasty "red nose": differential diagnosis and treatment by laser, Plast Reconstr Surg 67:661, 1981.
7. Shelley WB: Essential progressive telangiectasia, JAMA 210:1343, 1971.
8. Anderson RL and Smith JG Jr: Unilateral nevoid telangiectasia with gastric involvement, Arch Dermatol 111:617, 1975.
9. Duffy DM: Small vessel sclerotherapy: an overview, Adv Dermatol 3:221, 1988.
10. Sadick N: Treatment of varicose and telangiectatic leg veins with hypertonic saline: a comparative study of heparin and saline, J Dermatol Surg Oncol 16:24, 1990.
11. Pratt AG: Birthmarks in infants, Arch Dermat Syph 67:302, 1953.
12. Jacobs AH and Walton RG: The incidence of birthmarks in the neonate, Pediatrics 58:218, 1970.
13. Cosman B: Clinical experience in the laser therapy of port-wine stains, Lasers Surg Med 1:133, 1980.

14. Hobby LW: Treatment of port-wine stains and other cutaneous lesions, Contemp Surg 18:21, 1981.
15. Shelley WB and Livingood CS: Familial multiple nevi flammei, Arch Dermat Syph 59:343, 1949.
16. Kaplan P, Hollenberg RD, and Fraser FC: A spinal arteriovenous malformation in hereditary cutaneous hemangiomas, Am J Dis Child 130:1329, 1976.
17. Nova HR: Familial communicating hydrocephalus, posterior cerebellar agenesis, mega cisterna magna, and port-wine nevi, J Neurosurg 51:862, 1979.
18. Zaremba J et al: Hereditary neurocutaneous angioma: a new genetic entity? J Med Genet 6:443, 1979.
19. Barsky SH et al: The nature and evolution of port-wine stains: a computer-assisted study, J Invest Dermatol 74:154, 1980.
20. Finley JL et al: Port-wine stains: morphologic variations and developmental lesions, Arch Dermatol 120:1453, 1984.
21. Glovicki P et al: Surgical implications of Klippel-Trenaunay syndrome, Ann Surg 19:353, 1983.
22. Servelle M et al: Haematuria and rectal bleeding in the child with Klippel-Trenaunay syndrome, Ann Surg 183:410, 1976.
23. Vollmar JF et al: Aneurysmatische Transformation des Venensystems bei venosen Angiodysplasien der Gliedmassen, Vasa 18:96, 1989.
24. Colver GB: The clinical relevance of abnormal cutaneous vascular patterns and related pathologies. In Ryan J and Cherry GW, editors: Vascular birthmarks: pathogenesis and management, New York, 1987, Oxford University Press.
25. Bean WB: Vascular spiders and related lesions of the skin, Springfield, Ill, 1958, Charles C Thomas Publisher.
26. Pasyk KA: Classification and cinical and histopathological features of haemangiomas and other vascular malformations. In Ryan J and Cherry GW, editors: Vascular birthmarks: pathogenesis and management, New York, 1987, Oxford University Press.
27. Reed WB et al: Cutaneous manifestations of ataxia-telangiectasia, JAMA 195:126, 1966.
28. Martini GA and Staubesand J: Zur morphologie der gefäcbspinnen ("vascular spider") in der Haut Leverknankev, Virchows Archiv 324:147, 1953.
29. Marriott P, Munro D, and Ryan TJ: Angioma serpiginosum — familial incidence, Br J Dermatol 93:701, 1975.
30. Kumakiri M: Angioma serpiginosum, J Cutan Pathol 7:410, 1980.
31. Young AE, Ackroyd AE, and Baskerville P: Combined vascular malformations. In Mulliken JB and Young AE, editors: Vascular birthmarks, Philadelphia, 1988, WB Saunders Co.
32. Lewis RJ and Ketcham AS: Maffucci's syndrome: functional and neoplastic significance, J Bone Joint Surg 55:1465, 1973.
33. Cremer H, Gullotta F, and Wolf L: Maffucci-Kast syndrome, J Cancer Res Clin Oncol 101:231, 1981.
34. Cheng FC: Maffucci's syndrome with fibroadenomas of the breasts, J R Coll Surg Edinb 26:181, 1981.
35. Silver HK: Rothmund-Thomson syndrome: an oculocutaneous disorder, Am J Dis Child 111:182, 1966.
36. Ochshorn M, Ilie B, and Blum I: Multiple telangiectasias preceding the appearance of undifferentiated bronchiogenic carcinoma, Dermatologica 165:620, 1982.
37. Draelos ZK, Hansen RC, and Hays SB: Symmetric progressive telangiectatic nevi with hemorrhagic angiokeratomas, Pediatr Dermatol 3:212, 1986.
38. Ayers S Jr, Burrows LA, and Anderson NP: Generalized telangiectasia and sinus infection: report of a case with cure by treatment of chronic sinusitus, Arch Dermat Syph 26:56, 1932.
39. Shelley WB and Shelley ED: Essential progressive telangiectasia in an autoimmune setting: successful treatment with acyclovir, J Am Acad Dermatol 21:1094, 1989.
40. Girbig P and Voigtlander V: Besenreiservarizen im Rahmen progressiver essentieller Telangiektasien, Phlebol und Proctol 17:116, 1988.
41. McGrae JD and Winkelmann RK: Generalized essential telangiectasia: report of a clinical and histologic study of 13 patients with acquired cutaneous lesions, JAMA 185:909, 1963.
42. Paller AS: Vascular disorders, Dermatol Clin 5:239, 1987.
43. Way BH et al: Cutis marmorata telangiectatic congenita, J Cutan Pathol 1:10, 1974.
44. Powell ST and Su WPD: Cutis marmorata telangiectatica congenita: report of nine cases and review of the literature, Cutis 34:305, 1984.
45. Picascia DD and Esterly NB: Cutis marmorata telangiectatica congenita: report of 22 cases, J Am Acad Dermatol 20:1098, 1989.

46. South DA and Jacobs AH: Cutis marmorata telangiectatica congenita (congenital generalized phlebectasia), J Pediatr 93:944, 1978.

47. Andreev VC and Pramatarov K: Cutis marmorata telangiectatic congenita in two sisters, Br J Dermatol 101:345, 1979.

48. Kurczynski TW: Hereditary cutis marmorata telangiectatic congenita, Pediatrics 70:52, 1982.

49. Van Lohuizen CHJ: Uber eine seltene angeborene Hautanomalie (Cutis marmorata telangiectatica congenita), Acta Derm Venerol (Stockh) 3:202, 1922.

50. Cohen PR and Zalar GL: Cutis marmorata telangiectatica congenita: cliniopathologic characteristics and differential diagnosis, Cutis 42:518, 1988.

51. de Lorimier AA: Hepatic tumors of infancy and childhood, Surg Clin North Am 57:443, 1977.

52. Hurwitz S: Clinical pediatric dermatology: a textbook of skin disorders of childhood and adolescence, Philadelphia, 1981, WB Saunders Co.

53. Azizkhan G et al: Mast cell heparin stimulates migration of capillary endothelial cells in vitro, J Exp Med 152:931, 1980.

54. Ryan TJ and Kurban AK: New vessel growth in the adult skin, Br J Derm 82(suppl):92, 1970.

55. Fried SZ and Lynfield L: Unilateral facial telangiectasia macularis eruptiva perstans, J Am Acad Dermatol 16:250, 1987.

56. Tretbar LL: The origin of reflux in incompetent blue reticular/telangiectasia veins. In Davy A and Stemmer R, editors: Phlebologie '89, Montrouge, France, 1989, John Libby Eurotext Ltd.

57. Merlen JF: Telangiectasies rouges, telangiectasies bleues, Phlebologie 23:167, 1970.

58. Thibault P and Bray A: Cosmetic leg veins: evaluation using duplex venous imaging, J Dermatol Surg Oncol, 1990 (in press).

59. Curri GB and Lo Brutto ME: Influenza dei mucopolisaccaridi e dei loro costituenti sulla neoformazione vascolare, Riv Pat Clin Sper 8:379, 1967.

60. David M et al: Keratosis lichenoides chronica with prominent telangiectasia: response to etretinate, J Am Acad Dermatol 21:1112, 1989.

61. Margolis MH, Cooper GA, and Johnson SAM: Keratosis lichenoides chronica, Arch Dermatol 105:739, 1972.

62. Miller SS: Investigation and management of varicose veins, Ann R Coll Surg Engl 55:245, 1974.

63. Mullane DJ: Varicose veins of pregnancy, Am J Obstet Gynecol 63:620, 1952.

64. Goodrich SM and Wood JE: Peripheral venous distensibility and velocity of venous blood flow during pregnancy or during oral contraceptive therapy, Am J Obstet Gynecol 90:740, 1964.

65. Keates JS and Fitzgerald DE: An interim report on lower limb volume and blood flow changes during a normal menstrual cycle, 5th Europ Conf Microcirculation, Gothenburg, 1968, Bibl Anat 10:189, Basle, Switzerland, 1969, Karger.

66. McPheeters HO: The value of estrogen therapy in the treatment of varicose veins complicating pregnancy, J Lancet 69:2, 1949.

67. Davis LT and Duffy DM: Determination of incidence and risk factors for post-sclerotherapy telangiectatic matting of the lower extremity: a retrospective analysis, J Dermatol Surg Oncol 16:327, 1990.

68. Jensen EV et al: Receptors reconsidered: a 20-year perspective, Rec Prog Horm Res 38:1, 1982.

69. Colburn P and Buonossisi: Estrogen binding sites in endothelial cell cultures, Science 201:817, 1978.

70. Sadick NS and Niedt G: A study of estrogen receptors in spider telangiectasia of the lower extremities, J Dermatol Surg Oncol 16:620, 1990.

71. Wilkin JK: Unilateral nevoid telangiectasias, Arch Dermatol 113:486, 1977.

72. Leyden JJ, Thew M, and Kligman AM: Steroid rosacea, Arch Dermatol 110:619, 1974.

73. Katz HI and Prawer SE: Morphologic diagnosis of pre-atrophy of the skin. Scientific exhibit presented at the American Academy of Dermatology, New Orleans, December 6-11, 1986.

74. Zheng P et al: Morphologic investigations on the rebound phenomenon after corticosteroid-induced atrophy in human skin, J Invest Dermatol 82:345, 1984.

75. Katz HI et al: Preatrophy: covert sign of thinned skin, J Am Acad Dermatol 20:731, 1989.

76. Hogan DJ and Rooney ME: Facial telangiectasia associated with long-term application of a topical corticosteroid to the scalp, J Am Acad Dermatol 20:1129, 1989.

77. O'Brian JP: Solar and radiant damage to elastic tissue as a cause of internal vascular disease, Aust J Dermatol 21:1, 1980.

78. Kumakari M, Hashimoto K, and Willis I: Biologic changes due to long wave ultraviolet irradiation on human skin, J Invest Dermatol 69:392, 1977.

79. Engel A, Johnson M-L, and Haynes SG: Health effects of sunlight exposure in the United States: results from the first national health and nutrition examination survey, 1971-1974, Arch Dermatol 124:72, 1988.

80. Dvorak HF: Tumors: wounds that do not heal: similarities between tumor stroma generation and wound healing, New Engl J Med 26:1650, 1986.
81. Ryan TJ: Factors influencing the growth of vascular endothelium in the skin, Br J Derm 82(suppl 5):99, 1970.
82. Okada N: Solitary giant spider angioma with an overlying pyogenic granuloma, J Am Acad Dermatol 5:1053, 1987.
83. Folkman J and Klagsbrun M: Angiogenic factors, Science 235:442, 1987.
84. Ryan TJ and Barnhill RL: Physical factors and angiogenesis. In Nugent J and O'Connor M, editors: Development of the vascular system, Ciba Foundation Symposium. London, 1983 Pitman.
85. Smahel J: The healing of skin grafts, Clin Plast Surg 4:409, 1977.
86. Myers MB: Attempts to augment survival in skin flaps — mechanism of the delay phenomenon. In Grabb WC and Myers MB, editors: Skin flaps, Boston, 1975, Little, Brown & Co Inc.
87. Garcia FN, Ojta T, and Hoover RL: Stimulation of human umbilical vein endothelial cells (HUVEC) by Bartonella bacilliformis (BB), FASEB J A1189, 1988.
88. Becker SW: Generalized telangiectasia, Arch Dermatol Syph 14:387, 1926.
89. Ayers S Jr, Burrows A, and Anderson NP: Generalized telangiectasia and sinus infection: report of a case with cure by treatment of chronic sinusitis, Arch Dermat Syph 26:56, 1932.
90. Shelley WB: Essential progressive telangiectasia: successful treatment with tetracycline, JAMA 216:1343, 1971.
91. Shelley WB and Fierer JA: Focal intravascular coagulation in progressive ascending telangiectasia: ultrastructural studies of ketoconazole-induced involution of vessels, J Am Acad Dermatol 10:876, 1984.
92. Jimenez-Acosta F, Fonseca E, and Magallon M: Response to tetracycline of telangiectasias in a male hemophiliac with human immunodeficiency virus infection, J Am Acad Dermatol 19:369, 1988.
93. Fallon T Jr et al: Telangiectasias of the anterior chest in homosexual men, Ann Intern Med 105:679, 1986.
94. Cockerell CJ and LeBoit PE: Bacillary angiomatosis: a newly characterized, pseudoneoplastic infectious, cutaneous vascular disorder, J Am Acad Dermatol 22:501, 1990.
95. Clarke D, Martinez A, and Cox RS: Analysis of cosmetic results and complications in patients with stage I and II breast cancer treated by biopsy and irradiation, Int J Radiat Oncol Biol Phys 9:1807, 1983.
96. Goldschmidt H and Sherwin WK: Reactions to ionizing radiation, J Am Acad Dermatol 3:551, 1980.
97. Dover JS, Phillips TJ, and Arndt KA: Cutaneous effects and therapeutic uses of heat with emphasis on infrared radiation, J Am Acad Dermatol 20:278, 1989.

# 5 Noninvasive Examination of the Patient Before Sclerotherapy

*Helane S. Fronek*

The simplicity of sclerotherapy treatment of varicose vein disease invites certain problems. Physicians unfamiliar with the anatomy and pathophysiology of the venous system can easily feel otherwise well-prepared to simply "inject veins" and are thus lured into treating patients who may actually have very complicated conditions. Unfortunately, evidence of venous disease on examination is very subtle. For this reason, it is quite possible, and frequently the case, that an asymptomatic patient with no grossly visible varicose veins actually has significant venous disease that will either lead to treatment failure with a rapid recurrence of symptoms or to serious complications or worsened venous function if it goes unrecognized. Imaging of 83 limbs with clinical evidence of only telangiectatic vessels demonstrated that nearly 25% had insufficiency of the long or short saphenous veins, which was not apparent on physical examination.[1] Incomplete appreciation of the actual condition of the patient's venous system can thus subject the patient to avoidable risks and unnecessary treatment. As with any medical procedure, a great deal of thought, examination, and treatment planning is essential to achieve success. Therefore, a screening evaluation of the venous system should be performed before undertaking sclerotherapy. More involved examinations may also be necessary based on the initial findings.

## MEDICAL HISTORY

The approach to the patient who seeks treatment is to begin with a directed medical history. The duration of the known venous disease and the course of its evolution are important factors to consider in understanding both the severity of the disease in that patient and in planning treatment. Patients who noted the onset of large varicose veins by their early 20s, especially those with a strong family history of varicose vein disease, will undoubtedly have aggressive disease. These patients require a thorough examination of their venous system since long-standing varicose veins may be not only the result of but also the cause of venous valvular insufficiency in both the superficial and perforating veins and may be the sole cause of serious problems including venous ulceration.[2-4]

Worsening of varicose veins or the symptoms attributed to them following a period of immobilization, travel, or an operation suggests the occurrence of a clinically unrecognized deep venous thrombosis (DVT). These patients should be examined for calf muscle pump function, perforator vein valvular insufficiency, and deep venous valvular insufficiency. Persons with a confirmed history of DVT or superficial thrombophlebitis are also at risk for these complications since the thrombus or the inflammatory reaction may spread to perforating and deep veins, leading to valvular damage at these sites. A rapid or simply progressive increase in the size of the varicose veins or the recent onset of edema may be indicative of an abdominal or pelvic tumor compressing the inferior vena cava, interfering with venous outflow; therefore, abdominal and pelvic physical examination, supplemented with radiologic studies such as ultrasound, computerized axial tomography, or magnetic resonance imaging should be considered.

## Prior Treatment

It is important that prior treatment for venous disease be discussed. However, the physician must realize that although proper ligation, with or without stripping of the main saphenous trunks, implies that reflux through the saphenofemoral (SFJ) and saphenopopliteal (SPJ) junctions has been prevented, this is not always the case. In up to 27% of people there is a duplication of the long saphenous vein (LSV),[5-7] thus the removal of the LSV may be followed by the development of varicosity in the remaining LSV. In 20% to 40% the short saphenous vein (SSV) has an aberrant termination,[8-10] either not in the popliteal vein or in the popliteal vein above the popliteal fossa. Therefore, the actual SPJ may easily be missed, leading to an apparent rapid recurrence with varicose changes occurring in the remaining segment of the SSV and its tributaries. Lastly, in a number of patients a recurrence of varicose veins in the upper thigh may be the result of incomplete ligation and division of the other tributaries arising at the level of the SFJ or failure to accomplish the ligation flush with the femoral vein. In fact, in a review of 341 extremities reoperated on for varicose veins, Lofgren, Myers, and Webb[11] found that 61% had inadequate ligation. These facts make it imperative that, even in the patient with a history of ligation, division, and stripping, an examination for reflux through the SFJ and SPJ be performed.

## Symptoms

It is well known that the presence and severity of symptoms does not correlate with the size or severity of the varicose veins present. Symptoms usually attributable to varicose veins include feelings of heaviness, tiredness, aching, burning, throbbing, itching and cramping in the legs (see box below). These symptoms are generally worse with prolonged sitting or standing and are improved with leg elevation or walking. A premenstrual exacerbation of symptoms is also common. Generally, patients find relief with the use of compression, either in the form of support hose or an elastic bandage. Weight loss may also be accompanied by a diminution in the severity of varicose vein symptoms, as may the commencement of a regular program of lower extremity exercise. Clearly, these symptoms are not specific, as they may also be indicative of a variety of rheumatologic or orthopedic problems. However, their relationship to lower extremity movement and compression is usually helpful in establishing a venous origin for the symptoms. Significant symptoms suggestive of venous disease should prompt further evaluation for valvular insufficiency and calf muscle pump dysfunction.

The recent development of an extremely painful area on the lower leg asso-

---

**SYMPTOMS ATTRIBUTABLE TO VARICOSE VEINS**

Aching
Heaviness, tiredness
Pain (throbbing, burning, sharp, tingling)
Itching
Cramping

ciated with an overlying area of erythema and warmth may be indicative of lipo-dermatosclerosis caused by the insufficiency of an underlying perforator vein, and examination for this lesion should be performed.

## Complications of Varicose Vein Disease

Complications such as ulceration and hemorrhage should be discussed with the patient, since this will provide additional insight into both the severity and the probable locations of abnormality within the venous system. A history of ulcer-ation of the medial aspect of the lower leg should prompt further examination of the LSV trunk,[2] whereas involvement of the lateral aspect of the lower leg sug-gests an abnormality in the SSV, in addition to the deep and perforating vein sys-tems. A history of hemorrhage from telangiectasia in a particular area will sug-gest further examination for underlying incompetent perforators and is an indica-tion to treat all suspicious telangiectasias.[12]

## PURPOSE OF VENOUS EVALUATION

More extensive evaluation can provide essential information regarding both venous anatomy and function. Abnormalities of the superficial, perforating, or deep systems can be diagnosed, and the exact sites of valvular insufficiency within the various systems (and therefore the sites where treatment must be di-rected) can be determined. The hemodynamic significance of each of these ab-normalities may be defined, and the effect of correcting each site of reflux may be assessed. Insufficiency at a particular site within the venous system may be found to have no importance in the patient's pathologic venous hypertension or symp-toms and, therefore, may be ignored in the treatment plan, preventing unneces-sary treatment. Using the following examination techniques, the result of sclero-therapy may be documented in a more accurate and sensitive manner than with simple observation and palpation. Therefore, treatment success may be signifi-cantly enhanced since treatment can be continued until its endpoint, sclerosis and restoration of normal venous flow, is evident. Lastly, the presence of DVT and deep venous valvular insufficiency, absolute and relative contraindications to sclerotherapy, respectively, may be diagnosed, thus allowing for improved pa-tient selection and avoidance of serious complications.

## PHYSICAL EXAMINATION

The best way to approach the examination of the venous system before sclero-therapy is a matter of personal preference since many methods are available. Each has something to contribute, and each has limitations.

Using no special equipment, one can obtain a degree of information regard-ing overall venous outflow from the leg, the sites of valvular insufficiency, the presence of primary versus secondary varicose veins, and the presence of DVT.

The screening physical examination consists of careful observation of the legs. Any patient with large varicose veins; bulges in the thigh, calf, or the in-guinal region representative of incompetent perforating veins or a saphena varix;[13] signs of superficial venous hypertension such as an accumulation of telangiecta-sias in the ankle region; or any of the findings suggestive of venous dermatitis (pigmentation, induration, eczema) should be examined more fully. This also in-cludes patients with obvious cutaneous signs of venous disease such as venous ulceration, atrophie blanche, or lipodermatosclerosis. An obvious, but often for-gotten, point is the necessity of observing the entire leg and not confining the examination to simply the area that the patient feels is abnormal. The importance of this is demonstrated by Fig. 5-1. The patient came for treatment of an obvi-

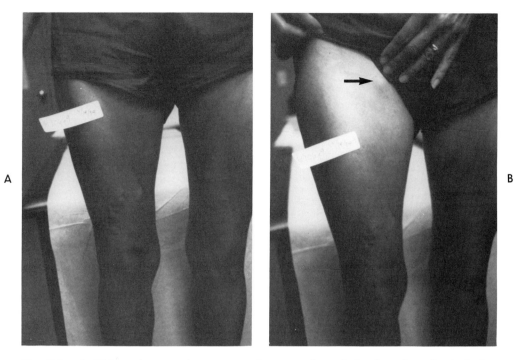

**Fig. 5-1** A, This patient sought treatment because of an obviously enlarged vein in her thigh. B, Further inspection revealed a saphena varix *(arrow)* indicative of SFJ insufficiency. (Courtesy Anton Butie, M.D.)

ously dilated anterior thigh vein, but further inspection revealed a saphena varix, indicative of incompetence at the level of the SFJ, thus defining the first step in her treatment. Similarly, patients will often seek treatment of specific clusters of telangiectasia and will not notice the underlying reticular veins that should be treated before or at the same time as the telangiectasia (see Chapter 11). Finally, since the veins of the leg empty into the pelvic and abdominal veins, inspection of the abdomen is also very important, since dilation of veins on the abdominal wall or across the pubic region suggests an old iliofemoral thrombus[14] or, rarely, a developmental anomaly of the venous system.[15]

A tourniquet may be placed around the patient's proximal thigh while the patient is standing. The patient then assumes the supine position with the affected leg elevated 45 degrees. The tourniquet is removed and the time required for the leg veins to empty, which is indicative of the adequacy of venous drainage, is recorded.

When compared with the contralateral leg, this method may demonstrate a degree of venous obstructive disease. Another approach is to elevate the leg while the patient is supine and observe the height of the heel in relation to the level of the heart that is required for the prominent veins to collapse (Fig. 5-2). Unfortunately, neither procedure is sufficiently sensitive nor accurate, and they do not differentiate acute from chronic obstruction and thus are of minimal assistance in current-day medical practice. However, there are several physical examination maneuvers that can provide information on the competence of the venous valves.

## Cough Test

One hand is placed gently over the LSV or the SFJ, and the patient is asked to cough or perform a Valsalva maneuver (Fig. 5-3). Simply palpating an impulse

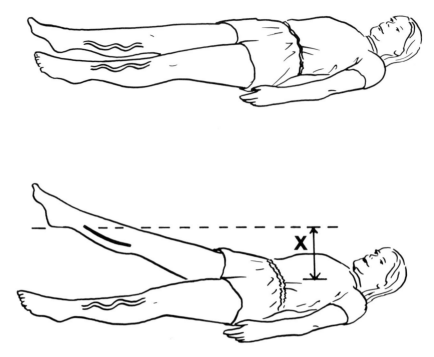

**Fig. 5-2**    Venous outflow may also be assessed by elevating the leg until the superficial veins collapse and then measuring the distance *(X)* from heart to the heel and comparing this measurement with the other leg.

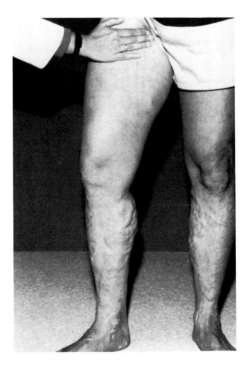

**Fig. 5-3**    Cough test. The SFJ is palpated while the patient coughs. Palpation of an impulse is indicative of SFJ insufficiency.

over the vein being examined is indicative of insufficiency of the valve at the saphenofemoral junction and also below to the level of the palpating hand. This test is not, however, applicable to the examination of the SSV and SPJ (see below).[8]

## Percussion/Schwartz Test

One hand is placed over the SFJ or SPJ while the other hand is used to tap very lightly on a distal segment of the LSV or SSV (Fig. 5-4). The production of an impulse in this manner implies insufficiency of the valves in the segment between the two hands. Confirmation of the valvular insufficiency can be achieved by tapping proximally while palpating distally. This test can also be used to detect whether an enlarged tributary is in direct connection with the LSV or SSV by palpating over the main trunk and tapping lightly on the dilated tributary, or vice versa. The presence of a direct connection will result in a palpable impulse being transmitted from the percussing to the palpating hand. As might be expected, these tests are far from infallible. In a study of 105 limbs, Chan, Chisholm, and Royle[16] found that these clinical examination techniques correctly identified SFJ incompetence in only 82%. False negatives were felt to be caused primarily by previous groin surgery with resultant scarring and by obesity, whereas false positives were the result of variations in venous anatomy, such as a dilated tributary emptying into the common femoral vein adjacent to the LSV or the absence of valves in the otherwise normal common femoral vein and the external iliac vein (seen in 5% to 30% of persons).[17,18] Another source of error with the cough test is simply a misinterpretation of the muscle contraction that occurs with coughing as a reflux impulse.

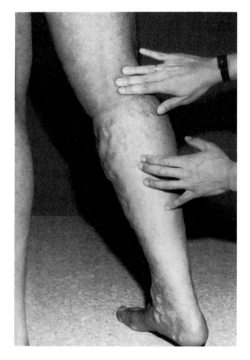

**Fig. 5-4**  Percussion test. The SPJ is palpated while the SSV is gently percussed. Palpation of an impulse is indicative of SPJ insufficiency.

## Brodie-Trendelenburg Test

The well-known Brodie-Trendelenburg test traditionally involves the manual obstruction of the proximal end of the LSV (or SSV), while the patient lies supine with the leg elevated, after stroking the vein in a cephalad direction to empty it of blood.[14,19-22] The patient then assumes the standing position, and the leg is observed for 30 seconds (Fig. 5-5). A "nil" test is one in which there is slow filling of the veins from below and the release of the compression does not result in rapid filling from above, indicating competence of valves in deep and perforating veins as well as at the SFJ (Fig. 5-6, *A*). Rapid filling of the LSV or more distal tributaries that occurs only after release of the compression constitutes a "positive" test, indicating the presence of an insufficient valve at the SFJ (Fig. 5-6, *B*). The "double-positive" test is one in which there is some distension of the veins

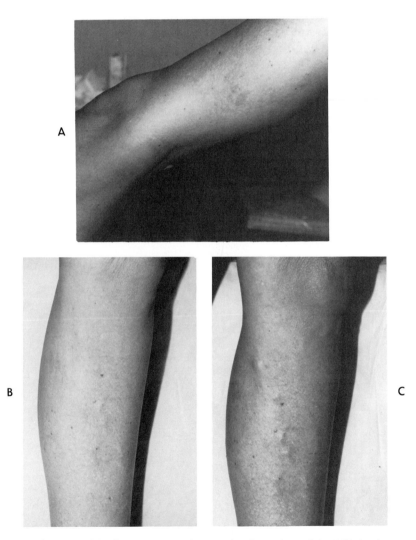

**Fig. 5-5** Brodie-Trendelenburg test. **A,** The proximal portion of the LSV is obstructed after the veins have emptied with the leg elevated. **B,** The distal veins are then observed after the patient stands. **C,** The veins are further inspected after the tourniquet is released. In this case, filling of the veins on standing and additional filling after tourniquet removal constitutes a double-positive test.

within the initial 30 seconds while the compression is maintained, as well as additional filling once the compression is released (Fig. 5-6, *C*). This is taken as evidence of incompetent deep and perforating veins as well as reflux through the SFJ. A "negative" test occurs when the veins fill within the initial 30 seconds with no increased filling after the compression is released, implying only deep and perforating valvular insufficiency (Fig. 5-6, *D*). The reverse may not be true, that

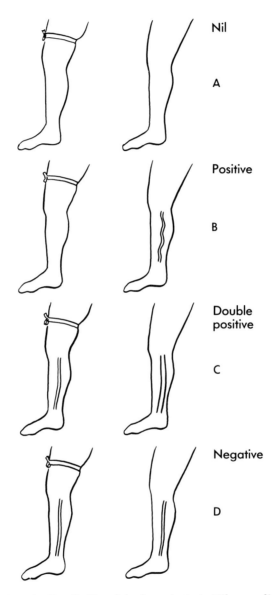

**Fig. 5-6**  Interpreting the Brodie-Trendelenburg test. **A,** Nil — no distension of the veins for 30 seconds both while the tourniquet remains on and also after it is removed implies a lack of reflux. **B,** Positive — distension of the veins only after the tourniquet is released implies reflux only through the SFJ. **C,** Double positive — distension of the veins while the tourniquet remains on and further distension after it is removed implies reflux through perforating veins as well as the SFJ. **D,** Negative — distension of the veins while the tourniquet remains on and no additional distension once it is removed implies reflux only through perforating veins.

is, filling in greater than 30 seconds does not imply competence of perforating veins. In a study of 901 extremities, Sherman[23] found that 95% had a nil Trendelenburg test, but surgical exploration later showed incompetent perforators in 90% of these patients. The Brodie-Trendelenburg test can thus be an important method of localizing the most proximal site of reflux in most dilated superficial veins by obstructing either the LSV, SSV, or whichever vein is suspected of refluxing into a more distal vein. Also, by placing the examining finger over palpable fascial defects in the leg while the patient is supine and then releasing the obstructions one by one once the patient is standing, the sites of insufficient perforators, or "points of control" (considered so crucial in Fegan's technique of sclerotherapy), may be defined, since the superficial veins distal to the insufficient perforator fill rapidly once the obstructing fingers are removed (see Chapter 9).[24,25]

With this technique, described well in many papers,[13,24-27] one first marks on the leg the sites of all dilated varicosities in the leg. The patient then assumes the supine position with the leg elevated to approximately 60 degrees to empty the veins. After at least 20 seconds, or when the distended veins are flattened, the leg is gently and rapidly palpated to detect any defects in the fascia. With experience these can be easily detected as places that allow the entrance of the examining finger without the use of any pressure. Since fascial defects can be caused by many abnormalities other than perforating veins, one continues the examination by compressing the individual fascial defects with one's fingers and then having the patient stand. The fingers are then released, one by one, starting with the most distal defect, and rapid filling of more distal varicosities is noted (Fig. 5-7). Those defects that, when released, result in distal filling are assumed to correspond to sites of incompetent perforating veins. In the presence of a dilated LSV or SSV, these points of reflux must first be controlled with either digital compression or a tourniquet to evaluate the lower volume reflux through the perforators. Compression of the defects must first result in sustained flattening of the varicosities when the patient initially stands for the evaluation to be helpful. If the veins fill before any of the fingers are released, the test must be restarted and other sites compressed until the sites responsible for the reflux are located. This examination is associated with a 50% to 70% accuracy[26-29] compared with findings at surgical exploration. Repeated examination at different times and improvement of edema will allow detection of increased numbers of perforators.

**Bracey variation.** A clever variation of the Brodie-Trendelenburg technique was proposed by Bracey[30] in 1958 (Fig. 5-8). He used a flat rubber tourniquet 3.8 cm wide and two rubber rings covered with latex, with inside diameters of 7 cm and 8.2 cm. The small ring is used between the ankle and knee and may also be used for the thigh if the patient is thin. If not, the larger ring is used for the thigh. With the patient standing, the small ring is rolled over the foot to just above the ankle, and the rubber tourniquet is then placed below the ring to obstruct any upward flow of blood through the superficial veins. The small ring is then slowly rolled upwards, emptying the superficial veins as it moves. As soon as it passes an incompetent perforating vein, the blood will enter the superficial vein connecting with it, causing a dilation of the vein. The exit site of the perforating vein may then be marked. This reflux of blood can be accentuated by asking the patient to repetitively dorsiflex the foot. When the ring reaches the knee, the tourniquet is moved up to the knee, just below the ring. Either the small or larger ring is then used to similarly examine the thigh.

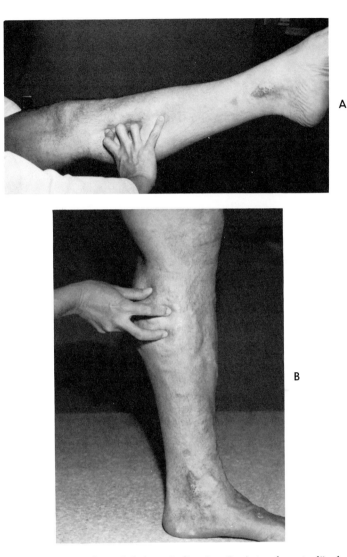

**Fig. 5-7**   **A,** Compression of fascial defects indicating "points of control" of an incompetent perforating vein with the leg elevated. **B,** When the patient stands, the varicose vein remains collapsed while pressure is maintained over control points and distends when the control point is released.

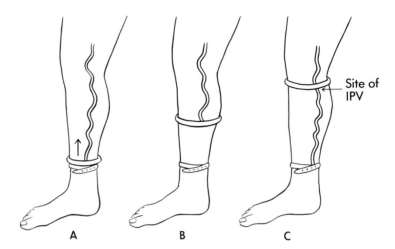

Site of
IPV

A          B          C

**Fig. 5-8**    Device for the detection of incompetent perforating veins (IPV). **A,** Two rubber rings are placed around the ankle, and, **B,** the more proximally placed ring is slowly rolled upward. **C,** As it rolls above an IPV the reflux of blood through the IPV results in an immediate distension of a superficial varix or the formation of a large bulge at the site of the IPV.

Table [ 5-1 ]    Perthes' test

| Finding | Interpretation |
|---|---|
| Decreased diameter of varicose veins | Primary varicose veins |
| No change in diameter of varicose veins | Secondary varicose veins<br>Impairment of calf muscle pump<br>Deep venous patency |
| Increased diameter of varicose veins | Deep venous obstruction |

## Perthes' Test

The Perthes' test[14,21,31] has several uses including distinguishing between venous valvular insufficiency in the deep, perforator, and superficial systems and screening for DVT (Table 5-1). To localize the site of valvular disease, one places a tourniquet around the proximal thigh with the patient standing. When the patient ambulates, a decrease in the distension of varicose veins suggests a primary process without underlying deep venous disease since the calf muscle pump effectively removes blood from the leg and the varicose veins empty. Secondary varicose veins do not change calibre (if there is patency of the deep venous system) because of the inability to empty blood out of the veins as a result of impairment of the calf muscle pump. In the setting of a current DVT, they may increase in size. If there is significant chronic or acute obstructive disease in the iliofemoral segment, the patient may note pain (venous claudication)[32-34] as a result of the obstruction to outflow through both the deep and superficial systems. Information regarding the presence of deep venous valvular insufficiency and thrombosis is important to note in patient selection to avoid causing catastrophic complications such as pulmonary embolism resulting from an undiagnosed and worsened DVT or venous claudication caused by further impairment of venous return. Indeed, these two complications are serious enough to warrant use of a

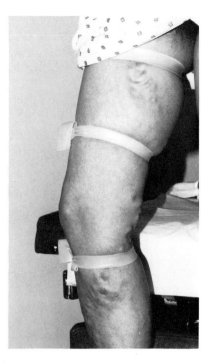

**Fig. 5-9**  Comparative tourniquet test. Distension of the varices in each segment of the leg when the patient ambulates implies the presence of IPVs in each segment.

much more sensitive and accurate method, and therefore, the Perthes' test is now of more historical rather than actual clinical importance.

To test for perforator valvular defects, one may embellish the traditional Perthes' test by placing a tourniquet around the calf just below the popliteal fossa.[24] If the dilated superficial veins in the calf and ankle become less prominent as the patient ambulates, this implies that the blood is being drawn into the deep system through competent perforating veins. However, if the veins become increasingly dilated, the perforating veins must be incompetent. A more involved test, the Mahorner-Ochsner comparative tourniquet test,[22] similarly localizes the site(s) of reflux by observing the leg while the patient walks with the tourniquet placed at various levels on the leg (upper, middle, and lower thigh) (Fig. 5-9).

## NONINVASIVE DIAGNOSTIC TECHNIQUES

The preceding three decades have been very fruitful and have provided us with a wealth of noninvasive technology that has revolutionized vascular diagnosis. A thorough description of all these techniques is certainly beyond the scope of this book, but those not presented here may be found in several excellent texts.[7,35,36] Some of the new technologies have real utility in the everyday performance of sclerotherapy, and the following discussion will attempt to acquaint you with their uses and limitations.

### Doppler Ultrasound

Probably the most useful, practical instrument for evaluating patients with venous disease is the Doppler ultrasound. Its first vascular application came in 1960 when Satomura and Kaneko[37] described a method of studying changes in blood flow in peripheral arteries using an ultrasonic blood rheograph. Its use in the field of venous disease was promoted by many groups, including Sumner, Baker, and Strandness,[38] Strandness et al.,[39] Felix and Sigel,[40] and Sigel et al.[41-45] The instrument is based on the principle of the Doppler effect and consists of an emitting crystal and a receiving crystal. Sound waves are directed into the limb and reflected off of the blood cells traveling through the vessel being examined (Fig. 5-10). The input picked up by the receiving crystal may be connected to a variety of audio or graphic recording systems. Dopplers come with either continuous or pulsed-wave ultrasound beams; the continuous-wave Doppler is adequate for venous examination even though the signal represents a composite of the flow in all vessels in the path of the ultrasound beam. Thus selective examination of one particular vessel may not always be possible. Pulsed Dopplers are used in sonar systems as well as medical ultrasound imaging and are required when the intent is to focus the beam at a particular depth. Dopplers are also available in either directional or nondirectional forms. The directional type is capable of determining the direction of blood flow and depicts the direction on the tracing as either a positive (toward the probe) or negative (away from the probe) deflection (Fig. 5-11). Although the directionality greatly simplifies the interpretation of the tracing, experience with a nondirectional Doppler will allow one to easily make this determination based on certain augmentation maneuvers.

The transmission frequency of the ultrasound beam may range from 2 to 10 MHz; the depth of penetration varies inversely with the frequency. Therefore, a frequency of 4 MHz produces a broad beam with deep penetration, especially useful for examining the deep veins in the pelvis and abdomen. A frequency of 8 MHz is much better suited to the examination of more superficial veins, including superficial segments of the deep veins of the legs, since it produces a narrower beam with relatively less penetration. Dopplers used for evaluation of the venous system generally permit detection of flow rates as low as 6 cm/sec.[42]

**Characteristics of Doppler waveform.** Venous Doppler signals display five characteristics (see box below). In a normal patient, there should be a *spontaneous* signal over any vessel not otherwise vasoconstricted, and the flow should only be *unidirectional.* This signal will diminish in intensity with inspiration as descension of the diaphragm results in a rise in intraabdominal pressure, thus decreasing venous outflow from the leg. It will be augmented similarly with exhalation. This waxing and waning of the intensity of the signal with the respiratory cycle is a phenomenon known as *phasicity.* Venous signals are continuous except for their respiratory variation and are *not pulsatile,* except in the setting of elevated right heart pressure such as congestive heart failure or tricuspid insufficiency[46] or in the normal common femoral vein (CFV).[47] Finally, and most important to their usefulness in evaluation of patients with varicose veins, venous signals may be *augmented* with certain compression maneuvers. It is the re-

---

**VENOUS DOPPLER CHARACTERISTICS**

Spontaneous
Unidirectional
Phasic with respiratory cycle
Nonpulsatile
Augmentation

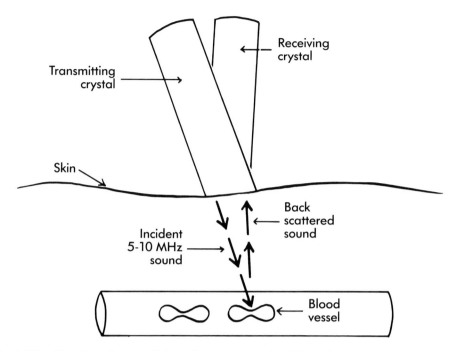

**Fig. 5-10**   Doppler ultrasound. Soundwaves are emitted from the transmitting crystal, reflected by moving particles (blood cells) within the vessel being examined, and picked up by the sensing crystal.

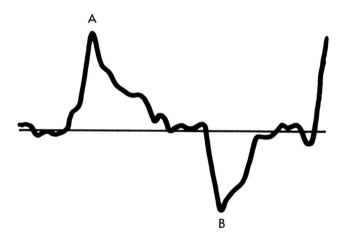

**Fig. 5-11**   Bidirectional Doppler tracing. *A,* Positive deflection indicates flow toward the probe; *B,* negative deflection indicates flow away from the probe.

sponse to these maneuvers that provides information regarding the sites of valvular insufficiency and obstruction of the venous system.

By compressing the limb distal to the Doppler probe (Fig. 5-12), one increases the flow through the vein, and an immediate increase in the signal intensity should be heard if there is no proximal obstruction. In the presence of a hemodynamically significant DVT, the augmented response would be weaker and delayed compared with the contralateral side. With the patient in the upright position, release of distal compression should be followed by silence as the valves close in response to the downward pressure of the blood being pulled by gravity. With the patient in the supine position, release of the compression should normally be followed by the return of the lower intensity spontaneous signal or by silence in the smaller veins. In the setting of valvular insufficiency at the level of the Doppler probe, a loud reflux flow signal can be heard on release of distal compression as blood is pulled in a caudad direction by gravity. To quantitate this reflux flow, the compression used may be standardized by using a pneumatic cuff inflated to a standard pressure (e.g., 80 to 120 mm Hg), and the amplitude and duration of reflux may be read off of the tracing obtained. Although this number has no actual significance, the two sides may be compared, and the evolution of the reflux with time or after treatment may be followed with serial examinations.

The other method of augmentation is that of the release of proximal compression (Fig. 5-13). Proximal compression produces a transient obstruction to outflow and thus causes an accumulation of blood distally, with an associated interruption of the Doppler signal. On its release, the large bolus of blood flowing past the Doppler probe will result in a loud signal. This has also been found to be the more sensitive maneuver in diagnosing DVT, even that limited to calf veins, with a diminished or delayed signal indicative of a significant thrombosis.[48,49] Valvular insufficiency is easily discovered since proximal compression will, instead of resulting in silence, yield a loud reflux flow.

In early descriptions of Doppler ultrasound use for detection of venous disease, Sigel et al.[42] named the various sounds "S" for spontaneous and "A" for augmented. They further specified A sounds as *distal* (if the compression was distal to the probe) or *proximal* (if the compression was proximal to the probe) and *positive* if the A sound was heard directly with compression or *negative* if the A sound was heard on release of the compression. This notation thus makes it possible for four A sounds to be generated at each site being examined. Table 5-2 summarizes these sounds and their significance. This schema provides a useful method of categorizing these sounds, however, the "S" and "A" nomenclature has not found generalized acceptance. Instead, sounds are referred to as manifesting flux or reflux, antegrade or retrograde flow, patency or incompetence, etc.

**Table 5-2** Interpretation of A sounds

| Type of A sound | Condition if present | Condition if absent |
| --- | --- | --- |
| Distal positive | Normal | Venous obstruction |
| Distal negative | Valvular insufficiency | Normal |
| Proximal positive | Valvular insufficiency | Normal |
| Proximal negative | Normal | Venous obstruction or marked valvular insufficiency |

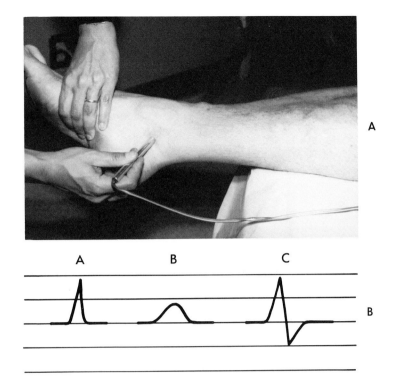

**Fig. 5-12**   **A,** Method of producing augmentation of flow in the posterior tibial vein by distal (foot) compression. **B,** Shows, *A,* normal flow; *B* venous obstruction; *C,* valvular insufficiency.

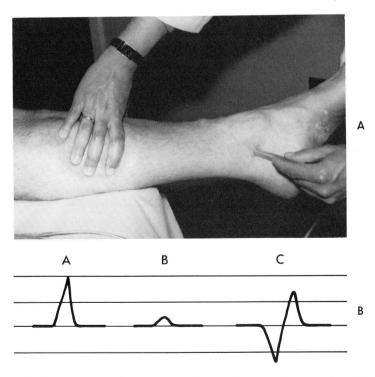

**Fig. 5-13**   **A,** Method of producing augmentation of flow in the posterior tibial vein by release of proximal (calf) compression. **B,** Shows, *A,* normal flow; *B,* venous obstruction; *C,* valvular insufficiency.

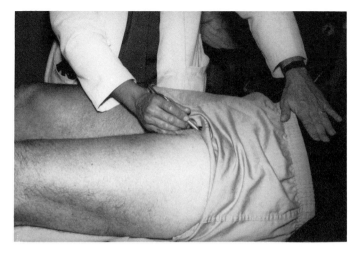

**Fig. 5-14** Augmentation of flow in the common femoral vein or through the SFJ with intermittent compression of the abdomen or with Valsalva maneuver and release (not shown).

Augmentation of the most proximal portion of the LSV and of the more proximal deep veins is accomplished either by compressing the abdomen or by using a variation of the proximal compression and release, the Valsalva maneuver (Fig. 5-14). The rise in intraabdominal pressure caused by descension of the diaphragm is accentuated by contraction of the intercostal muscles. In the normal patient an abrupt closure of the valves will result in silence. However, over 38% of normal persons will have a brief period of reflux at the commencement of the Valsalva.[50] Also, with a weak effort by the patient, a slow retrograde flow may pass through the valve and produce a Doppler flow signal since sufficient force to cause valve closure has not been generated. Visualization of the valves using ultrasound demonstrates that these valves do eventually close and that they are not actually insufficient.[51] Therefore, the continuation of reflux through at least half of the period of compression or at least 0.5 seconds (usually 1 to 4 seconds) is important in diagnosing pathologic valvular incompetence.[4] A less sensitive, but perhaps more specific, response may be elicited simply with deep breathing. With valvular insufficiency, instead of hearing the cessation of flow as the patient takes a deep breath, flow will be reversed and a continuous signal will be heard, which will show a reverse deflection on a directional Doppler tracing (Fig. 5-15). When using the Valsalva maneuver to produce reflux while listening over more distal veins, it is important to realize that the path of the reflux may be either straight down the superficial vein or via the deep vein to the perforating vein to the superficial vein (Fig. 5-16).[52] Therefore, additional testing is necessary to further delineate the exact site of abnormality. This is easily accomplished by manually obstructing the superficial vein, and if reflux is still heard, the retrograde flow is assumed to be traveling through the deep and perforating systems.

**Doppler examination technique.** The Doppler examination of the patient is begun with the deep veins, several of which are easily accessible.[53]

*Femoral vein.* With the patient supine and the hips slightly flexed and externally rotated, one first locates the pulsatile signal of the femoral artery in the groin. If desired, the examination can also be performed with the patient stand-

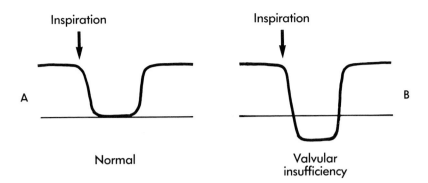

**Fig. 5-15**  Venous Doppler tracings. **A,** Normal phasic flow. **B,** Reflux with deep inspiration in the setting of valvular insufficiency.

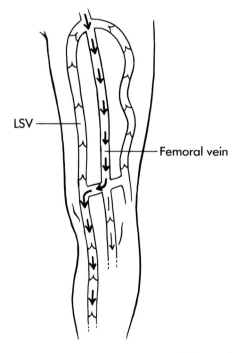

**Fig. 5-16**  Pathways of reflux may be typically through the SFJ but also through atypical channels such as via a deep vein through a perforating vein into a superficial vein (shown). Reflux may also travel via a superficial vein through a perforating vein into another superficial vein (not shown). (Redrawn from Schultz-Ehrenburg U and Hubner H-J: Reflux diagnosis with Doppler ultrasound. In Findings in angiology and phlebology, vol 35, New York, 1989, FK Schattauer Verlag.)

ing, which may provide a more physiologic evaluation since most symptoms occur when the patient is upright and reflux is more easily elicited in this position. The Doppler probe is then gradually angled medially until the spontaneous, continuous sound of the femoral vein, suggestive of a windstorm, is heard. Clear phasicity with respiration should be easily detected. Patency can be further tested by manually compressing the thigh or the calf and listening for a strongly augmented signal. Valvular competence may be assessed by listening first for the phasic waxing and waning of the signal that, in severe cases of insufficiency, will show a decrease in intensity of the signal followed by a reversal of flow direction as inspiration progresses, rather than the expected silence. The patient is then asked to perform a Valsalva maneuver; alternatively, one may press on the abdomen. These latter maneuvers should result in an abrupt closure of the valve and silence, followed by a more intense antegrade flow on release if the valves are competent. A loud reflux flow heard through the Valsalva maneuver is pathognomonic of valvular insufficiency, which may be present in 5% to 30% of normal patients and in one study was found in 100% of patients with bilateral LSV varicosities.[44] The effort invested in the Valsalva maneuver may be standardized to ensure the proper force and reproducibility by asking the patient to blow into a tube connected to a mercury manometer such that the mercury column rises to 30 mm.

*Differentiation of femoral from saphenous veins.* Since the SFJ is located in close proximity to the femoral artery pulsation, valvular incompetence at the junction can sometimes be mistaken for common femoral vein insufficiency. Several techniques can be used to aid in making this important differentiation. Since the saphenous vein is much more easily compressed than the femoral vein, manual compression using the Doppler probe may occlude the saphenous vein and allow the physician to listen selectively to the femoral vein. A separate occlusive device such as the other hand or a tourniquet may be used to compress the LSV distal to the Doppler probe and thus prevent reflux through it. Any reflux still heard is then assumed to be through the femoral vein. Lastly, moving or angling the Doppler probe in a cephalad direction may enable the physician to direct the ultrasound beam away from the saphenous vein to a more proximal segment of the femoral vein. Still, there are a small number of patients in whom differentiation of femoral from junctional signals may be impossible using only the continuous-wave Doppler, and an imaging procedure such as Duplex scanning, which uses a pulsed ultrasound beam, may be necessary.[54,55]

*Popliteal vein.* For the next site of examination, the popliteal vein, the patient may be in the supine, prone, or standing position. It is important to have the knee slightly flexed, however, since full extension of the knee joint may cause a functional obstruction of the popliteal vein. Also, if the examination is performed while the patient is standing, the weight should be borne on the opposite foot (Fig. 5-17). The pulsatile arterial signal is located, generally, in the popliteal crease just lateral to the midline, and the Doppler probe may be angled medially to find a softer, though spontaneous, venous signal, or it may be left over the popliteal artery. Augmentation with either calf compression or thigh compression and release will, as described above, disclose both obstruction and valvular insufficiency. The Valsalva maneuver will only disclose reflux if the more proximal deep veins (common femoral vein) are also incompetent. As with reflux heard at the femoral level, reflux at the popliteal level may actually be caused by reflux through the SPJ. Therefore, in any patient who appears to have reflux through the popliteal vein, the test should be repeated while firm manual compression is applied to the SSV. Obliteration of the reflux in this manner will localize the site of reflux to the SPJ and not the popliteal vein itself. Another method consists of slightly compressing an uninvolved portion of the calf with one finger, which will cause flow through the popliteal vein and not the short saphenous vein.[52] Popliteal vein reflux can be detected in this way with a sensitivity of 100% and a specificity of 92%, with most false positives being the result of variations in the anatomy of the SSV (see Chapter 1).[4,9,56] The presence of popliteal valvular in-

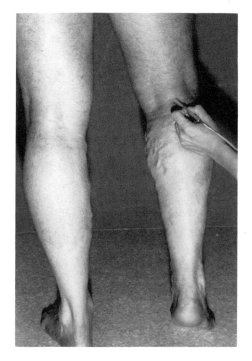

**Fig. 5-17**    The popliteal vein is examined with the knee flexed and the weight borne on the opposite foot.

sufficiency is an important finding since it is associated with diminished calf muscle pump function and may be the most important prognostic factor in the development of venous ulceration.[4,57,58] This relationship is not, however, absolute, since one study showed that popliteal incompetence was found in only 20% of patients with ulceration and 31.2% of postphlebitic legs.[50]

*Posterior tibial vein.* The final deep vein that should be examined is the posterior tibial vein, located just posterior to the medial malleolus and beside the posterior tibial artery, whose pulsatile signal is easily located. This vein is frequently vasoconstricted, except if the patient is examined in a warm room, and therefore a spontaneous signal may not be noticeable. Augmentation maneuvers are as described for the other deep veins. Again, although the Doppler is generally not felt to be sufficiently sensitive in the diagnosis of DVT below the knee, the response of posterior tibial venous flow to release of calf compression has been found to allow an 87% accuracy in this diagnosis.[48,49]

*Superficial veins.* After the above mentioned deep veins are examined, attention is then turned to the superficial and perforating systems. The major saphenous trunks and their junctions with the deep veins may be examined with the patient in the standing position. Because of the lower flow rate in these vessels, a spontaneous signal may only rarely be audible. The presence of a saphena varix, or a visible bulge over the SFJ, is nearly pathognomonic of valvular incompetence. The junction is easily located with the Doppler approximately two fingerbreadths below the inguinal ligament. Alternatively, one may first locate the LSV in the thigh and then gradually move the Doppler probe superiorly and laterally while repetitively compressing the LSV until its location is reached. A positive cough or percussion test may also help to localize the site of the SFJ. The presence of reflux on release of more distal compression is indicative of SFJ insufficiency. The magnitude of the compression can, again, be standardized for serial comparisons by using a pneumatic cuff inflated to a specific level. Also, the Valsalva maneuver may be employed to elicit reflux, although manual compression of the SFJ by the inguinal ligament may occur during a forceful Valsalva, thus creating the false impression of a competent valve.

If no reflux is heard over the SFJ, it should not be assumed that the entire LSV is competent since the perforator(s) in Hunter's canal may frequently be the first abnormality to develop, leading to dilation and incompetence beginning just below the level of the middle thigh (see Chapters 1 and 3).[23,59] Reflux may also originate in branches of the LSV, the "atypical refluxes" described by Schultz-Ehrenburg and Hubner.[52] Incompetence of the LSV that is limited to the calf suggests insufficiency of the geniculate or lower leg perforators. It is, therefore, important to test the LSV for reflux in the groin, at the level of the knee, and in the lower leg, not assuming it is normal until all sites fail to demonstrate reflux.

Examination of the SSV and the SPJ is best carried out with the patient standing or prone and the knee slightly flexed, as previously described. The SSV is more easily felt with the knee flexed and the popliteal fossa relaxed.[8] When enlarged, the SSV is generally still not visible but is easily palpable as a spongy tubular structure leading inferiorly from the popliteal crease. By listening over the popliteal vein and tapping the leg very gently 5 to 10 cm below the probe, one will selectively compress and thus listen to the SSV and not the popliteal vein, which requires a much stronger force. Since the termination of the SSV is variable, the exact location of the probe cannot be known for certain, and therefore, it is difficult to determine if any reflux heard is originating from the SPJ or is simply within a dilated SSV. The Valsalva maneuver or compression of the thigh will aid in this differentiation, since it will result in reflux only if the SPJ is incompetent. Distinction between flow through the SPJ and popliteal vein can also be difficult but is facilitated by manually compressing the SSV below the probe while compressing the calf as described previously. Abolition of the reflux is evidence that the source was the SPJ.[9] Another method is to listen over a more distal segment of the SSV, along the posterolateral calf, and to compress and release the SSV at the popliteal crease. Reflux or only augmentation after release will easily be detected.

*Perforating veins.* The examination of perforating veins is, at best, only 80% accurate using the Doppler,[60-62] and many believe that physical examination, that is, palpation of fascial defects where the incompetent perforator meets a dilated superficial vein at the depth of the superficial fascia, is perhaps even more helpful.[63] In fact, published studies document that palpation is accurate only 51% (27) to 69% (29) of the time. This technique, which is discussed more fully in Chapter 9, yields a large number of false-positive results, since a fascial defect may result merely from dilation of a superficial varicosity or even from a separate pathologic process, such as a muscle hernia. In these situations the Doppler will afford increased reliability. In fact, Doppler examination for incompetent perforating veins is advised after preliminary clinical localization of suspected sites, listening for the characteristic to and fro movement of blood over sites of palpable defects in the fascia. Some authors have advocated placing tourniquets at 4-inch increments along the course of the lower leg before listening for flux and reflux at the sites of fascial weakness while the calf or thigh is repetitively compressed.[60-62] A simpler approach is to place one tourniquet at the level of the ankle and to compress the foot while listening over each marked fascial defect. Any audible signal will thus represent flow proximally through the deep system and outward through an incompetent perforating vein. This provides greater specificity since it interrupts the flow through the superficial veins, thus allowing selective examination of the perforating veins. Fig. 5-18 provides a rational method of recording the venous Doppler examination findings.

**Posttreatment evaluation.** Follow-up examinations of injected veins using the Doppler contribute more precise information regarding the response to treatment than physical examination since a vein that has been sclerosed will lose both spontaneous and augmented flow signals. However, the Doppler detects flow through any vessel passing within the sound wave beam and thus does not allow the examiner to be certain that the signal is from a particular vessel. Also, the Doppler will not differentiate thrombus from fibrosis because both will lead to an absence of a flow signal. These limitations are precisely the advantages of the recently introduced Duplex scanners (Table 5-3).[64-67]

## Duplex Scanners

Duplex scanners are ultrasound machines that generally use a 7.5- or 10-MHz imaging probe along with a 3-MHz pulsed Doppler to enable them to visualize the superficial venous system as well as determine the direction of blood flow within the examined veins. Anatomy, flow within the veins, and the movement of the valves may also be studied (Fig. 5-19). Newer scanners employ a computer-generated color system in which antegrade and retrograde flow may be coded to appear as different colors (red or blue), with varying intensities (brighter with lower velocities, paler with higher velocities), thus allowing immediate integration of this information by the examiner (Fig. 5-20). Visual ultrasound images have found their greatest use within the field of venous disease in the diagnosis of DVT and have now all but replaced venography in centers in which the instrumentation is available (Fig. 5-21).[68-73] More recent alterations in the frequency range of the probes have enabled clear resolution of superficial and deep veins, thus introducing what may be an entirely new era in the treatment of varicose veins by sclerotherapy.

**Table 5-3** A comparison of Doppler ultrasound and Duplex scanning in the presclerotherapy evaluation

|  | Doppler | Duplex |
|---|---|---|
| Portability | Portable | Not easily portable<br>"Luggable" units available |
| Ease of use | Requires short period of training and experience | Requires longer period of training |
| Cost (approx.) | Unidirectional—$300<br>Bidirectional—$2500 | Grey scale—$40,000 and up<br>Color—$150,000 and up |
| Information obtained | 1. Patency, competence of venous valves<br>2. DVT in thigh (?calf) | 1. Patency, competence of venous valves<br>2. DVT w/greater accuracy<br>3. Velocity of reflux<br>4. Anatomy and anomalies of venous system<br>5. Termination of SSV<br>6. Thrombosis vs. sclerosis |
| Reliability | Less reliable because of blind, non-pulsed sound beam | More reliable because of actual visualization of vein being examined |

## PRESCLEROTHERAPY EXAMINATION

| Deep Veins | | Right | Left |
|---|---|---|---|
| Common femoral | Phasicity | | |
| | Reflux w/inspiration | | |
| | Reflux w/Valsalva | | |
| | Duration | | |
| Popliteal | Reflux w/Valsalva | | |
| | Reflux w/thigh compression | | |
| | Reflux w/calf release | | |
| Posterior tibial | Reflux w/calf compression | | |
| | Reflux w/foot release | | |
| SFJ | Reflux w/Valsalva | | |
| | Reflux w/calf release | | |
| | Duration | | |
| | Trendelenburg test | | |
| LSV distal thigh | Reflux | | |
| | Diameter | | |
| LSV calf | Reflux | | |
| | Diameter | | |
| SPJ | Reflux | | |
| | Diameter | | |
| SSV | Reflux | | |
| | Diameter | | |

Tributary 1: Location _____ Diameter _____ LSV _____ SSV _____

Tributary 2: Location _____ Diameter _____ LSV _____ SSV _____

Tributary 3: Location _____ Diameter _____ LSV _____ SSV _____

Tributary 4: Location _____ Diameter _____ LSV _____ SSV _____

**Fig. 5-18** Chart for recording venous Doppler examination.

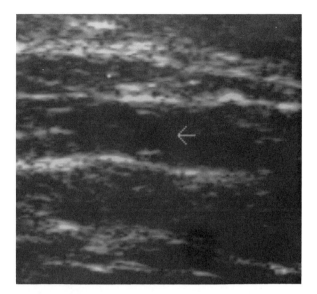

**Fig. 5-19** Duplex scanners may provide clear images of anatomic structures such as the SFJ and venous valves *(arrow)*.

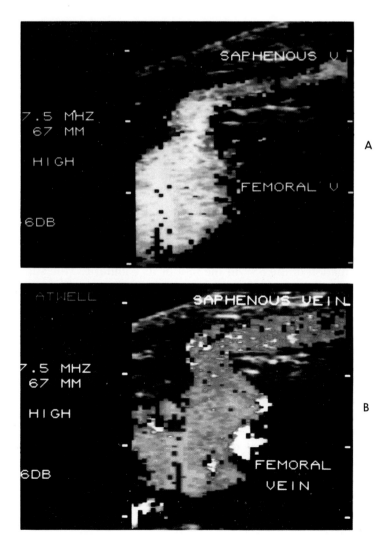

**Fig. 5-20** Color scanners display flow, **A,** in the normal direction in blue and **B,** reflux flow in red.

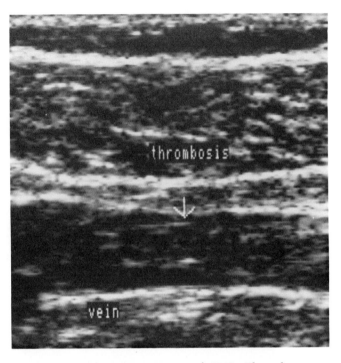

**Fig. 5-21** Ultrasound provides clear images of DVT. Thrombus may appear as an echogenic mass or simply result in the vein being noncompressible.

**As an aid to sclerotherapy.** If the Doppler is the "ears" of the phlebologist, the Duplex scanner may be considered both the ears and a pair of binoculars, because it allows the examiner to "see" much more than can be ascertained otherwise. The Duplex scanner allows for determination of the exact anatomy including the important saphenofemoral and saphenopopliteal junctions. Although the anatomy of the SFJ is generally believed to be similar in all persons, there is actually significant variation. Duplication of the LSV can be found in up to 27% of persons[5-7] and is easily demonstrable with this technology (Fig. 5-22). Since the termination of the SSV is so variable, the exact location of the SPJ or the termination of the SSV in the LSV or its tributaries (the superficial or common femoral veins) or in tributaries of the internal iliac veins[74] can be seen on the Duplex scan. Before operating on the SSV, selective venography was previously advised to determine the exact site of termination of the SSV.[74-76] Now the Duplex scanner may noninvasively provide this piece of information. Injections into the SFJ or SPJ, if performed under ultrasonic guidance,[77] confer an added degree of accuracy and safety to this procedure (Fig. 5-23). Finally, the anatomic basis for proximal recurrences following LSV or SSV ligation may be found through Duplex scanning. If the recurrent varicosities are found to communicate directly with the common femoral or popliteal veins, repeat ligation may be indicated.

**Posttreatment evaluation.** Another major use of the Duplex scanner with sclerotherapy is in the follow-up of patients. As mentioned above, the Doppler does not allow differentiation between thrombus and fibrosis, both of which yield abolition of flow through the involved vein segment. The Duplex scanner can more clearly diffentiate these two situations. Depending on its age, thrombus may appear as a variably echogenic space associated with soft tissue swelling and

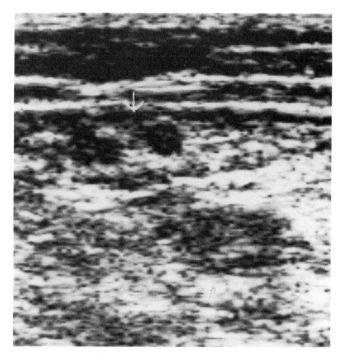

**Fig. 5-22**    Anomalies such as this duplication of the LSV *(arrow)* may be visualized with a Duplex scanner.

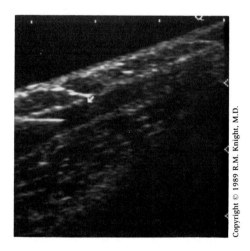

**Fig. 5-23**    Injection into the SFJ may be performed under ultrasonic guidance. The needle is seen inside of the SFJ. (Courtesy Robert M. Knight, M.D.)

inflammation, whereas fibrosis will appear more often as a dense line with no associated inflammatory reaction (Fig. 5-24). Since patient response to treatment is so variable, one can now more accurately determine if the treatment rendered has been completely effective, producing fibrosis, or if the vessel is only occluded by thrombus, thereby necessitating additional treatment. Many apparent treatment failures with early recurrence will likely be found to be the result of inadequate treatment and not inadequate response. One might surmise, therefore, that

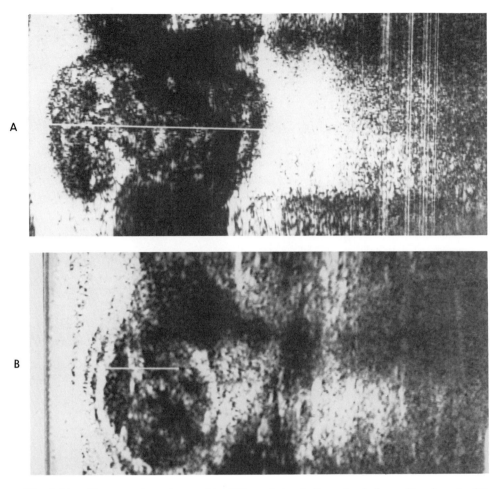

**Fig. 5-24** Ultrasound can be used to differentiate, **A**, thrombosis from, **B**, sclerosis. (Horizontal white line indicates the diameter of the vessel.) (Courtesy Pauline Raymond-Martimbeau, M.D.)

exact assessment of the presence or absence of fibrosis will allow the technique of sclerotherapy to progress to a science instead of the art that now dominates this field.

Another important advantage of the Duplex scanner over the Doppler is its ability to quantitate venous reflux. This parameter has been found to have some prognostic potential. The flow in milliliters per second at peak reflux was measured in 47 limbs of patients who presented with chronic venous problems. It was found that dermatitis or ulceration did not develop if the sum of the peak refluxes in the LSV, SSV, and popliteal vein was less than 10 ml/sec. A sum of greater than 15 ml/sec was associated with a high incidence of these sequelae.[4] In addition, superficial venous reflux alone may result in ulceration if the peak flow is greater than 7 ml/sec.[78]

In summary, advantages provided by Duplex scanning include the ability to evaluate the anatomy of the main saphenous trunks and recurrences, inject difficult areas under ultrasonic guidance, determine the presence of fibrosis, and quantitate reflux. Unfortunately, both the Doppler and Duplex scanner leave the actual hemodynamic effect of the various abnormalities unknown. Therefore, especially in the setting of deep as well as superfical venous insufficiency or when

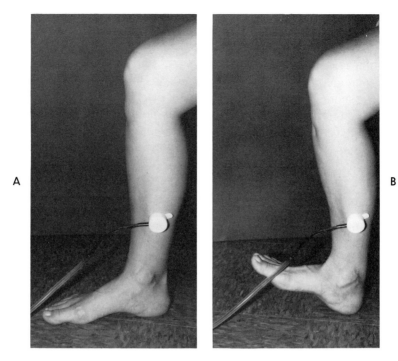

**Fig. 5-25**  A, Photoplethysmography measures venous emptying during and refilling after exercise of the calf and foot muscles. B, Emptying is accomplished with 5 to 10 dorsiflexions of the foot.

multiple segments of the superficial system are incompetent (e.g., both the SFJ and lower leg perforators), a functional study is necessary.

## Photoplethysmography

The most widely used functional evaluation for presclerotherapy purposes is photoplethysmography (PPG).[79-82] Various forms of plethysmography have been used to evaluate venous function since 1956,[83] and they have been shown to correlate well with venographic findings[84] and ambulatory venous pressure (AVP) measurements. In one study of 338 paired measurements of PPG and AVP, the correlation coefficient was 0.9.[79] The principle of PPG is quite simple, and the test is very easy and quick to perform. An infrared light source and sensor are attached with adhesive to the medial aspect of the lower leg approximately 10 cm proximal to the medial malleolus. The infrared light is transmitted into the leg to a depth of approximately 0.5 to 1.5 mm, within the subdermal venous plexus, where it is absorbed by hemoglobin in red blood cells. Any light not absorbed is reflected, some returning to the sensor. Therefore, the amount of infrared light reflected is inversely proportional to the volume of blood in the skin. Once a baseline level is reached, the patient is asked to actively dorsiflex the foot 5 to 10 times resulting in activation of the calf muscle pump, producing venous outflow (Fig. 5-25). With a reduced volume of blood in the calf and the subdermal plexus, more light is reflected, and the tracing shows a gradual deflection (the direction of the deflection depends on the electronics of the particular instrument). At the conclusion of exercise the patient is asked to relax, and the tracing then returns to either the original baseline value or levels off at a new value of light transmission. The time required for this value to be reached, the venous refilling time (VRT), provides information on the presence and degree of reflux of blood through either superficial or deep veins (Fig. 5-26).

VRT has been found to correlate well with AVP measurements that have long been considered the gold standard in the functional evaluation of venous hemodynamics. AVP measurements show a linear relationship between their value and the incidence of venous ulceration.[4] In the normal person, refilling of blood occurs only through the arterial circuit and takes at least 20 to 25 seconds. Therefore, a value less than 20 seconds is indicative of the presence of an abnormal refilling channel, namely retrograde flow through incompetent superficial or deep veins. Repeating the test while firmly compressing a particular vein allows one to assess the degree of hemodynamic disturbance contributed by that vein. Specifically, if the venous refilling time lengthens from 15 to 35 seconds when the vein is compressed, one can be assured that this vein is contributing significantly to the patient's problem. Similarly, in the setting of both superficial and deep venous incompetence, by compressing the superficial veins one can theoretically prevent reflux of blood through these veins and observe the effect of the deep venous system alone. If the VRT lengthens significantly when a tourniquet is placed around the thigh to occlude the superficial veins, this implies the dominance of the superficial system in the patient's pathology. If the VRT remains essentially unchanged, one can assume that the deep veins are the primary problem. A word of caution must be mentioned, however, relating to the method of compression of the vein(s). A simple tourniquet such as that used in phlebotomy is often used and has the advantage of compressing all of the superficial veins, even those that one may not suspect are enlarged and insufficient. However, one must be aware that this type of compression may not adequately compress all of the superficial veins, particularly large, thick-walled varicosities.

This is especially true in the obese patient but is also true in patients of normal weight. By using a Duplex scanner to visualize the flow through the LSV, McMullin, Coleridge Smith, and Scurr[85] found that the pressure within a 2.5-cm-wide tourniquet required to prevent reflux through the vein varied between 40

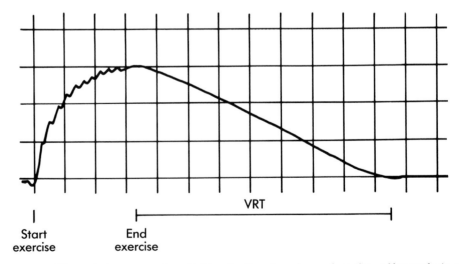

**Fig. 5-26**   Photoplethysmography. Light reflection is enhanced as the calf muscle is exercised and blood is pumped out of the leg. A reduction in light reflection is seen once the leg is allowed to rest. The venous refilling time *(VRT)* is indicative of the degree of reflux although it is not quantitative.

and 300 mm Hg in the 40 patients studied. Therefore, manual compression applied directly to the vein being considered is the preferred method as it is allows one to more reliably interrupt the flow and obtain reproducibly accurate results.

## Light Reflection Rheography

The accuracy of the PPG is felt to be somewhat inferior to a related technique, light reflection rheography (LRR), which uses both superior electronics and three light-emitting diodes, as opposed to the single diode used in the PPG.[86,87] The result is a light beam with deeper penetration, thus avoiding the problem encountered by the PPG in evaluating patients with pigmented skin. Dermal pigment, such as that commonly found in patients with chronic venous insufficiency, is concentrated in the more superficial layers of the skin and interferes with light transmission, yielding inaccurate and variable values. By focusing its light beam on the deeper tissues, the LRR bypasses the tissues containing the majority of the pigment.

The PPG may also be used to quantify the blood changes within the subdermal plexus, thus quantifying the degree of reflux. This involves performing an in vivo calibration maneuver that allows one to assign a numerical value to the deflections on the tracing.[88,89] The transducer is placed on the leg in its usual location while the patient rests in the supine position, and the tracing on the recorder is set to a zero baseline. The patient then stands, bearing weight on the opposite leg, and after the tracing levels off, the gain is adjusted so that the deflection reflects the calculated hydrostatic pressure in the superficial veins, as measured by the distance from the right atrium to the site of the transducer on the leg. This maneuver is repeated until the zero baseline and standing levels of subdermal plexus blood content reproducibly reflect the hydrostatic pressures. The decrement in the tracing is then proportional to the degree of fall in AVP, as measured by invasive venous pressure recordings. The LRR, on the other hand, more easily measures both venous emptying and venous refilling time (VRT) without time-consuming calibration maneuvers, and a newer digital version is now available that automatically calibrates these parameters.[90]

That PPG is useful in assessing venous valvular insufficiency is undisputed, however, the claims that it is accurate in diagnosing DVT are controversial. The general statement that a "picket fence" pattern (Fig. 5-27) produced by the 10 dorsiflexions with essentially no vertical movement off of the baseline is diagnostic of DVT certainly is incorrect, because there are many false positives using this

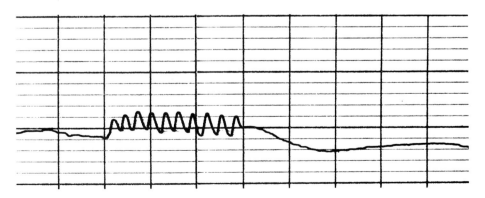

**Fig. 5-27**   A "picket fence" pattern may indicate DVT but may also be seen with chronic venous insufficiency without thrombosis.

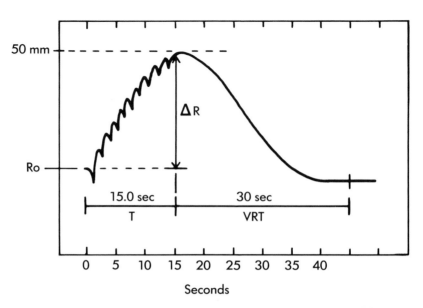

**Fig. 5-28** Usefulness of PPG in the diagnosis of DVT may be improved by examination of the slope R/T; <.31 mm/sec predicts the presence of DVT with a 96% sensitivity.

criterion. In a study of 30 limbs, the correlation coefficient between venous emptying and AVP was only 0.73.[86] However, in a study performed at the University of Miami,[91] the slope of the deflection correlated well with the presence of acute DVT as documented by venography. As in Fig. 5-28, the finding of a slope (R/T) of less than 0.31 mm/sec predicts the presence of DVT with a 96% sensitivity. Still, at this time, LRR alone is not considered sufficient to make the diagnosis of DVT, and at least one other noninvasive test would be required to confirm the diagnosis.

## Air Plethysmography

Another technology that is just as simple to use and potentially supplies a great deal of additional information is the air plethysmograph (APG),[93] which consists of a 14-inch long tubular polyvinylchloride air chamber that surrounds the leg from knee to ankle. This is inflated to 6 mm Hg and connected to a pressure transducer, amplifier, and recorder. A smaller bag placed between the air chamber and the leg is used for calibration by injecting a certain volume of air or water and measuring the change in the recording associated with that volume (Fig. 5-29). Parameters assessed include (a) functional venous volume (VV), the volume in the leg while the patient stands; (b) venous filling time 90 (VFT 90), the time required to achieve 90% of the VV; (c) venous filling index (VFI), 90% VV/VFT 90; (d) ejection volume (EV), the volume expelled from the leg with one tip-toe motion; (f) residual volume (RV), the volume at the end of 10 tip-toe motions; (g) residual volume fraction (RVF), RV/VV 100 (Fig. 5-30). In a study of 22 patients with superficial venous insufficiency and 9 patients with deep venous disease,[93] it was found that VV was elevated in 80% of patients. VFT 90 was greater than 70 seconds in normal limbs, 8 to 82 seconds in limbs with superficial venous insufficiency, and 9 to 19 seconds in limbs with deep venous disease. VFI was less than 1.7 ml/sec in normal limbs, 2 to 30 ml/sec in limbs with superficial venous insufficiency, and 7 to 28 ml/sec in limbs with deep venous dis-

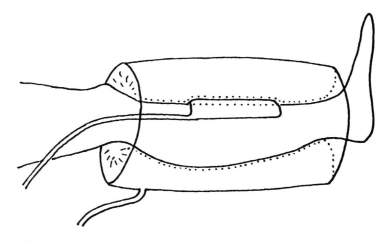

**Fig. 5-29** The air plethysmograph consists of a long tubular polyvinyl chamber that surrounds the entire leg. This chamber is inflated to 6 mm Hg and is connected to a pressure transducer, amplifier, and recorder. A smaller bag is placed between the air chamber and the leg for calibration. (From Christopoulos DG et al: J Vasc Surg 5(1):148, 1987.)

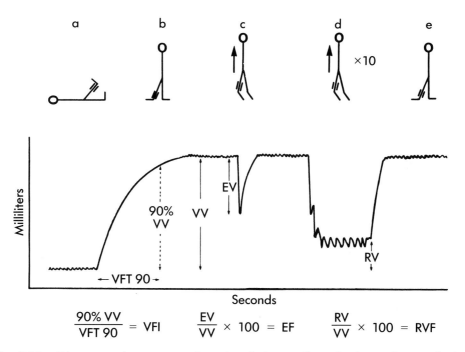

**Fig. 5-30** Diagrammatic representation of typical recording of volume changes during standard sequence of postural changes and exercise using the air plethysmograph. Patient in supine position with leg elevated 45 degrees *(a)*; patient standing with weight on nonexamined leg *(b)*; single tiptoe movement *(c)*; ten tiptoe movements *(d)*; single tiptoe movement *(e)*. *VV* = functional venous volume; *VFT* = venous filling time; *VFI* = venous filling index; *EV* = ejected volume; *RV* = residual volume; *EF* = ejection fraction; *RVF* = residual volume fraction. (From Christopoulos DG et al: J Vasc Surg 5(1):148, 1987.)

ease. Ejection fraction (EF) appeared to show better descrimination than EV. The RVF was 20% in normal legs, 45% in legs with superficial venous insufficiency, and 60% in legs with deep venous disease (Fig. 5-31).

A linear correlation with r = 0.83 was present between RVF and AVP. In another study of 104 patients,[78,94] VFI was found to correlate with the incidence of sequelae of venous disease such as chronic swelling, skin changes, and ulceration, as seen in Table 5-4. In a third study of 205 limbs,[95] the same authors found an increasing incidence of ulceration in patients with diminished EF and elevated VFI (Table 5-5) and that the RVF showed a good correlation (r = 0.81) with the incidence of ulceration and AVP measurements. The real advantages of this method are its ability to quantitate reflux with the VFI and thus to determine prognosis and its ability to measure calf muscle pump function through the determination of the EF.[78,92-96]

## Foot Volumetry

Yet another method for evaluation of the functional state of the venous system is foot volumetry.[97-102] First introduced in the early 1970s, this technique has not earned a prominent place in phlebology, most likely because of certain logistics in performing the test. The patient stands with his feet in an open water-filled plethysmograph (Fig. 5-32). The water level is monitored by a photo-electric sensor and changes in foot volume are continuously measured, first while the patient is standing still, then during the performance of 20 knee bends, and again while standing still. The parameters measured include the volume of blood expelled from the foot during exercise, the flow rate after exercise, and the time required for half and then full refilling to occur. Norgren et al.[100] have shown good correlation between foot volumetry and invasive venous pressure measurements in control subjects (r = 0.662) and in patients with varicose veins (r = 0.760) but poor correlation in patients with deep venous valvular insufficiency (r = 0.410). In their study, venous pressure measurements were significantly different in patients with varicose veins and controls, but were similar in patients with primary varicose veins and those with deep venous valvular insufficiency.

**Table 5-4** Venous filling index and sequelae of venous disease

| VFI (ml/sec) | Chronic swelling (%) | Ulceration (%) | Skin change (+/− ulcer) |
|---|---|---|---|
| <3 | 0 | 0 | 0 |
| 3-5 | 12 | 0 | 19 |
| 5-10 | 46 | 46 | 61 |
| >10 | 76 | 58 | 76 |

**Table 5-5** Effect of VFI and EF on incidence of venous ulceration

| | EF >40% | | | EF <40% | | | |
|---|---|---|---|---|---|---|---|
| | Total no. of limbs | Limbs w/ulcers No. | % | Total no. of limbs | Limbs w/ulcers No. | % | p |
| VFI < 5 | 41 | 1 | 2 | 19 | 6 | 32 | <0.01 |
| 5 < VFI < 10 | 37 | 11 | 30 | 19 | 12 | 63 | <0.02 |
| VFI > 10 | 32 | 13 | 41 | 27 | 19 | 70 | <0.05 |

From Christopoulos DG et al: Surgery 106(5):829, 1989.

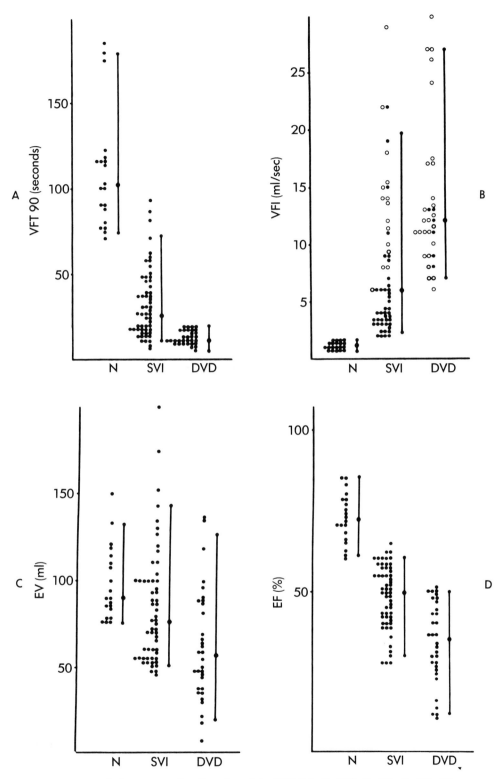

**Fig. 5-31**    Air plethysmography. Results of **A**, VFT/90; **B**, VFI; **C**, EV, **D**, EF. ($N$ = normal limbs; $SVI$ = limbs with superficial venous incompetence; $DVD$ = limbs with deep venous disease.) (From Christopoulos DG et al: J Vasc Surg 5(1):148, 1987.)

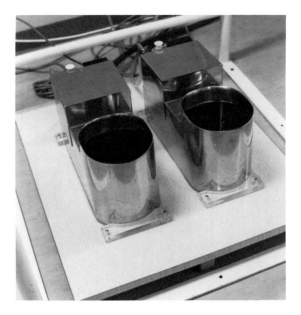

**Fig. 5-32**   The apparatus for foot volumetry consists of an open water-filled plethysmograph that allows continuous measurement of foot volume at rest and during exercise via monitoring of the water level by a photo-electric floatsensor. (Courtesy Lars Norgren, M.D.)

**Table** ⟦ **5-6** ⟧   Functional venous studies

|  | **PPG** | **Foot volumetry** | **APG** |
|---|---|---|---|
| Ease of use | Easy | Easy | Requires practice by patient |
|  | Hygienic<br>5 min test | Communal bath<br>5-10 min test | Hygienic<br>5-10 min test |
| Cost | $2500 and up |  | $7500 |
| Information obtained | 1. Presence of reflux | 1. Presence and degree of reflux | 1. Presence and degree of reflux |
|  | 2. Superficial vs deep | 2. Calf muscle pump function | 2. Superficial vs. deep |
|  | 3. ?DVT |  | 3. Calf muscle pump function |

However, using foot volumetry, there were significant differences between all three groups. Thus although it is possible that foot volumetry is inaccurate in this important categorization, it is quite likely that this technique is actually more sensitive in distinguishing between these groups than are venous pressure measurements.[101] It has been shown that the volume expelled with exercise and the refilling time both increase after treatment of varicose veins.[102] Therefore, this test could be used to evaluate the success of a particular treatment, to follow the effect of different stages in treatment, and to monitor the severity of chronic venous insufficiency. It does not, however, allow localization of a particular site of reflux, thus limiting its usefulness for presclerotherapy evaluation compared with other methods (Table 5-6).

# Venography

Venography is still felt by many clinicians to represent the "gold standard" in the evaluation of venous obstructive disease, and the results of all studies evaluating newer methods for the diagnosis of DVT are compared with those of venography. The most serious disadvantages of venography are its invasive method, the frequent development of superficial phlebitis as a result of the procedure; and a 5% to 10% incidence of allergy to the contrast medium. The latter complications have been significantly reduced through the introduction of newer nonionic contrast media,[7] and venography continues to find frequent use in the diagnosis and treatment planning of venous disease. It also has great utility in the evaluation of groin and pelvic recurrences including vulvar varicosities.[103] Four techniques have been described: ascending, descending, intraosseous venography, and varicography.

A variation of venography involving the injection of fluorescein into a vein on the dorsum of the foot has been used for the localization of incompetent ankle perforating veins.[104] This simple bedside test is performed by placing a 2.5-cm cuff, inflated to 80 mm Hg, just above the malleoli. The leg is elevated to 90 degrees, and the patient is asked to plantarflex the foot 10 times. A second 13-cm cuff is then inflated to 120 mm Hg just above the knee, and the leg is lowered. Acqueous fluorescein, 5 ml, is then injected into the distal later portion of the foot, and an ultraviolet light is directed toward the leg in the darkened room. A second set of 10 plantarflexions is performed, drawing the solution into the deep veins and outward through any incompetent perforators. This is reflected on the skin surface as a circle of yellow-green fluorescence, 1 to 2 cm in diameter, within 30 seconds to 2 minutes. In 37 legs studied, this method had a 96% accuracy, identifying 50 of the 52 perforating veins later found to be incompetent at surgery, with two false negatives and four false positives.

**Ascending venography.** Ascending venography[7] is performed by injecting the contrast medium into a superficial vein on the dorsum of the foot after a 2.5-cm tourniquet is placed around the ankle to prevent flow through the superficial venous system. This forces the contrast to enter only the deep veins and allows clearer visualization of the deep system. Fluoroscopic imaging with the patient in various positions allows examination of the deep veins from the foot to the lower segment of the inferior vena cava for the presence of thrombi (Fig. 5-33, *A*). Passage of the contrast into the perforating veins is abnormal and diagnostic of valvular insufficiency (Fig. 5-33, *B*).[28] The addition of a Valsalva maneuver will show competent venous valves and define bicuspid structures with a concentration of contrast media in their sinuses and may obviate the need for descending venography if this procedure was to be considered later. Ascending functional venography requires the patient to plantarflex the foot, thus forcing the contrast into the superficial veins through any incompetent perforating veins during muscle relaxation.[4]

**Descending venography.** Descending venography involves injection of the contrast into the femoral or the popliteal vein with the patient supine or tilted head up and performing a Valsalva maneuver. Valvular insufficiency is readily demonstrated since the contrast flows rapidly in a retrograde direction. Five grades of reflux have been described (Fig. 5-34).[50,105] One of the disadvantages of this technique is that the demonstration of reflux at a given level relies on the presence of reflux at the higher levels. Therefore, using descending venography

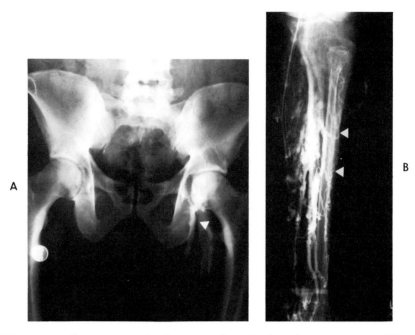

**Fig. 5-33**  Ascending venography demonstrating, **A**, thrombus as a space filling defect *(arrowhead)* and, **B**, incompetent perforating vein *(arrowheads)*.

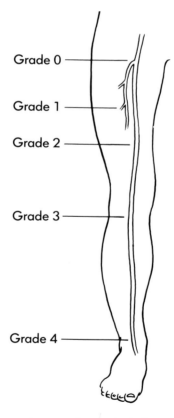

**Fig. 5-34**  Descending venography may demonstrate 5 grades of reflux: *Grade 0—* no reflux below the confluence of the superficial and profunda femoris veins; *Grade 1—* reflux into the superficial femoral vein but not below the middle of the thigh; *Grade 2—* reflux into the superficial femoral vein but not through the popliteal vein; *Grade 3—* reflux to just below the knee; *Grade 4—* reflux to the ankle level.

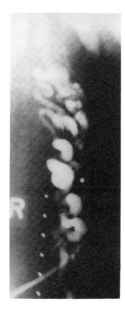

**Fig. 5-35**   Varicography. Injection directly into the varix may demonstrate the origin of a recurrence in the groin after vein stripping. (From Lea Thomas M and Mahraj RPM: Phlebology 3:155, 1988.)

alone, one might miss isolated incompetence of tibial veins or gastrocnemius veins, both of which have been shown to be responsible for the production of significant symptoms (see Chapters 3 and 4).[106,107]

**Intraosseus venography.** Intraosseus venography is simply a variation of ascending venography in which the contrast is injected not directly into a vein but instead into bone, with rapid distribution throughout the deep venous system. This technique may be significantly easier to perform in patients with edema[108] and may be especially helpful in diagnosing incompetent perforating veins,[28] yet it has not found any significant recent use.

**Varicography.** Varicography (Fig. 5-35) is a very helpful technique in which the contrast agent is injected directly into the dilated varix, showing the extent of the varicosities and their connection with other superficial, perforating, and deep veins.[7,103,109,110] The direction of blood flow and therefore the competence of valves is not discernible, although other criteria have been found to correlate with valvular insufficiency. For instance, if a perforator is greater than 3 mm in diameter and is seen to be tortuous, it is assumed to be incompetent.[7]

## Thermography

Infrared thermography is based on the fact that infrared waves radiate from the skin surface in proportion to the temperature of that surface.[111,112] It is possible to scan the surface with an infrared detector and create an image where gradations of white and black or color reflect degrees of heat. Two identical symmetric skin areas of the body should be at the same temperature unless certain factors are present. These factors include structural abnormalities of vessels (dilation and incompetence), abnormalities of vascular control, local effects on vessels, changes in thermal conductivity of the tissues, or increased heat production of the tissues. When veins are dilated, such as with varicose veins or with an underlying arteriovenous communication, the overlying skin will be warmer because of the accumulation of the extra volume of blood in the dilated vein. Similarly, when venous valves are incompetent, the reflux of blood from the more central common femoral vein down the LSV when the limb is lowered or outward from the warmer deep veins through a perforating vein when the calf muscle is activated will produce a rise in skin temperature, and this may be visualized on the thermograph as a white, or "hot," spot (Fig. 5-36). In fact, this technique may be used to localize the site of an incompetent perforating vein (see Chapter 3).[29] After recording the general distribution of thermal patterns in the standing position, the leg is elevated for 1 minute to drain the veins, and the leg temperature is lowered by cooling with a cold, wet towel or a fan for 5 minutes. A tourniquet is placed around the proximal thigh to occlude the superficial veins, and the patient is asked to stand. Areas of rapid rewarming suggest possible sites of incompetent perforating veins. These areas are reexamined after placing tourniquets above and below each site. The segment in question is again cooled, and the appearance of a hot area within 60 seconds of standing (in the case of a thigh perforator) or of calf muscle action (in the case of a lower leg perforator) identifies the site of an incompetent perforator. Of 84 incompetent perforating veins later found at operation, thermography correctly identified 79 (94%). The five that were missed by thermography were found at surgery to be very small in diameter or in close proximity to a larger incompetent perforator that was correctly identified. Of the 12 false positives, 4 were caused by inadequate surgical exploration of the area, and the others were the result of heat changes from communicating sites of superficial veins or from the penetration of the LSV into the deep fascia of the thigh.

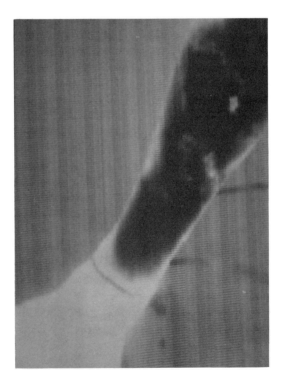

**Fig. 5-36** Positive thermograph. The presence of an IPV may be indicated by a "hot" spot. (Courtesy K. Lloyd Williams, M.D., CHIR, FRCS.)

## USE OF NONINVASIVE TECHNIQUES

Each of the above described techniques has advantages, limitations, and use in specific situations. Prohibitive cost or limited access may preclude the use of the most sensitive and accurate method. Therefore, the following section discusses a reasonable use of various noninvasive techniques for a variety of situations commonly encountered in the everyday practice of sclerotherapy (Table 5-7).

### Examination of Deep Veins

One of the simplest techniques available for the detection of valvular competence in the deep venous system also happens to be quite sensitive and accurate. The Doppler ultrasound can be used to completely examine the common femoral, popliteal, and posterior tibial veins in less than 5 minutes, as described above, giving information on the presence and specific location of incompetent valves. Pitfalls occur in the differentiation of the femoral from the SFJ and the popliteal from the SPJ, yet these can generally be sorted out by compressing the superficial vein and repeating the test. If confusion still exists, a limited Duplex scan will easily provide the answer. Venography will, similarly, provide accurate information on the state of the deep venous valves, but its invasiveness and associated risks and pain make it a much less attractive option. PPG will detect the presence of valvular insufficiency, and compression of the superficial veins, either manually or with a tourniquet, will allow differentiation between superficial and deep venous reflux, however, it still cannot localize the reflux to the level within the deep system (femoral versus popliteal, etc.). When both superficial and deep venous reflux are present, the PPG will allow the determination of the relative importance of each segment. Ascending venography is still considered the gold standard for the diagnosis of acute or chronic deep venous obstructive disease, although most institutions now use B-mode ultrasound in everyday clinical prac-

**Table** 5-7   Preferred methods of evaluation

| | Preferred method | Pitfalls | Additional methods |
|---|---|---|---|
| Deep veins | Doppler ultrasound | Differentiation SFJ vs CFV, SPJ vs popliteal vein | PPG/LRR Venography Duplex |
| Saphenous trunks | Doppler ultrasound | Same as above | Percussion Trendelenburg Venography Duplex |
| Tributaries of saphenous trunks | Doppler ultrasound | | Percussion Duplex |
| Perforating veins | Clinical exam + Doppler | 50%-80% accurate | Venography Duplex Thermography Fluorescein |
| Contribution of superficial vs deep reflux | PPG/LRR | | AVP Duplex velocities |
| Functional evaluation | PPG/LRR | | AVP Foot volumetry |
| Vulvar varices | Clinical exam for LSV reflux | | Varicography |

tice. Descending venography will detect deep venous valvular reflux but, again, the Duplex scanner offers the additional advantage of quantifying the reflux by determining flow velocities. The finding of deep venous valvular insufficiency is worrisome, for it may be associated with chronic obstructive disease that may give rise to venous claudication,[32-34] since there are a certain small number of patients who rely on their dilated superficial channels for venous return. This was determined using strain gauge plethysmography[113] and may most likely be assessed with PPG as well. Impairment of VRT with the tourniquet might caution one to avoid treatment. Alternatively, the simplest and most practical test is to place a 30 to 40-mm Hg compression stocking on the patient for 24 hours. The development of pain while walking would contraindicate sclerotherapy. Deep venous valvular insufficiency has also been found to reduce the likelihood of successful long-term sclerosis of the main saphenous trunk.[52]

## Examination of Saphenous Vein Trunks

Although many physicians use percussion and Trendelenburg tests as their first maneuver in assessing the competence of the saphenous trunks, Doppler ultrasound is probably the most useful preliminary technique for this examination. In most cases it will provide an accurate evaluation of competence in the long and short saphenous trunks as described previously. However, Lea Thomas and Bowles[114] found that it grossly overdiagnosed incompetence when compared with venography, and they actually recommended that all LSVs be examined with venography before ligation and stripping. One reason for this is the fact that Doppler examination is "blind," and thus dilated tributaries or duplications may easily be mistaken for the LSV. This was addressed in two studies[54,55] that compared the results of Doppler examination with those obtained with Duplex scanning. The researchers found that in the examination of the LSV, Doppler was no better than 77% sensitive and 83% specific compared with the Duplex scan.

On the basis of this data, it might be argued that all patients with LSV varicosity should undergo Duplex scanning to confirm the Doppler findings. However, the cost of this testing is high. Therefore, at this time Doppler examination affords the physician the most practical approach to this important segment of the venous system, and certainly, the Duplex scan may be obtained if there is any doubt as to the diagnosis.

The Doppler examination of the junction of the saphenous trunks with the deep veins (SFJ and SPJ) and the distinction between reflux through these junctions versus reflux through the deep veins themselves is often difficult and a common source of error. In fact, studies using Doppler ultrasound have quoted an incidence of deep venous valvular reflux from 5% to 30%,[17,18,52] a range partially determined most likely by the difficulty of the examination and not solely by differences between the populations examined. The importance of being able to distinguish junctional from actual deep venous reflux is illustrated by the finding of Schultz-Ehrenburg[17,52] that patients with deep venous valvular incompetence fared far better with a surgical approach to their disease. This makes the accuracy of this portion of the examination quite important, since it has direct application to the treatment plan. The technique of examination is quite simple. The Doppler probe may be placed over the site of the SFJ or over the femoral vein with the patient standing or supine, and the patient is asked to perform the Valsalva maneuver. The procedure is then repeated with the LSV firmly compressed below the Doppler probe. If reflux can still be heard after compression is applied, one assumes that the reflux is in the femoral vein. In contrast, if the reflux is obliterated with this maneuver, the retrograde flow is only through the SFJ and not through the femoral vein itself.

## Examination of Tributaries of the Saphenous Trunks

The examination of the tributaries of the saphenous trunks focuses on two major questions: (1) to which saphenous trunk does the tributary belong, and (2) is there reflux of blood from the deep vein directly into the tributary? Both answers may be obtained by either physical examination maneuvers or with the Doppler. The origin of any tributary may be assessed with the percussion test, in which the palpating hand is placed gently over the tributary while the LSV or SSV is percussed with the other hand (or vice versa). The palpation of an impulse with percussion of a particular trunk localizes the origin of the tributary to that trunk. Alternatively, a modified Trendelenburg test will supply this information. The patient is asked to lie down with the leg elevated to nearly 90 degrees. The proximal LSV or SSV is then firmly compressed and the patient is asked to stand. If the varicose tributary remains empty and only fills when the compression is released from the LSV, this localizes the origin of the tributary to that system. The presence of reflux from the deep system may then be discovered by using the cough test, in which the palpation of an impulse over the tributary when the patient coughs implies reflux of blood from the deep system through incompetent valves into the tributary.

As mentioned previously, although the Trendelenburg test is reasonably accurate, the cough and percussion tests are now considered confirmatory, since the Doppler provides a more accurate answer to these questions. Placement of the Doppler probe over the tributary while intermittently compressing or percussing either the LSV or SSV allows determination of the origin of the tributary (Fig. 5-37). Listening for reflux while the patient coughs or performs the Valvalva maneuver uncovers connections to the deep system (since there should be no reflux unless there is a pathway directly to the deep vein that is unobstructed by competent valves). The applicability of the first piece of information is obvious since

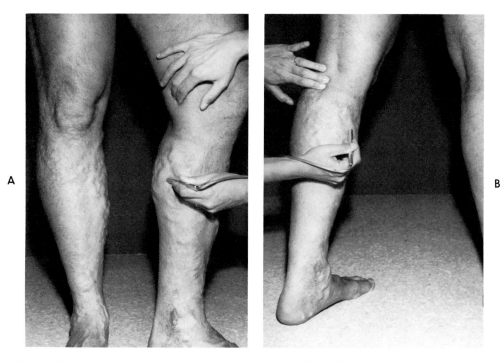

**Fig. 5-37** The origin of a particular varicosity may be defined by listening over the dilated vein while alternately compressing the, **A,** LSV and, **B,** SSV trunks.

treatment must then be directed at that particular saphenous trunk to achieve sclerosis of the tributary as well. However, the connection of the tributary to the deep system must be explored further, because the exact route that the blood has taken from the deep to the superficial system must be defined. If the connection is simply through the SFJ or SPJ, again, the treatment directive is apparent. On the other hand, if the connection is actually through a perforating vein or another tributary,[52] then treatment must be aimed at that particular vein and, perhaps, treatment of the saphenous trunk may not be necessary. Manual occlusion of the involved saphenous trunk at its proximal end followed by repeat examination will afford this important differentiation. If this occlusion results in the obliteration of reflux with the cough or Valsalva maneuver, then the blood must have flowed through the SFJ or SPJ. If, on the other hand, this maneuver does not change the result of the test, then the saphenous trunk is not an important conduit, and the perforating vein must be the important route.

## Examination of Perforating Veins

The perforator segment of the venous system is probably the most mysterious because of its variability, the difficulty of locating perforators even under direct visualization in the operating room, and the overwhelming importance ascribed to perforating veins in the development of varicose veins and the skin changes associated with chronic venous insufficiency.[115] It is no wonder, therefore, that there is no consensus as to what constitutes the "best" method for examination of perforating veins and their valvular competence. Nearly every technique including venography, Doppler, Duplex, thermography, fluorescein injection, and physical examination of fascial defects has been employed, with varying degrees of success. Complicating the evaluation of each method is the fact that all are compared with later surgical findings, which most likely also miss many incompetent perforating veins and which are impossible to standardize. Underscoring the current difficulties in this aspect of venous diagnosis are data that show that the number of incompetent perforating veins detected per limb in studies of the various diagnostic methods may be one to four, whereas anatomic studies have shown a range of one to fourteen, with an average of seven.[22] Thus the exact sensitivity and accuracy of each method is still not possible to test. Therefore, at best one may still miss a great deal of important pathology. In spite of the pitfalls and limitations of current diagnostic methods, examination for incompetent perforating veins is still crucial and is usually productive. As mentioned previously, in a study of 901 limbs with varicose veins,[22] 90% were found to have incompetent perforators. Of interest, only 9% of the perforators were found in the thigh. Thigh perforators may be either single or multiple and may occur anywhere from just proximal to the patella to just below the SFJ, with most being single and located in the middle third of the thigh.[116] In evaluating patients with incompetent perforating veins in the lower leg, Dodd[117] found that 45% were associated with incompetence of the LSV, 15% with incompetence of the SSV, and 2% with an incompetent perforating vein in Hunter's canal. Therefore, any patient with significant truncal varicosities as well as those with signs of chronic venous insufficiency should undergo evaluation for perforator valvular insufficiency.

Historically, the most important and probably the most commonly employed technique is that of clinical examination. With its ability to detect 50% to 70% of incompetent perforating veins, clinical examination should be the first step in the evaluation. Other techniques have been studied extensively, such as thermography,[26,29,118,119] fluorescein injection,[120,121] and ascending[26,27,120] and intraosseus[29] venography, generally demonstrating accuracies in the range of 60% to

90%. Unfortunately, the instrumentation required makes these techniques impractical for most practicioners. They can, however, be used when perforator disease is strongly suspected but has escaped localization by other methods.

Ultrasound technology can also be helpful and is associated with greater ease and lower risks than these other methods. Doppler evaluation of perforator incompetence provides a diagnostic accuracy of 60% to 90%[27,60-62,121] and definitely improves with experience. In one study of 39 legs,[27] its accuracy improved from 60% to 87% when it was combined with clinical examination, thus making this combination of techniques well suited for routine clinical practice. Duplex scans are extremely useful in visualizing the site(s) of incompetent perforating veins and may be considered along with venography or fluorescein injection or thermography if one is otherwise unable to localize a vein in a suspected area and has the necessary equipment available.

## Differentiation of the Relative Contribution of Deep and Superficial Reflux

The PPG, with and without compression, is especially useful in the setting of both deep and superficial venous disease; it is also simple and inexpensive to use. If the Doppler examination has disclosed that the superficial (LSV or SSV) and deep veins (CFV or popliteal) are both incompetent, this test will help to determine the relative importance of each segment of the venous system and whether correction of the superficial problem will afford the patient sufficient benefit, given the persistent deep vein reflux, to be worth the potential risks of treatment. This is exemplified by the case of a 40-year-old woman with congenital absence of valves within her femoral veins and a history of bilateral leg edema, lymphedema, and more recently the progressive enlargement of varicosities of her main long saphenous trunks. Although it was felt that her main problem was her deep venous defect, the application of this relatively simple examination scheme allowed a more precise understanding of her condition. By manually compressing her LSV, her initial refilling time of 8 seconds lengthened to 19 seconds, indicating a significant contribution by her superficial system to her pathologic hemodynamics. To further test these findings, a Duplex scan was performed, showing that the peak velocity of reflux flow through the LSV was greater than 33 cm/sec, whereas that through her CFV was only 9.5 cm/sec. She underwent high ligation and division of her LSVs and postoperative sclerotherapy. Marked improvement in the discomfort and the edema in her legs resulted, such that she was able to reduce the usage of her lymphapress and periodically wear hose with less compression without the disabling aching in her legs that she had experienced previously.

Other examples of the usefulness of the PPG are illustrated below:

J.S., a 59-year-old woman, sought treatment for dilated veins in her left calf. These connected with a minimally enlarged LSV in her thigh, and reflux was heard with the Doppler through her SFJ, whereas her deep veins all displayed valvular competence. The refilling time with PPG was found to be 15 seconds and lengthened to 25 seconds with obstruction of her LSV, thus indicating that obliteration of the flow through her SFJ would provide her with significantly improved hemodynamics.

R.S., on the other hand, a 72-year-old woman having a similar picture of dilated veins, only in her right calf, had a different etiology of her problem. The Doppler examination revealed reflux through her SFJ and normal deep vein valvular function as well. However, her refilling time of 15 seconds did not improve with obstruction of her LSV, thus implicating her perforating veins as the origin of her problem. By further varying the location at which the LSV was obstructed, the exact location of the responsible perforator was found.

If obstruction of the LSV just above the knee results in improvement in the refilling time, the Hunterian perforator must be involved. If the refilling time is not improved until the LSV is obstructed just below the knee, the geniculate perforator must be responsible. If this fails to improve the refilling time, the Boyd or Cockett perforators may be implicated.

As mentioned previously, the method of compression of the superficial vein(s) is of extreme importance since one must assure that adequate pressure is achieved to prevent flow through the vein. When attempting to compress a particular vein, manual pressure directly over the vein is probably most effective. On the other hand, when there are multiple veins, placement of a tourniquet might be a more appropriate method.

### Evaluation of the Origin of Recurrences after Ligation and Stripping

It is indeed disconcerting for both patient and physician alike to have to approach the treatment of varicosities that have developed in the groin or the popliteal fossa after previous ligation or ligation and stripping. Again, there are several noninvasive or minimally invasive methods that will provide information crucial to understanding the remaining connections and therefore the necessary sites of

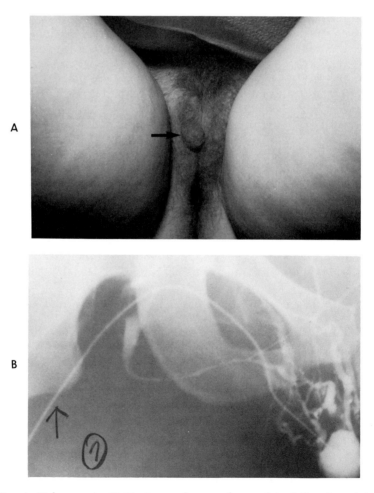

**Fig. 5-38**  A, Vulvar varix. B, Varicography may be used to define its origin. (Courtesy Jeffry Weisfeld, D.O.)

treatment. As found by Lofgren[11] in his study of 510 operations performed on patients with recurrence after ligation and stripping, most of these recurrences will be found to be the result of inadequate surgery. Either treatment of a dilated tributary with the actual saphenous trunk left untouched or ligation distal to the SFJ/SPJ are the usual findings.

He felt strongly that all patients with recurrence should be explored surgically, thus obviating the need for an imaging procedure. Since many of these patients will be found to have problems amenable to sclerotherapy alone, this is not a very satisfying approach, and one should first attempt to define the anatomy of the recurrence before proceeding with treatment decisions.

The approach to such a patient begins in the same way as the approach to any patient with involvement of the saphenous trunk. The palpation of the LSV or SSV is attempted, followed by the Doppler examination for reflux. It is always possible that the dilated vein noticed by the patient may, in fact, be simply a collateral that is functioning normally and does not need to be treated. Once reflux through the vein has been documented, a Valsalva maneuver will demonstrate whether this vein is still in connection with the deep venous system. If not, sclerotherapy may generally be successfully employed. If reflux is heard with a Valsalva maneuver, the patient may then be approached as if he or she were presenting de novo with SFJ or SPJ reflux. Venography has historically been used in this situation and will provide a good image of the exact connection of the recurrent varix. However, Duplex scanning provides excellent images, without the associated risks of the contrast media and radiation.

## Evaluation of Vulvar Varices

Vulvar varices generally arise from the pudendal or iliac veins and require treatment only of the varices themselves. In some cases, however, they connect directly with the long saphenous system. Therefore, before treatment the presence of an incompetent SFJ should be sought, since long-term control of these varices will require control of the SFJ if blood is refluxing through it into the vulvar veins. The technique for this determination is as previously described. The exact connection may also be determined by varicography (Fig. 5-38).

### REFERENCES

1. Thibault P, Bray A, and Wlodarczyk J: Cosmetic leg veins — evaluation using Duplex venous imaging, J Derm Surg Oncol, 1990 (in press).
2. Hoare MC et al: The role of primary varicose veins in venous ulceration, Surgery 92(3):450, 1982.
3. Sethia KK and Darke SG: Long saphenous incompetence as a cause of venous ulceration, Br J Surg 71:754, 1984.
4. Nicolaides A, Christopoulous D, and Vasdekis S: Progress in the investigation of chronic venous insufficiency, Ann Vasc Surg 3(3):278, 1989.
5. Haeger D: The anatomy of the veins of the leg. In Hobbs JT, editor: The treatment of venous disorders, Philadelphia, 1977, Lancaster MTP Press.
6. May R and Nissl R: Surgery of the veins of the leg and pelvis. In May R, editor: Anatomy, Stuttgart, 1979, Thieme.
7. Browse NL, Burnand KG, and Leo TM: Diseases of the veins: pathology, diagnosis, and treatment, London, 1988, Arnold.
8. Dodd H: The varicose tributaries of the popliteal vein, Br J Surg 52(5):350, 1965.
9. Hoare MC and Royle JP: Doppler ultrasound detection of saphenofemoral and saphenopopliteal incompetence and operative venography to ensure precise saphenopopliteal ligation, Aust N Z J Surg 54:49, 1984.
10. Sherman RS: Varicose veins: anatomy, reevaluation of Trendelenburg tests, and an operative procedure, Surg Clin North Am 44:1369, 1964.

11. Lofgren KA, Myers TT, and Webb WD: Recurrent varicose veins, Surg Gynecol Obstet 102:729, 1956.
12. Tretbar LL: Bleeding from varicose veins: treatment with injection sclerotherapy. Presented at tenth World Congress of Phlebology, Abstract 3G 15, Strasbourg, Sept 25-29, 1989.
13. Nabatoff RA: Simple palpation to detect valvular incompetence in patients with varicose veins, JAMA 159:27, 1955.
14. Dodd H and Cockett FB: The pathology and surgery of the veins of the lower limb, ed 2, London, 1986, Churchill Livingstone Inc.
15. Knudtzen J, Gudmundsen TE, and Svane S: Congenital absence of the entire inferior vena cava, Acta Chir Scand 152:541, 1986.
16. Chan A, Chisholm I, and Royle JP: The use of directional ultrasound in the assessment of saphenofemoral incompetence, Aust N Z J Surg 53:399, 1983.
17. Schultz-Ehrenburg U: Functional sclerotherapy. Presented at second annual Congress of the North American Society of Phlebology, New Orleans, Feb 25-26, 1989.
18. Schadeck M: Personal communication, Sept, 1989.
19. Brodie B: Lecture illustrative of various subjects in pathology and surgery, London, 1846, Longman.
20. Trendelenburg F: Ueber die Unterbindung der Vena Saphena magna bei Unterschendelvaricen, Beitr Z Klin Chir 7:195, 1891.
21. Steiner CA and Palmer LH: A simplification of the diagnosis of varicose veins, Ann Surg 127(2):362, 1948.
22. Mahorner HR and Ochsner A: The modern treatment of varicose veins as indicated by the comparative tourniquet test, Ann Surg 107:927, 1938.
23. Sherman RS: Varicose veins: further findings based on anatomic and surgical dissections, Ann Surg 130(2):218, 1949.
24. Fegan WG: Compression sclerotherapy, Ann R Coll Surg Engl 41(4):364, 1967.
25. Fegan G: Varicose veins: compression sclerotherapy, London, 1967, Heinemann Medical.
26. Beesley WH and Fegan WG: An investigation into the localization of incompetent perforating veins, Br J Surg 57(1):30, 1970.
27. O'Donnell TF Jr et al: Doppler examination vs clinical and phlebographic detection of the location of incompetent perforating veins, Arch Surg 112:31, 1977.
28. Townsend J, Jones H, and Williams JE: Detection of incompetent perforating veins by venography at operation, Br Med J 3:583, 1967.
29. Patil KD, Williams JR, and Williams KL: Thermographic localization of incompetent perforating veins in the leg, Br Med J 1:195, 1970.
30. Bracey DW: Simple device for location of perforating veins, Br Med J 2:101, 1958.
31. Perthes G: Über die Operation der Unterschenkelvaricen nach Trendelenburg, Deutsche Med Wehrschr 21:253, 1895.
32. Killewich LA et al: Pathophysiology of venous claudication, J Vasc Surg 1(4):507, 1984.
33. Anastasios JT: The physiology of venous claudication, Am J Surg 139:447, 1980.
34. Tripolitis AJ et al: The physiology of venous claudication, Am J Surg 139:447, 1980.
35. Fronek A: Noninvasive diagnostics in vascular disease, New York, 1989, McGraw-Hill Inc.
36. Bernstein EF, editor: Noninvasive diagnostic techniques in vascular disease, ed 3, St Louis, 1985, The CV Mosby Co.
37. Satomura S and Kaneko Z: Study of the flow patterns in peripheral arteries by ultrasonics, J Acoust Soc Japan 15:151, 1959.
38. Sumner DS, Baker DW, and Strandness DE Jr: The ultrasonic velocity detector in a clinical study of venous disease, Arch Surg 97:75, 1968.
39. Strandness DE Jr et al: Ultrasonic flow detection: a useful technique in the evaluation of peripheral vascular disease, Am J Surg 113:311, 1967.
40. Felix WR and Sigel B: Doppler ultrasound diagnosis in vascular disease, Penn Med 75:67, 1972.
41. Sigel B et al: A Doppler ultrasound method for diagnosing lower extremity venous disease, Surg Gynecol Obstet 127:339, 1968.
42. Sigel B et al: Augmentation flow sounds in the ultrasonic detection of venous abnormalities: a preliminary report, Invest Radiol 2:256, 1967.
43. Sigel B et al: Diagnosis of venous disease by ultrasonic detection, Surg Forum 18:185, 1967.
44. Sigel B et al: Comparison of clinical and Doppler ultrasound evaluation of confirmed lower extremity venous disease, Surgery 64(1):332, 1968.
45. Sigel B et al: Evaluation of Doppler ultrasound examination, Arch Surg 100(5):535, 1970.
46. Krahenbuhl B, Restellini A, and Frangos A: Peripheral venous pulsatility detected by Doppler method for diagnosis of right hear failure, Cardiology 71:173, 1984.
47. Folse R: The influence of femoral vein dynamics on the development of varicose veins, Surgery 68(6):974, 1970.

48. Barnes RW et al: Accuracy of Doppler ultrasound in clinically suspected venous thrombosis of the calf, Surg Gynecol Obstet 143:425, 1976.
49. Sumner DS and Lambeth A: Reliability of Doppler ultrasound in the diagnosis of acute venous thrombosis both above and below the knee, Am J Surg 130(2):218, 1979.
50. Ackroyd JS, Lea Thomas M, and Browse NL: Deep venous reflux: an assessment by descending venography, Br J Surg 73:31, 1986.
51. Bishop C: Personal communication, Sept, 1989.
52. Schultz-Ehrenburg U and Hubner H-J: Reflux diagnosis with Doppler ultrasound. In Findings in angiology and phlebology, vol 35, New York, 1989, FK Schattauer Verlag.
53. Barnes RW, Russell HE, and Wilson MR: Doppler ultrasonic evaluation of venous disease — a programmed audiovisual instruction, ed 2, Iowa City, 1975, University of Iowa Press.
54. Stonebridge PA et al: Comparison of Doppler and Duplex scanning for the evaluation of valvular reflux within the veins of the lower limb, Abstract 4S 09:20. Presented at the tenth World Congress of Phlebology, Strasbourg, Sept 25-29, 1989.
55. Bishop C et al: Real time color Duplex scanning following sclerotherapy of the greater saphenous vein. Submitted to the Society for Vascular Surgery, June 1990.
56. Vasdekis S et al: A comparison of Duplex scanning, Doppler ultrasound, and peroperative venography in assessing the termination of the short saphenous vein, Abstract 25 ii2. Presented at the fourth European-American Symposium on Venous Diseases, Washington DC, Mar 31-Apr 2, 1987.
57. Partsch H: Investigations on the pathogenesis of venous leg ulcers, Acta Chir Scand Suppl 544:25, 1988.
58. Shull KC et al: Significance of popliteal reflux in relation to ambulatory venous pressure and ulceration, Arch Surg 114:1304, 1979.
59. Rettori R: Recurrence of varicose veins due to the incompetence of the perforating veins at the medial aspect of the thigh, Abstract W 51-18. Presented at the ninth World Congress of Phlebology, Kyoto, 1986.
60. Folse A and Alexander RH: Directional flow detection for localizing venous valvular incompetency, Surgery 67(1):114, 1970.
61. Miller SS and Foote AV: The ultrasonic detection of incompetent perforating veins, Br J Surg 61:653, 1974.
62. Foote AV and Miller SS: Ultrasonic flow probe detection of incompetent perforating veins, Scott Med J 14:96, 1969.
63. O'Donnell TF et al: Doppler examination vs clinical and phlebographic detection of the location of incompetent perforating veins, Arch Surg 112:31, 1977.
64. Zweibel WJ, editor: Introduction to vascular ultrasonography, ed 2, Philadelphia, 1986, WB Saunders Co.
65. Knight RM and Zygmunt JA: Ultrasonic detection of the efficacy of injection sclerotherapy of the saphenofemoral junction, Abstract 3G 15. Presented at the tenth World Congress of Phlebology, Strasbourg, Sept 25-29, 1989.
66. Schadeck M: Sclerotherapy of the long saphenous veins: methodology and results controlled by Echo-Doppler on 400 patients, Abstract 2 S 15:30. Presented at the tenth World Congress of Phlebology, Strasbourg, Sept 25-29, 1989.
67. Raymond-Martimbeau P: Duplex ultrasonography, color flow Doppler and magnetic resonance imaging in phlebology, Abstract 1 T 15:50. Presented at the tenth World Congress of Phlebology, Strasbourg, Sept 15-19, 1989.
68. Day TK, Rish PJ, and Kakkar VV: Detection of deep vein thrombosis by Doppler angiography, Br Med J 1:618, 1976.
69. Sullivan ED, Peter DJ, and Cranley JJ: Real-time B-mode venous ultrasound, J Vasc Surg 1:465, 1984.
70. Raghavendra BN et al: Deep venous thrombosis: detection by probe compression of veins, J Ultrasound Med 5:80, 1986.
71. Talbot SR: Use of real time imaging in identifying deep venous obstruction: a preliminary report, Bruit 1:41, 1982.
72. Hannan LJ et al: Venous imaging of the extremities: our first 2500 cases, Bruit 10:29, 1986.
73. Flanagan LD, Sullivan ED, and Cranley JJ: Venous imaging of the extremities using real-time B-mode ultrasound. In Bergan JJ and Yao JST, editors: Surgery of the veins, Orlando, 1984, Grune & Stratton Inc.
74. Hobbs JT et al: Comparison of clinical examination, Doppler ultrasound, and color Duplex scanning with peroperative venography in the assessment of the short saphenous vein termination. Presented at the second annual Congress of the North American Society of Phlebology, New Orleans, Feb 25-26, 1989.
75. Hobbs JT: Peroperative venography to ensure accurate saphenopopliteal vein ligation, Br Med J 280:1578, 1980.

76. Corcos L et al: Intra-operative phlebography of the short saphenous vein, Phlebology 2:241, 1987.

77. Knight RM, Vin F, and Zygmunt JA: Ultrasonic guidance of injections into the superficial venous system, Abstract 4S 14:50. Presented at the tenth World Congress of Phlebology, Strasbourg, Sept 25-29, 1989.

78. Christopoulos D, Nicolaides AN, and Szendro G: Venous reflux: quantitation and correlation with the clinical severity of chronic venous disease, Br J Surg 75:352, 1988.

79. Abramowitz HB et al: The use of photoplethysmography in the assessment of venous insufficiency: a comparison to venous pressure measurements, Surgery 86(3):434, 1979.

80. Pearce WH et al: Hemodynamic assessment of venous problems, Surgery 93(5):715, 1983.

81. Barnes RW et al: Photoplethysmographic assessment of altered cutaneous circulation in the post phlebitic syndrome, Proc AAMI thirteenth annual meeting, Washington DC, Mar 28-Apr 1, 1978.

82. Killewich LA et al: An objective assessment of the physiologic changes in the post thrombotic syndrome, Arch Surg 120:424, 1985.

83. Dohn K: Plethysmography during functional states for investigation of the peripheral circulation. Proc second Int Congress Phys Med, Copenhagen, 1957.

84. Bygdeman S, Aschberg S, and Hindmarsh T: Venous plethysmography in the diagnosis of chronic venous insufficiency, Acta Chir Scand 137:423, 1971.

85. McMullin G, Coleridge Smith P, and Scurr J: An assessment of pneumatic tourniquets. Personal communication, 1990.

86. Shepard AD et al: Light reflection rheography (LRR): a new non-invasive test of venous function, Bruit 8:266, 1984.

87. Hubner K: Is the light reflection rheography (LRR) suitable as a diagnostic method for the phlebology practice? Phlebol Proctol 15:209, 1986.

88. Barnes RW and Yao JST: Photoplethysmography in chronic venous insufficiency. In Bernstein EF, editor: Noninvasive diagnostic techniques in vascular disease, ed 2, St Louis, 1982, The CV Mosby Co.

89. Norris CS, Beyrau A, and Barnes RW: Quantitative photoplethysmography in chronic venous insufficiency: a new method of noninvasive estimation of ambulatory venous pressure, Surgery 94(5):758, 1983.

90. Kerner J, Schultz-Ehrenburg U, and Blazek V: First clinical experiences on two new plethysmographic measuring systems: digital-PPG and computer aided gravimetric plethysmography (CGP), Abstract 5 T 08:40. Presented at the tenth World Congress of Phlebology, Strasbourg, Sept 25-29, 1989.

91. Hemodynamics Inc: Guidelines for measuring venous emptying with LRR as validated by the University of Miami. Personal communication, 1989.

92. Christopoulos D and Nicolaides AN: Air plethysmography in the assessment of the calf muscle pump in man, J Phys 374:11, 1986.

93. Christopoulos DG et al: Air-plethysmography and effect of elastic compression on venous hemodynamics of the leg, J Vasc Surg 5(1):148, 1987.

94. Nicolaides AN and Christopoulos D: Diagnosis and quantitation of venous reflux. In Baccolon H: Angiologie Paris, 1988, John Libbey Eurotext.

95. Christopoulos D et al: Pathogenesis of venous ulceration in relation to calf muscle pump function, Surgery 106:829, 1989.

96. Christopoulos DG and Nicolaides AN: Noninvasive diagnosis and quantitation of popliteal reflux in the swollen and ulcerated leg, J Cardiovasc Surg 29:535, 1988.

97. Norgren L: Functional evaluation of chronic venous insufficiency by foot volumetry, Acta Chir Scand Suppl 444:1, 1974.

98. Kakkar VV and Lawrence DA: Venous presure measurement and foot volumetry in venous disease, Int Angiol 1:87, 1982.

99. Thulesius O, Norgren L, and Gjores JE: Foot-volumetry, a new method for objective assessment of edema and venous function, Vasa 2(4):325, 1973.

100. Norgren L et al: Foot-volumetry and simultaneous venous pressure measurements for evaluation of venous insufficiency, Vasa 3(2):140, 1974.

101. Lawrence D and Kakkar VV: Post-phlebitic syndrome — a functional assessment, Br J Surg 67:686, 1980.

102. Norgren L: Foot-volumetry before and after surgical treatment of patients with varicose veins, Acta Chir Scand 141:129, 1975.

103. Lea Thomas M and Mahraj RPM: A comparison of varicography and descending phlebography in clinically suspected recurrent groin and upper thigh varicose veins, Phlebology 3:155, 1988.

104. Chilvers AS and Thomas MH: A method for the localization of incompetent ankle perforating veins, Br Med J 2:577, 1970.
105. Herman RJ, Neiman HL, and Yao JST: Descending venography: a method of evaluating lower extremity valvular function, Radiology 137:63, 1980.
106. Moore DF, Himmel PD, and Sumner DS: Distribution of venous valvular incompetence in patients with post phlebitic syndrome, J Vasc Surg 3(1):49, 1986.
107. Thiery L: Varicose veins as a result of gastrocnemial vein pathology: a 20-year survey. Presented at the second annual Congress of the North American Society of Phlebology, New Orleans, Feb 25-26, 1989.
108. Begg AC: Intraosseus venography of the lower limb and pelvis, Br J Radiol 27:318, 1954.
109. Lea Thomas M and Posniak HV: Varicography, Int Angiol 4:475, 1985.
110. Lea Thomas M and Keeling FP: Varicography in the management of recurrent varicose veins, Angiology 37:570, 1986.
111. Rosenberg N and Stefanides A: Thermography in the management of varicose veins and venous insufficiency, Ann NY Acad Sci 122:113, 1964.
112. Williams KL: Infrared thermography as a tool in medical research, Ann NY Acad Sci 121:99, 1964.
113. Barnes RW, Ross EA, and Strandness DE Jr: Differentiation of primary from secondary varicose veins by Doppler ultrasound and strain gauge plethysmography, Surg Gynecol Obstet 141:207, 1975.
114. Lea Thomas M and Bowles JN: Descending phlebography in the assessment of long saphenous vein incompetence, Am J Radiol 145:1255, 1985.
115. Burnand KG et al: The relative importance of incompetent communicating veins in the production of varicose veins and venous ulcers, Surgery 82(1):9, 1977.
116. Papadakis K et al: Number and anatomical distribution of incompetent thigh perforating veins, Br J Surg 76(6):581, 1989.
117. Dodd H: The diagnosis and ligation of incompetent ankle perforating veins, Ann R Coll Surg Engl 34:186, 1964.
118. Noble J and Gunn AA: Varicose veins: comparative study of methods of detecting incompetent perforators, Lancet 1:1253, 1972.
119. Elem B, Shorey BA, and Williams KL: Comparison between thermography and fluorescein test in the detection of incompetent perforating veins, Br Med J 4:651, 1971.
120. Lea Thomas M et al: A simplified technique of phlebography for the localization of incompetent perforating veins of the legs, Clin Radiol 23:486, 1972.
121. Miller SS, Crossman JA, and Foote AV: The ultrasound detection of incompetent perforating veins, Br J Surg 58:872, 1971.

# 6 Compression Hosiery and Elastic Bandages

*Their Use in the Prevention and Treatment of Varicose and Telangiectatic Leg Veins*

## HISTORICAL DEVELOPMENTS

Compression therapy of the leg is not a new procedure. Ancient Egyptians used paste bandages in the treatment of leg ulcers. Orbach[1] points out that the use of compression therapy for treatment of venous disease is mentioned in the Old Testament (book of Isaiah, Chapter 1, Verse 6), placing its use in the eighth century BC. It was practiced by Hippocrates in the fourth century BC. Celcus discovered plaster and linen bandages. Virgo refers to compression treatment with circular bandages after application of caustic agents, white lead and litharage.[2] Roman soldiers in 20 BC allegedly noted that leg fatigue could be reduced by applying tight strappings to the legs.[3]

The physicians of the middle ages used compression bandages, plaster dressings, and laced stockings made from dog leather. Theden, one of Fredrick the Great's three surgeons in the late 1700s, used a modification of lace-up dog leather stockings described by Fabrizio d'Aquapendente (1537-1619).[4] Theden reported in 1771 that he had cured a woman of varices in the eighth month of pregnancy by enveloping her legs to the abdomen with 20 ell-long bandages.[2]

The development of elastic medical compression bandages and stockings began in the middle 1800s with the discovery by Charles Goodyear in 1839 of a heating process for rubber that would increase its elasticity and durability. This, after much investigation, led to the manufacturing of rubber threads into stockings by William Brown in England in 1848. These stockings, made exclusively from rubber threads, were uncomfortable. It was not until Jonathan Sparks patented a method for winding cotton and silk around the rubber threads that elastic stockings became popular.[4]

During the late 1800s and early 1900s, technical advances in the manufacturing process led from the development of the frame-knitting to the flat-knitting method. Ultra-fine rounded latex yarns became available that permitted the construction of seamless stockings. Two-way-stretch stockings were then developed. Finally, the development of synthetic elastomers in the 1960s gave rise to rubberless compression stockings.

## MECHANISM OF ACTION

External compression can benefit the patient with venous insufficiency by augmentation of the body's natural muscle pump through application of a graduation of pressure in the leg forcing blood towards the heart.[5] This effect has been demonstrated in ambulatory patients with superficial venous insufficiency while wearing a graduated compression stocking with an ankle pressure of as little as 18 mm Hg.[5] In addition, venous flow is improved by returning the distended veins to normal size, rendering incompetent nonfunctioning venous valves competent. This summarizes the present theory. However, other benefits of compression may be realized with future research. For example, the vein diameter alone, irrespective of valvular function, may be important. This later effect is demonstrated in patients with postthrombotic venous stasis whose valves are destroyed but who achieve an improvement in hemodynamic function with the use of external compression. Also, other as yet unknown effects may stimulate an improvement in microcirculation. Studies have demonstrated that after 90 days of elastic compression with a 30-to-40 mm Hg graduated compression stocking, patients with cutaneous manifestations of venous stasis, including leg ulcerations, had remarkable changes in the structural pattern of dermal connective tissue. New capillaries are formed with a reduction in the diameter of existing capillaries and efferent venular systems.[6] Finally, external compression counterbalances the lost elasticity of the tissues to help lymph flow by "graduated" compression. Lymphatic flow is also augmented through an increase in hydrostatic pressure that discourages reaccumulation of edema.[7]

The adaptation of compression in the treatment of varicose veins has only been used with sclerosing treatment within the last 30 years. Postsclerosis compression initially described by Sigg[8] and Orbach[9] in the 1950s and Fegan in the 1960s[10] is perhaps the most important advance in sclerotherapy treatment of varicose veins since the introduction of relatively safe synthetic sclerosing agents in the 1940s.

## PHARMACOLOGIC VENOUS CONSTRICTION

As an addition to graduated compression stockings that produce a mechanical constriction of superficial veins via external pressure, venous constriction can also be induced pharmacologically. Dihydroergotamine (DHE), when given intravenously to patients with varicose veins, has been shown to produce venous constriction and changes in local venous hemodynamics comparable to that caused by compression bandages and stockings.[11] DHE exerts a relatively selective effect on smooth muscle stimulation of capacitance vessels in the peripheral circulation.[12] This effect can be demonstrated experimentally and visualized clinically when 1 mg of DHE is given intravenously, producing a mean reduction of 20.4% in the volume of blood in the legs.[11] This dose of DHE has been estimated to equal the compressive effect of a 25-mm Hg graduated compression stocking. The vasoconstrictive effect also occurs in the arms and the abdomen with a simultaneous increase in thoracic blood volume. Unfortunately, the frequency of side effects, especially headaches, limits its practical use. An oral preparation of DHE is being evaluated that would increase the efficiency of the calf muscle pump.[13]

This chapter examines the rationale for the use of compression in both the prevention and treatment of varicose and telangiectatic veins. An evaluation of the various compression stockings available including an in-depth discussion regarding their production and composition follows.

## THE USE OF COMPRESSION ALONE IN PREVENTING VARICOSE AND TELANGIECTATIC LEG VEINS

Varicose and telangiectatic leg veins progress when the volume and subsequent pressure of blood within the vessel lumen exceeds the vessel's capacity to enclose that volume. The deep venous system, by virtue of its position within a musculofibrous sheath, can accommodate such changes by pumping more blood towards the heart. The superficial venous system is not enclosed in a rigid sheath. Thus, to accommodate the increase in flow, the vessel lumen increases in diameter. When this increase in diameter is supraphysiologic, the one-way valve cusps no longer meet, and then become incompetent. This causes excessive pressure

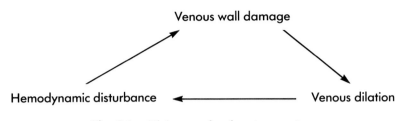

**Fig. 6-1**   Vicious cycle of varicose veins.

and blood volume to be routed into smaller branching vessels producing an abnormal dilation. This hemodynamical explanation of varicose vein development is best regarded as a vicious cycle (Fig. 6-1).

The primary method of reversing these changes is to first normalize the pressure and quantity of blood within the vessel lumen. This can be accomplished by sealing off incompetent perforator veins or junctions between the deep and superficial systems through surgical ligation or sclerotherapy-induced endofibrosis. When this is not possible, blood must be pushed from the superficial venous system to the heart. This is accomplished by restoring the competency of valves within the vessel lumen or by establishing a sheath around the vessel so that blood flow will be propelled upwards towards the heart instead of laterally against the vein wall. Bandages and graduated compression stockings provide the external support needed to produce this effect.

## External Pressure Provided by Medical Support Stockings

The principle governing the magnitude of the applied pressure to the external leg is Laplace's law:

$$\text{Pressure} = \frac{\text{Tension (force of the bandage)}}{\text{Radius (of the leg)}}$$

In general, pressure is calculated for the circumference of the limb at a specific level. Since the leg is oval and not circular (in cross section), the applied point pressures vary at different locations around the leg. Using this formula, it is evident that the effective pressure is greatest at the point of maximum radius and least at the point of minimum radius in inverse proportions. Thus, when a stocking is applied, the anterior and posterior aspects of the leg receive the greatest amount of pressure and the lateral and medial sides of the leg the least compression pressure. Therefore, to achieve uniform pressure around the leg circumference, the lateral and medial aspects should be padded to make the contour more circular (Fig. 6-2). This is especially important in the malleolar area where the greatest degree of compression occurs because the medial and lateral surfaces are flat or hollow (Fig. 6-3). Also, as is obvious from Laplace's law, a very thick leg requires more tension to achieve the optimum cutaneous and subcutaneous pressure. This factor should be considered when treating large-legged people.

All elastic compression stockings do not reduce ambulatory superficial venous pressure. This is because of the lack of graduated compression, which is caused by ankle-calf disproportion — narrow ankles and wide calves.[14] Therefore, a graduated compression stocking is only effective if it has been properly measured and fitted to a patient's limb (customized). When properly fitted, graduated compression stockings have been demonstrated to reduce ambulatory venous pressures by as much as 20 to 30 mm Hg.[14] Even in recumbency, a graduation in pressure produced by stockings (18 mm Hg at the ankle falling to 8 mm Hg at

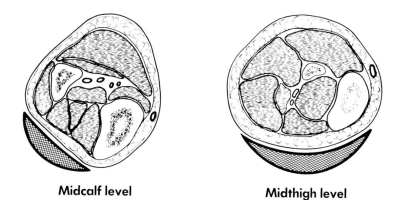

**Midcalf level**  **Midthigh level**

**Fig. 6-2**  Schematized cross section at the midcalf and midthigh levels after application of compression pads and stocking. The pads are placed to create both increased compression over the treated vein and rounding out of the otherwise oval calf or thigh to more uniformly distribute the graduated compression from the stocking.

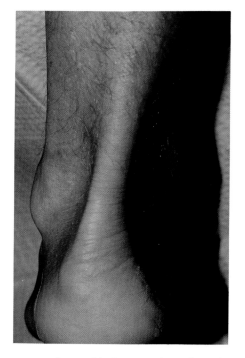

**Fig. 6-3**  Typical appearance of an ankle in posterior orientation. Note the bulging malleoli and the resulting concavity produced on the lateral and medial aspects.

the thigh) results in a significantly increased deep femoral vein flow velocity when uniform compression (11 mm Hg) is applied.[15] In the future, pressure-sensing devices used at the time of fitting of a stocking may allow for a more accurate graduation of pressure to be obtained.[16]

Fegan has demonstrated that incompetent venous valves can become competent with the application of external pressure. However, if the valves are allowed to remain incompetent for prolonged periods of time, fibrosis of the cusps may occur causing irreversible damage.[17] This effect is commonly noted in multiparous women who first note the temporary development of varicose veins during their first or second pregnancy. When the factors responsible for dilation of pregnancy-induced varicose veins (excessive blood volume, hormonally induced relaxation of the vein wall, etc.) resolve, the veins return to normal. However, after repeated pregnancies varicose veins may become permanent. This progression is probably related to recurrent insult on the valves resulting in fibrosis and permanent incompetence. Therefore, the use of graduated compression stockings for pregnancy-induced varicose veins should be considered preventative medicine, the goal being to maintain valvular competence and prevent sustained valvular damage.

At the first indication of pregnancy, patients should initially be fitted with a 20-to-30 mm Hg panty hose. In multiparous women, or in those with a previous history of varicose veins, a stronger 30-to-40 mm Hg panty hose should be worn. In women with large legs or in patients who are too uncomfortable with a 30-to-40 mm Hg panty hose, a calf length 20-to-30 mm Hg compression stocking can be worn over a 20-to-30 mm Hg panty hose. Using these guidelines, compression stockings worn during pregnancy can prevent or lessen the development of venous insufficiency.

The above rationale also applies to most other forms of venous stasis disease. External pressure restores the calf muscle pump, thereby alleviating the increase in superficial venous pressure and thus preventing the sequelae of venous hypertension. In addition to increasing deep venous flow and decreasing the caliber of superficial veins, compression stockings counteract the lateral expansion and dilation of superficial veins during muscle contraction (venous systole) by encasing the veins in a semirigid elastic envelope.[18]

Besides restoring the calf muscle pump function, graduated compression stockings or bandages correct venous hypertension by increasing the interstitial fluid pressure that both assists in transporting excess fluid back into circulation and prevents the leakage of fluid into the interstitium. Unfortunately, this effect is not always beneficial. Increasing the interstitial pressure forces the arterial circulation to increase its pressure to effect the release of interstitial fluid. When this occurs, the syndrome of intermittent claudication (pain in a limb, produced by exercise and relieved by rest) is produced. Therefore, if pain worsens when walking during compression therapy, the stocking should be removed, and an evaluation for arterial disease should be undertaken.

## Compression Bandaging Versus Graduated Compression Stockings

For most patients, there is no such thing as an attractive or comfortable compression stocking; there are only degrees of ugliness and discomfort. This is not true for compression bandages. Patients note that a bandage is worn only for a short time and is perceived as a sign of illness. It is therefore regarded with sympathetic understanding. A stockinged leg, however, is seen as an infirmity, a defect, and arouses only pity. This perception must be discussed with every patient if one is to ensure compliance with medical instruction.

**Compression bandages.** The primary difference between bandages and stockings is that the effect of bandages can be modified by bandaging technique. Pressure can be altered by varying the strength of wrapping. The elasticity of bandages, although limited, changes somewhat according to the type used and functions as a fixed support. Stockings, however, with elastic properties and graduated pressures fixed at the time of manufacture, undergo no change until the stocking is worn out and no longer usable. In fact, stockings must be made of highly elastic materials to enable them to be pulled over the heel of the foot.

Bandages are therefore best indicated when temporary compression is required, such as with edema or inflammatory conditions associated with a predisposing condition. Another benefit of bandages is that they can be constantly reapplied as necessary as the edema in the affected limb is reduced. In this way, the optimum compression needed for efficient therapy is obtainable. Bandages, by providing a limited stretch, also act to reduce peripheral mean ambulatory venous pressure. This forces the deep system to increase its working pressure with muscular contraction; however, it also exerts a lower pressure during muscular relaxation, thus allowing a more intense retrograde refilling of superficial veins to occur. This explains the relative increase in upward flow of blood.[19]

A major drawback of bandages is their nonuniform application. A comparison of the range in pressures measured during application of an elastic bandage by skilled persons versus nursing students demonstrated that skilled bandagers applied the bandages with a pressure of 34 mm Hg +/− 4.7 versus 36.6 mm Hg +/− 15.6 for unskilled personnel.[20] The skilled bandagers' pressure ranged from 25 to 50 mm Hg and the unskilled bandagers' pressure ranged from 15 to 70 mm Hg. In addition, even when bandages are applied by physicians expert in their use, a true graduation in pressure may not always be obtained. If graduated compression does not occur, thrombosis of normal veins may occur instead because of stagnation of blood flow caused by a tourniquet effect.[21] Intracapillary pressure varies with posture and exercise. When a bandage is applied, it should be wrapped tighter at the foot and ankle and looser proximally. Unfortunately, the bandage tends to work loose with movement and only maintains the initial pressure in the posture in which it was applied.

Because the degree of compression with manual bandages is unknown, arterial ischemia can occur. This is of concern particularly in the presence of venous leg ulcers during treatment. Two studies estimated the frequency of unsuspected arterial insufficiency among patients with chronic leg ulcers at 21%[22] and 31%.[23] Callam et al.[24] surveyed consultants in general surgery in Scotland regarding their experience with compression therapy in the previous 5 years. Of these consultants, 32% reported at least one case of ulceration or cutaneous necrosis aggravated by compression bandages; 21% reported more than one experience. Compression bandages accounted for 73 of 147 cases reported, with elastic and antiembolism stockings accounting for 36 and 38 cases respectively. Also, eight patients were reported who required amputations of the digits or feet as a direct result of arterial ischemia caused by an excessively tight compression bandage or stocking.[22] Finally, it has been estimated that up to 50% of patients over 80 years of age with leg ulceration also have significant arterial disease.[22] Therefore, one should always check arterial pulses before and after applying a compression bandage or fitting a compression stocking, especially in the elderly.

**Compression stockings.** Graduated compression stockings are required for long-term therapy. Here they provide an external support to constrict dilated veins to restore valvular competency, thus impeding reflux of blood from the deep to the superficial veins. By virtue of their "graduation," they serve to help propel blood towards the heart (Fig. 6-4). Unlike nonelastic bandages, they do not lose compression with time, and they work well as part of the calf muscle pump. Compression stockings should be used only when the leg diameter has stabilized and edema is no longer a factor. When used in this manner, the stocking will correspond to the leg dimensions over a long period to prevent a re-

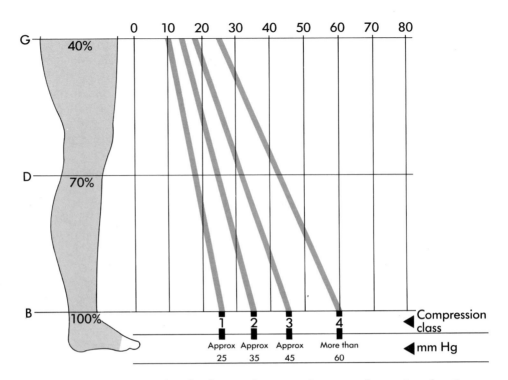

**Fig. 6-4** Diagram comparing the degree of compression exerted at various locations on the leg with different compression class stockings. *B* is the pressure generated at the ankle; *D* is the pressure generated at the knee; *G* is the pressure generated at the superior thigh. Note that there is a graduation of pressure with all classes of stockings with the highest pressure exerted at the ankle. Also note that the most significant difference in pressure generated by the different classes of stockings is at the ankle. (Courtesy Julius Zorn, Inc.)

newed increase in leg circumference. In addition, compression stockings function best when fitted early in the day when edema is reduced.

## CHARACTERISTICS OF MEDICAL GRADUATED COMPRESSION STOCKING

Compression stockings are almost exclusively two-way stretch stockings — elastic in both the longitudinal and transverse directions. This provides the necessary stretch needed to apply a stocking that has the smallest diameter at the ankle to be drawn over the heel. Two-way stretch stockings also have the characteristics of longitudinal bandages. The longitudinal elasticity of the stocking compensates for differences in limb length, thereby facilitating joint movements.

### Terminology

To understand the basic properties of the various compression stockings, the physician should be familiar with the following terms.

**Stretch resistance.** Stretch resistance is a measure of the tensile force required to elongate an elastic material. This represents the amount of resistance the wearer must overcome to don the support stocking. Of note is that an easy way to decrease the stretch resistance while increasing the degree of elastic support is to don two low-pressure stockings, one over the other. The end pressure will be equal to the pressure of both stockings added together, but each will be easier to don because of its individually lower stretch resistance.

**Stress relaxation.** Stress relaxation is the decrease in tensile force that occurs when an elastic yarn is held in an expanded state. This is a natural realignment of the molecular bonds within the framework of the elastomer. The amount of relaxation decay is different for each material and for the composition of the final elastic yarn.

**Holding power.** Holding power is the force exerted by an elastic material in an attempt to revert to its original length. This is the true reading of the support power available for applying pressure to a limb. The holding power is determined by the unloading portion of the stress/strain curve and is less than the stretch resistance.

**Hysteresis.** Hysteresis is a measure of the energy loss that occurs between loading (stretching) and unloading (relaxing). Yarns with minimal hysteresis are best since they have maximum holding power with minimal stretch resistance.

**Available stretch.** The available stretch is a measure of the amount of additional stretch available for donning and for joint mobility. It is a measure of the garment's ability to adapt to body movements.

**Modulus.** The ratio of change in the stress (force) to the change in the unit strain (percent stretch) is called the modulus. It is a measure of the rate of increased holding power with increased stretch.

**Stretch recovery.** Stretch recovery is the ability of an elastic material to return to its original shape after deformation and subsequent removal of an applied stress.

## Ready-Made or Customized, Made-To-Measure Stockings
### Ready-made stockings

Ready-made or off-the-shelf stockings are manufactured in fixed sizes. Most manufacturers have 12 sizes varying in both length and width at various points on the ankle, calf, and thigh (Table 6-1). Although the sizes are standardized to some degree by associations of stocking manufacturers, such as the Gutezeichengemeinschaft Medizinischer Gummistrumpfe e. V. (Quality Seal Association for Medical Compression Stockings) in Europe, there may be considerable variation between the sizing of different manufacturers (Fig. 6-5). Therefore, it may be prudent for distributors to carry multiple brands of stockings in the event that some patients experience a poor fit. One study has estimated that 90% of patients seeking treatment for venous disease could be fitted with ready-made stockings.[25]

### Made-to-measure stockings

*Prescription guidelines.* Made-to-measure stockings are custom-made according to the length and circumference measurements of the patient's leg. Adjustments are made either by hand on flat-knitting machines where shaping is achieved by altering the width of the knit or by machine in a circular-knit manner in which changes in the pressure and width are achieved by varying the tension of the weft and stitch size. Made-to-measure stockings should be prescribed under the following circumstances:
1. For very large or small patients
2. When there is a significant difference in the length between the right and left leg

**Table 6-1** Characteristics and care of graduated compression stockings

| Stocking brand name | Composition | Number of sizes Total/ankle/calf/foot/length | Toe Open/closed | Maintenance |
|---|---|---|---|---|
| Camp Classic 1600 | Nylon/spandex (natural rubber) | 12/3/2/1/2 | Open | Hand wash/ air dry |
| Camp 1800 | Nylon/spandex | 12/3/2/1/2 | Open | Hand wash/ air dry |
| Jobst | | | | |
| Vairox | Rubber/nylon (knee-length) | 12/3/2/1/2 | Open | Machine wash/ air dry |
| | (other lengths) | 12/3/2/1/1 | Open | Machine wash/ air dry |
| Vairox (Zipper) | Spandex/nylon | 6/3/1/1/2 | Open | Machine wash/ air dry |
| Fast fit | Spandex/nylon | 3/3/1/1/1 | Open/closed | Machine wash/ air dry |
| Ultimate | Lycra/nylon (uncovered) (knee-length) | 4/4/1/1/1 | Closed | Machine wash/ air dry |
| Sheer | Nylon (panty hose) | 6/6/1/1/1 | | |
| JuZo | | | | |
| Hostess | Syn elastomers (coated) | 12/6/1/1/2 | Closed | Machine wash/ dry |
| Varin Soft | Syn elastomers (coated) | 12/6/1/1/2 | Open/closed | Machine wash/ dry |
| Varin Super | Syn elastomers (coated) | 12/6/1/1/2 | Open/closed | Machine wash/ dry |
| Varilastic | Syn elastomers (coated) | 12/6/1/1/2 | Open | Machine wash/ dry |
| Legato | 35% Lycra 65% Nylon | 4/4/1/1/1 | Closed | Machine wash/ air dry |
| Medi 75 | Spandex/nylon (un-coated) | 12/6/1/2/2 | Closed | Machine wash/ dry |
| Medi Plus | Spandex/nylon (un-coated) | 12/6/1/2/2 | Open | Machine wash/ dry |
| Medi Lastex | Spandex/nylon (un-coated) | 12/6/1/2/2 | Open | Machine wash/ dry |
| Sigvaris 202 | Syn rubber (cotton-covered) | 12/3/2/1/2 | Open | Machine wash/ air dry |
| Sigvaris 503/504/505 | Natural rubber (nylon-covered) | 12/3/2/1/2 | Open | Hand wash/ air dry |
| Sigvaris 601 | Syn rubber (nylon-covered) | 12/3/2/1/2 | Open | Machine wash/ air dry |
| Sigvaris 801/802 | Syn rubber (nylon-covered) | 24/3/2/1/2 | Closed | Machine wash/ air dry |
| Sigvaris 902 | Syn rubber (nylon-covered) | 12/3/2/1/2 | Open/closed | Machine wash/ air dry |
| Venosan 1000 | Lycra 28% Nylon 72% | 12/3/2/1/2 | Open/closed | Machine wash/ air dry |
| Venosan 2000 | Lycra 25% Cotton 15% Nylon 60% | 12/3/2/1/2 | Open | Machine wash/ air dry |
| Venosan 3000 | Lycra 25% Cotton 75% | 12/3/2/1/2 | Open | Machine wash/ air dry |
| Venosan Boutique | Lycra 16% Nylon 84% | 4/4/1/1/1 | Closed | Machine wash/ air dry |

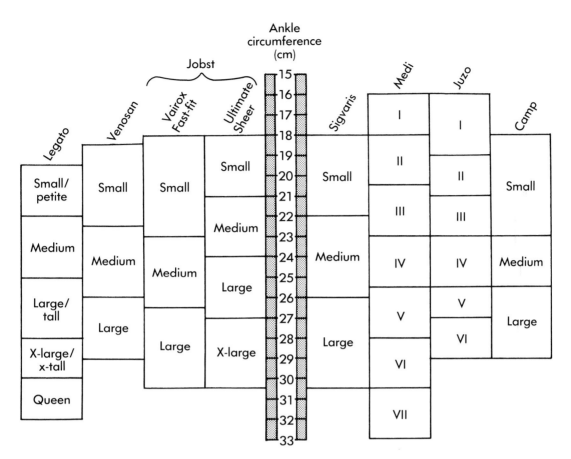

**Fig. 6-5**  Conversion chart based on the primary measurement around the smallest circumference above the ankle.

3. For patients with partial amputations or deformities of the leg or foot
4. When a special pressure gradient is required (e.g., increased pressure over the thigh)
5. When the measurements of ready-made stockings do not correspond to the leg length and girth measurements of a patient (e.g., when there is a difference of more than 3 cm between the lower leg length and the standard 39-cm length used for ready-made stockings); this may not be applicable for all brands of stockings
6. For patients who have very large instep to heel circumferences

**Measurement**

The most important measurement location is at the ankle (Fig. 6-6, point *b*) where a graduated stocking exerts the greatest degree of pressure. Therefore, all ready-made stockings include this point as one of the measuring points. Measurements taken at various levels of the calf and thigh must conform to the manufacturer's guidelines. If a calf or thigh diameter does not conform to the manufacturer's guide for that particular stocking size, then a made-to-order stocking should be used.

A common error made by the physician to avoid prescribing a made-to-measure stocking is that of prescribing the next larger size of a ready-made stocking. This results in a lower pressure being exerted at the ankle; in addition, the coun-

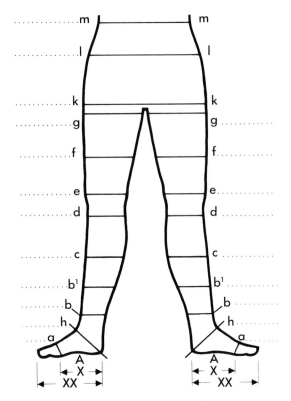

**Fig. 6-6** Diagram of the points of measurement for fitting of graduated support stockings. Measurement b is the most important measurement. Each stocking manufacturer has its own set of required measuring points to ensure proper fit of the ready-made stocking. Points c and f are usually required as well as the length points, a to f or a to g. Points k, l, and m are only required for fitting compression leotards. (Courtesy Julius Zorn, Inc.)

terpressures are altered since the wider stocking was designed at all levels for different leg measurements.

Proper measurement and fit of a compression stocking becomes increasingly important when higher compression classes are required. Therefore, made-to-measure stockings have particular application for compression classes above 40 mm Hg.

One should note that differences of over 15 mm Hg can occur among different stocking manufacturers not only by virtue of different types and strengths of elastic materials, but also by different methods of measuring the stocking to fit the leg.[26] Some manufacturers provide only three ankle sizes of stockings, whereas others provide up to 6 or more ankle sizes. Thus there may be a large variation of applied pressure for different-sized legs among different stocking brands as dictated by Laplace's law (see p. 160).

### Stocking lengths

Up to six styles of medical compression stockings are available depending on the manufacturer; knee-length, mid-thigh, thigh, panty hose or leotard, one-legged panty hose, thigh with waist attachment, and maternity panty hose (Fig. 6-7). Regardless of the style, most stockings are available in three lengths: knee-length, midthigh, and thigh length. According to the standardized figure, a knee-

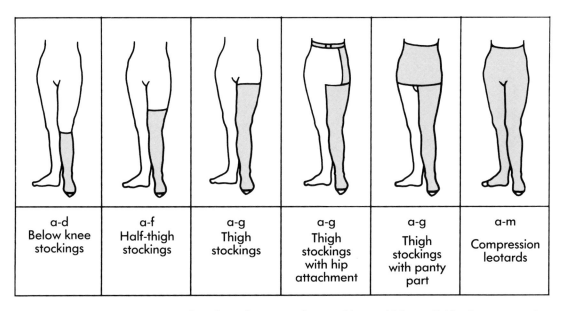

| a-d | a-f | a-g | a-g | a-g | a-m |
|---|---|---|---|---|---|
| Below knee stockings | Half-thigh stockings | Thigh stockings | Thigh stockings with hip attachment | Thigh stockings with panty part | Compression leotards |

**Fig. 6-7**   Six types of graduated compression stockings widely available. (Courtesy Julius Zorn, Inc.)

length stocking is designated as A-D, a mid-thigh stocking as A-F, and a thigh length stocking as A-G.

There are specific indications and contraindications for the various stocking lengths. Knee-length stockings should only be prescribed if the "c" circumference is about 2 cm greater than the "d" circumference; otherwise it will have no hold on the leg and tend to slide down (see Fig. 6-6). In addition, if the a to d length is too great, the excessive length will interfere with movement at the knee. Then the patient will usually fold the excess stocking down below the knee; this doubles the counterpressure at d and thus may reverse the "graduated pressure." Likewise, if the a to d length is too short, the patient will try to stretch the stocking beyond its natural point, thereby decreasing the effective circumferential pressure and thus defeating the purpose for wearing the stocking.

In patients with marked adiposity of the knee region, the upper edge of the stocking may produce skin bulging, which may be particularly bothersome on the inner aspect of the knee. In these cases it may be necessary to fit the patient with a midthigh stocking.

### Proper fit and position

Since the efficacy of any compression stocking is directly related to a proper fit, its adherence to the leg to prevent vertical movement is important. Panty hose stockings are the most expensive method used to ensure that the stocking remains in place by virtue of its attachment at the panty line. The only disadvantage is the increased constriction and heat generated by an additional undergarment.

With single-leg, thigh, or calf stockings, various inexpensive methods such as adhesive tape, glues, or garter belts serve to ensure proper positioning. Disadvantages include the pain on removal of tape from hairy legs, and irritation or allergy caused by the adhesive portion of the tape.

Garter belts comprise another more elegant yet out-of-fashion method for ensuring correct stocking placement. These belts may be built into the stocking as a waist attachment. Disadvantages include the digging in of the belt into an obese thigh if the belt is too narrow.

Finally, a new type of silicone top-band on thigh or midthigh length stockings is now available on the Medi USA stocking. It keeps the stocking in place without the disadvantages of glues or garter belts.

## THE RATIONALE FOR THE USE OF COMPRESSION IN VARICOSE VEIN SCLEROTHERAPY

Postsclerotherapy compression primarily eliminates a thrombophlebitic reaction and substitutes a "sclerophlebitis" with the production of a firm fibrous cord.[27] Compression serves at least six purposes:

1. Compression, if adequate, may result in direct apposition of the treated vein walls to produce a more effective fibrosis (Figs. 6-8 and 6-9).[9,36] Therefore, sclerosing solutions of lesser strength may be used successfully.

2. Compressing the treated vessel will decrease the extent of thrombus formation, which inevitably occurs with the use of all sclerosing agents,[28-31] hopefully decreasing the subsequent risk for recanalization of the treated vessel.[10,32,33]

3. A decrease in the extent of thrombus formation may also decrease the incidence of postsclerosis pigmentation.[34-36]

4. The limitation of thrombosis and phlebitic reactions may prevent the appearance of telangiectatic matting.[33]

5. The physiologic effect of a graduated compression stocking is to improve the function of the calf muscle pump, which is accompanied by subjective improvement.[37]

6. Compression stockings increase blood flow through the deep venous system.[38,39] This acts to rapidly clear any sclerosing solution that has inadvertently made its way into the deep venous system and thus prevent damage to valves in the deep venous system.

Externally supporting untreated varicose veins will narrow their diameter, restoring a competent valvular function and thereby decreasing retrograde blood flow.[40] External pressure will also retard the reflux of blood from incompetent perforating veins into the superficial veins.[41] Theoretically, since dermal collect-

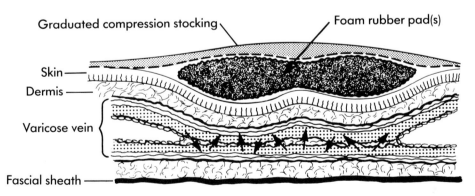

**Fig. 6-8** Schematic diagram demonstrating idealized compression of a treated varicose vein segment using foam rubber pads under a compression stocking. (Redrawn from Wenner L: Vasa 15:180, 1986.)

ing veins have been found histologically to contain one-way valves,[42] external pressure may also provide a normalization of cutaneous blood flow. In support of this theory, improvement in cutaneous oxygenation has been demonstrated with the use of compression in patients with venous stasis after only 10 to 15 minutes.[43]

Patients with varicose veins note relief of aching symptoms with all classes of compression stockings.[44,45] Patients with postphlebitic limbs find that the 30 to 40 and 40 to 50 mm Hg stockings control their edema and symptoms better than do the 20 to 30 mm Hg stocking. Interestingly, although symptoms are improved with all classes of compression stockings, patients with varicose veins only achieve physiologic improvement when 30 to 40 and 40 to 50 mm Hg compression stockings were worn. Therefore, 30 to 40 mm Hg graduated compression stockings are best used for conservative treatment of varicose veins and 40 to 50 mm Hg compression stockings are best used for conservative treatment of chronic venous insufficiency.

## How Much Pressure Is Necessary for Varicose Veins?

The optimum cutaneous pressure required to compress the varicose vein after sclerotherapy has yet to be defined. Venous ambulatory pressures of 48 mm Hg have been recorded from the superficial dorsal foot veins in patients with venous insufficiency.[41] A pressure of at least 30 mm Hg is required to reduce the capacity by 96% of a model distended to similar venous pressures.[41] Initial compression measurements taken during manual wrapping of the leg with Crevic crepe bandages by multiple surgeons using the technique of Fegan[10] average between 20 and 100 mm Hg with a mean of 54 mm Hg at calf level.[46] In addition, experimental varicose vein models have shown this level of compression to result in a reduction of the vessel lumina by 94% even in veins distended to 90 mm Hg.[46] Thus the classic technique for compression sclerotherapy is theoretically sound.

The posture of the patient should also be taken into consideration when pre-

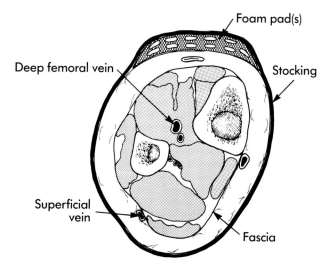

**Fig. 6-9** Schematic cross section of a superficial varicose vein compressed with a foam rubber pad under a compression stocking. Note that superficial varicosities lateral to the foam rubber pad are only slightly compressed, and veins deep to the fascia are not compressed. (Redrawn from Reid RG and Rothnie NG: Br J Surg 55:889, 1968.)

scribing compression stockings. If higher-compression pressures are used (through the use of double stockings), care must be taken to inform the patients to remove the outer stocking when not ambulatory. Ankle pressures greater than 20 mm Hg have been reported to produce an impairment of calf muscle and cutaneous blood flow in some nonambulatory patients.[47-49] Recent studies concerning peripheral blood circulation and skin temperature demonstrate a significant impairment of blood when external pressures above 30 mm Hg are applied to the leg of supine patients.[20] This may be perceived by the patient as achiness in the ankle area that occurs during sleep and resolves with walking after 30 to 40 mm Hg compression stockings are worn to bed after sclerotherapy is performed.

By having compression of 30 to 40 mm Hg at the ankle, the compressive strength at other locations on the leg may be between 10 and 20 mm Hg depending on the site and amount of underlying bone, adipose tissue, and muscle.[64] Experimental models have demonstrated that external pressures of 8.5 mm Hg reduce the capacity of the underlying varicose vein by only 22%.[46] Therefore, with the use of this degree of compression, one does not attempt to completely empty intravascular blood from the treated veins. However, any compression will decrease the effective vein diameter to some degree, thus theoretically minimizing subsequent thrombus formation. This hypothesis supports the rationale for the use of compression in the treatment of both varicose veins and leg telangiectasias.

## How Long Should Compression Be Maintained?

In addition to the degree of compression needed to effect optimal sclerotherapy, the time duration needed to maintain compression is also open for debate. The classic technique for sclerosis of varicose veins described by Fegan[10,32] and used by Hobbs[50] and Doran and White[51] is to continue compression for 6 weeks. This time period was not arrived at randomly, but through multiple histologic examinations of sclerotherapy-treated varicose veins at time intervals of 30 seconds; 1 and 5 minutes; 12, 24, and 36 hours; 6, 8, 12, and 14 days; 3, 4, 7, 10, 16, and 20 weeks; and ½, 1 and 5 years.[17] Fegan concluded that organization of the fibrous occlussion required at least 6 weeks. However, a randomized study found no difference in clinical results at 2 years when compression was maintained for 3 weeks as compared with 6 weeks.[52] Thus many phlebologists recommend a maximum of 3 weeks of compression.[53-57]

Recently studies have shown that compression bandages only maintain significant compression for 6 to 8 hours while patients are ambulatory[58] and lose up to 50% of their initial compression pressure in recumbent patients at 24 hours,[59] thus questioning the need for their prolonged use. Indeed, Raj and Makin[60] have shown that there was no significant clinical difference at 60 days between patients treated with either 8 hours or 6 weeks of compression after sclerotherapy of below the knee varices without saphenofemoral incompetence. Unfortunately, long-term follow-up examination of these patients to determine the ultimate success of therapy has not been reported. A study on the treatment of varicose veins less than 1.5 cm in diameter without saphenofemoral incompetence using compression with elastic bandages for 48 hours demonstrated good to excellent results at 1 and 5 year follow-up intervals.[61] Most recently, a randomized study on the use of compressive bandages in the treatment of varicose veins with a 3 month follow-up was reported.[62] Fraser, et al.[62] concluded through both subjective and objective findings that 3 days of compression equaled the results at 6 weeks. Unfortunately, this study used a Coban bandage dressing that may not maintain effective pressure beyond 8 hours.

A corollary to the amount of time necessary to effect adequate compression is whether it is necessary to continue compression while the patient is lying down or asleep. The author recommends that some degree of compression be maintained at all times to ensure optimal contraction of the treated vein. In fact, studies have demonstrated that veins become more distensible during sleep.[63] This has been postulated to occur as a result of respiratory factors or emotional factors during dream states. Finally, it may be impractical for a patient to remove and reapply the stocking at night if he or she must get out of bed for any reason. Therefore, if a high degree of compression is required after treatment, the use of double stockings appears practical since one of the stockings can be removed while the patient is lying down.

## Practical Considerations

To optimize patient acceptability and compliance, a medium-strength compression stocking of 30 to 40 mm Hg is recommended. One study demonstrated that approximately 80% of patients with varicose veins who use Sigvaris 30 to 40 mm Hg graduated compression stockings find them comfortable to wear, and symptoms are improved.[65] However, patients with varicose veins demonstrate a compliance of 67% when fitted with 30 to 40 mm Hg Medi Plus and a compliance of 41% when fitted with a 30 to 40 mm Hg Sigvaris graduated compression stocking.[66] Therefore, if patients refuse to wear the initially prescribed stockings, another brand of stockings should be recommended.

Some anatomic sites require inventive measures to effect compression of the underlying varicose veins. Perhaps the most difficult area on the "leg" to compress is the vulvar region. The author has found the "vulvar pad" described by Nabatoff to be effective in this region.[67]

## THE RATIONALE FOR THE USE OF COMPRESSION IN THE TREATMENT OF TELANGIECTASIAS

In short, compression sclerotherapy is now standard practice in the treatment of varicose veins. However, its use in the treatment of smaller abnormal leg veins and telangiectatic "spider" veins has never been studied. Theoretically, the same justification for the use of compression in larger veins should hold true for its use in smaller veins.

Duffy[68] has recently classified unwanted leg veins into six types based on clinical (and possibly functional) appearance (see p. 52). Types 1, 1A, and 1B are probably dilated venules, possibly with intimate and direct communication to underlying larger veins from which they are direct tributaries.[69] Both Bodian[70] and Faria and Moraes[71] have found on biopsy examination that such "telangiectasias" are actually ectatic veins. However, Duffy[68] and Biegeleisen[72] believe that the Duffy types 1, 1A, 1B, and 2 vessels may become dilated by virtue of their proximity to small arteriovenous communications. Indeed, multiple investigators[73-76] have demonstrated arteriovenous communications in association with larger varicose veins. However, serial histologic examination from 26 biopsies in 16 patients with telangiectatic leg veins (all but two with associated varicose veins) demonstrated an arteriovenous anastomosis in only one vein.[71] Thus the vast majority of telangiectasias arise from the venous system.

Therefore, since a significant percentage of smaller spider veins occur in direct communication with larger varicose or reticular superficial veins, compression of the "feeder" vein should decrease, if not eliminate, the blood flow to the smaller connected vessels. Thus, in addition to the effects of compression on the treated vessels themselves, compression of the entire leg should lead to a relatively stagnant blood flow in the feeder veins, which should allow for more effective endosclerosis of the treated vessel and a subsequent decreased risk of recanalization.

## How Much Pressure Is Necessary to Compress Telangiectasia?

The only reported study measuring the pressure necessary to empty superficial "capillaries" (telangiectasias) on the leg demonstrated that a sudden emptying of superficial cutaneous capillaries occurs between 40 and 60 mm Hg at a point 5 cm above the medial malleolus while the patient is recumbant.[77] However, 80 mm Hg was required to produce a complete emptying of blood with the patient in a standing position. Unfortunately, this degree of pressure is difficult to obtain with graduated compression stockings on areas of the leg above the ankle.

Interestingly, even graduated stockings with an ankle pressure of 7 to 8 mm Hg have been demonstrated in 6% of patients to control small superficial varices.[78] In this limited trial of women whose jobs entail standing for prolonged periods, this degree of ankle pressure was enough to produce a significant degree of symptomatic improvement in 74% of those studied. Whether these findings are real or merely a placebo effect await further study. However, they do emphasize that at the very least, graduated compression stockings, properly fitted and applied, can be perceived as being beneficial in a large number of people.

Compression of the leg should be applied in a *graduated* manner to ensure and aid in the optimal unidirectional flow of blood towards the heart and to avoid a proximal tourniquet effect.

Multiple studies have demonstrated a pressure drop of 26% to 59% from the ankle to the thigh with graduated medical stockings.[41,64,79] Indeed, studies using photoplethysmography to evaluate the efficiency of venous return from the lower leg demonstrate a significant worsening when nongraduated, commercially available "support" panty hose are worn.[80] Therefore, obtaining a pressure high enough to empty telangiectasias on the thigh would require a cutaneous pressure at least 30% higher at the ankle for the stocking to be graduated.[81,82] The degree of pressure required to completely empty a thigh telangiectasia would likely result in cutaneous ischemia, especially with recumbency, thereby increasing the likelihood of cutaneous ulcerations.[83]

Recently, studies have demonstrated that the use of narrow foam rubber pads under compression stockings will result in an increase in cutaneous pressure under the pad by 15%[46] to 50%[58] over compression with the stocking alone. Foam Sorbo pads are widely used in Great Britain.[27] In addition to producing an increase in cutaneous pressure, their use, especially in the popliteal region, has decreased the incidence of abrasions from pressure stockings and tape, thereby improving patient comfort. Thus a localized relative increase in pressure on areas of the leg above the ankle may be possible. However, efforts to increase local compression through the use of foam rubber pads to effect complete emptying of telangiectatic leg veins is rarely achieved. Follow-up of patients with Duffy type 1 and 2 veins treated with sclerotherapy and a combination of foam pads under a 30-to-40 mm Hg compression stocking demonstrates limited thrombus formation in the treated vessels.

## How Long Should Compression Be Maintained?

Formal studies on the use of compression in the treatment of leg telangiectasias have not been reported to my knowledge. However, a 3-day time period for compression of leg telangiectasias is chosen based on the empirical report of Ouvry and Davy,[33] who advised a minimum of 3 days to limit the development of pe-

**Table** 6-2  Adverse sequelae of sclerotherapy

|  | Pigmentation | Ankle edema | Calf edema |
|---|---|---|---|
| Compression | 28.5% | 33% | 0% |
| Noncompression | 40.5% | 66% | 40% |

Modified from Goldman MP et al: Compression in the treatment of leg telangiecta-sia, J Dermatol Surg Oncol 16:332, 1990.

ripheral inflammation and intravascular thrombosis. Without supporting infor-mation, Harridge[30] recommends a 1-week period of compression for spider veins, using a local pressure band of elastic adhesive only.

## Inadequacies of Compression

One limitation to the use of compression stockings in treating leg telangiectasias is the lack of complete emptying of the treated telangiectasias when only one stocking is used. Theoretically, the incorporation of foam pads directly over the injected vessels and a double layer of compression stockings for daytime use, with one stocking removed on recumbency, should produce a more complete vascular occlusion (see Figs. 6-8 and 6-9). It has been demonstrated that the ad-dition of a second stocking results in an effective pressure equal to or slightly higher than the sum of the individual stocking pressures.[19,84]

A multicenter, bilateral comparative study through the North American Soci-ety of Phlebology examined the necessity for the use of a single stocking when treating leg telangiectasias.[85] In short, 37 women with bilaterally symmetrical te-langiectatic leg veins less than 1 mm in diameter were evaluated. One set of ves-sels was compressed for 3 days with a 30-to-40 mm Hg compression stocking* over cotton ball dressing. The alternate set of vessels had a cotton ball dressing applied for 2 hours with no overlying compression stocking. A greater clinical resolution of vessels occurred after treatment with one sclerotherapy injection on vessels located on the distal leg, or when vessels were greater than 0.5 mm in diameter. Vessels located elsewhere or less than 0.5 mm in diameter showed no significant difference when this form of compression was used (Table 6-2).

The main benefit of compression treatment was noted in the evaluation of adverse sequelae. The most significant finding in this study was that compression produced a relative decrease in postsclerotherapy hyperpigmentation, which fell from an incidence of 40.5% to 28.5% with the use of compression. In addition, ankle and calf edema were lessened if a graduated compression stocking was worn immediately after sclerotherapy.

The major limitation to the above-mentioned study was the lack of complete emptying of the treated telangiectasia with the compression stocking used. Future studies may wish to incorporate different compression techniques to more com-pletely empty the treated vessels. Also, they should address the optimal length of time needed for postsclerosis compression of telangiectasias.

## DONNING MEDICAL COMPRESSION STOCKINGS

Before donning the stocking, the patient should be advised of the following con-siderations. To avoid damaging the stockings, hand jewelry should be removed. Fingernails should be smooth and relatively short. Rubber gloves are helpful in

---

*Medi USA, Arlington Heights, IL 60005.

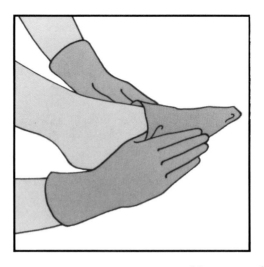

**Fig. 6-10**  Foot sock helpful for getting open-toe stocking over ankle. (Courtesy Julius Zorn, Inc.)

both preventing damage to the stockings from long fingernails and gripping the stocking. Talcum powder may be applied to the leg or a light perlon panty hose or stocking may be worn under the compression stocking to create a smoother leg over which to slide the stocking. Finally, satin foot "socks" provided by the stocking manufacturer are helpful in getting an open-toe stocking over the ankle (Fig. 6-10).

After preparing the foot and leg, turn the stocking inside out with the foot from the heel to the toe tucked into the stocking (Fig. 6-11, *A*). Stretch the foot opening with the fingers or thumbs of both hands and pull the stocking foot over the foot up to the instep. Draw the stocking upwards over the heel until pulling becomes difficult (Fig. 6-11, *B*). Push the fold that forms across the instep and heel of the stocking over the heel. Finally, pull the stocking up in sections, always remembering not to pull it over long distances all at once but to proceed in small steps (Fig. 6-11, *C*). When the stocking is applied without folds over the calf, the thigh section is then pulled over the knee (Fig. 6-11, *D*). Finally, remove the foot "sock" (Fig. 6-11, *E*).

It is very important for the physician or nurse to instruct and observe the patient applying the stocking. Effectiveness of compression will only occur when a correctly fitted stocking is applied correctly. If the patient encounters difficulties in applying the stocking because of age, obesity, arthritis, etc., arrangements should be made to have an experienced helper on hand when needed. It is important to note that if patients have difficulty in applying higher-compression class stockings, wearing two layers of lighter stockings, one over the other, should be helpful. As discussed previously, the compressive effects of stockings are additive. Zippers in stockings also make donning them easier.

Recently, an application aid for compression stockings has been produced by Medi USA. The "Butler" is a cleverly designed, simple metal support that makes donning compression stockings easier, even when the stockings must be placed over compression padding (Fig. 6-12). The compression stocking is pulled over the half circle bracket located on the front (open) side of the "Butler" so that the heel portion of the stocking is 2 to 3 inches below the top on the half circle bracket. The heel portion is positioned facing the user, the toe of the stocking is

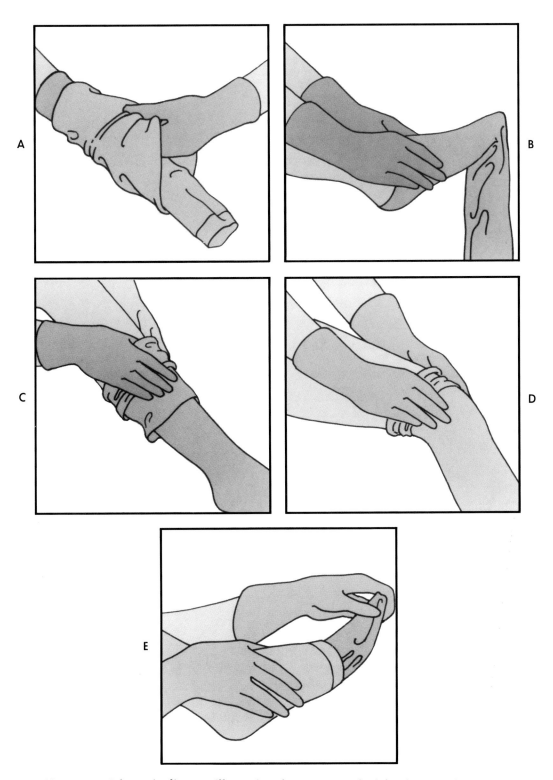

**Fig. 6-11**  Schematic diagram illustrating the proper method for donning the compression stocking. **A,** Turn the stocking inside out. Tuck in the foot from the heel to the toe. **B,** Using both hands, pull the stocking over the foot up to the instep, drawing it upwards over the heel. **C,** Continue pulling the stocking up in small sections. **D,** Pull the thigh section over the knee. **E,** Remove the foot sock. (Courtesy Julius Zorn, Inc.)

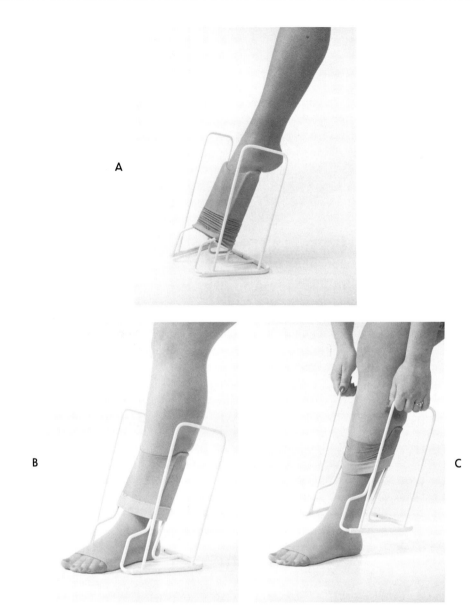

**Fig. 6-12** The Medi Butler. **A,** After putting the compression stocking on the bracket, insert the foot. **B,** Continue until the foot is completely on the floor, and heel is in place. **C,** Pull up on the metal side grips until the Butler is above the calf. Then remove it and continue until stocking is in place. (Courtesy Medi U.S.A.)

facing towards the open side of the "Butler." The foot is then placed into the foot part of the stocking until the foot is completely on the floor or until the heel is in place. The metal grips on either side are then used to pull the rest of the stocking onto the leg. Once the stocking is above the calf the "Butler" may be pulled away and the remainder of the stocking can then be easily pulled up.

## CARE OF THE MEDICAL COMPRESSION STOCKING

Since these stockings are worn on a daily basis in extremely close contact with the skin, they are subjected to considerable wear. The chemical stresses from sweat, soaps, creams, and body oils, in addition to the physical stresses of near continuous stretch and relaxation with movement of the leg, result in a gradual decline in the compressive effect of the stockings. Compression stockings, therefore, have a limited effective life. To ensure that they last as long as possible certain special care is required.

The first lesson in proper stocking care is to avoid excessive trauma. Therefore, rubber gloves should be worn when the stocking is put on to avoid tearing the threads with fingernails. Likewise, toenails should be trimmed and hard calluses, verruca, or other rough spots on the feet should be softened or removed. Also, the stocking should be eased onto the leg, not pulled on.

The stocking should not come into contact with ointments, creams, stain removers, or other solvents, especially if it is composed of rubber threads. These substances can damage the fine elastic yarns by causing them to swell and thus reduce the strength and elasticity of the fabric.

Regular and careful washing is necessary to maintain the elastic properties of the fabric. This is because of the harmful effects of sweat, skin oils, and environmental dirt that accumulate in the fabric while the stocking is worn. These substances will penetrate deeper into the elastic yarns if allowed to remain on the fabric for long intervals between washings. Environmental dust is damaging to the yarn by virtue of its abrasive action when the elastomers are stretched and relaxed.

Ideally, compression stockings should be washed every day. In fact a study of six stocking types machine-washed 15 times at 40° C demonstrated no decrease in the resting pressure and elasticity.[40] Therefore, if long-term use is required, it is best to provide the patient with two pairs that can be alternated between washings. Most compression stockings incorporating spandex can be machine washed on a fine/gentle cycle with warm (40° C) water. This gives a better cleansing action than hand washing. (Consult the manufacturer's guidelines for specific instructions.) Gentle detergents without bleach or alkali are best. Gentle spinning after the washing cycle is harmless to compression stockings and quickens the drying process. Rather than being hang-dried from a line, compression stockings should be laid flat on a drying rack or towel. Heat should not be used in the drying process. However, Medi USA permits machine drying. With normal wear and proper care, compression stockings should have an effective life of 4 to 6 months.

## REFERENCES

1. Orbach EJ: Compression therapy of vein and lymph vessel diseases of the lower extremities, Angiology 30:95, 1979.
2. Kohler H: Venous diseases of the leg and medical compression stockings and panty stockings, St Gallen, 1981, Ganzoni & Cie AG.
3. Johnson G Jr: The role of elastic support in venous problems. In Bergan J and Yao JST, editors: Surgery of the veins, 1985, Grune & Stratton Inc.
4. Hohlbaum GG: The history of medical compression hoisery. In Hohlbaum GG et al, editors: The medical compression stocking, New York, 1989, Stuttgart.
5. Christopoulos DG et al: Air-plethysmography and the effect of elastic compression on venous hemodynamics of the leg, J Vasc Surg 5:148, 1987.
6. Curri SB et al: Changes of cutaneous microcirculation from elasto-compression in chronic venous insufficiency. In Davy A and Stemmer R, editors: Phlebology '89, Montrouge, France, 1989, John Libby Eurotext Ltd.
7. Ryan TJ, Mortimer PS, and Jones RL: Lymphatics and the skin: neglected but important, Int J Dermatol 25:411, 1986.
8. Sigg K: The treatment of varicosities and accompanying complications, Angiology 3:355, 1952.
9. Orbach EJ: A new approach to the sclerotherapy of varicose veins, Angiology 1:302, 1950.
10. Fegan WG: Continuous compression technique of injecting varicose veins, Lancet 2:109, 1963.
11. Partsch H and Mostbeck A: Constriction of varicose veins and improvement of venous pumping by dihydroergotamine, Vasa 14:74, 1985.

12. Mellander S and Nordenfelt I: Comparative effects of dihydroergotamine and noradrenaline on resistance, exchange, and capacitance functions in the peripheral circulation, Clin Sci 39:183, 1970.
13. Partsch H: Personal communication, 1990.
14. Horner J, Fernandes E, and Nicolaides AN: Valve of graduated compression stockings in deep venous insufficiency, Br Med J 280:820, 1980.
15. Siegel B et al: Type of compression for reducing venous stasis: a study of lower extremities during inactive recumbency, Arch Surg 110:171, 1975.
16. Horner J, Lowth LC, and Nicolaides AN: A pressure profile for elastic stockings, Br Med J 280:818, 1980.
17. Fegan WG: Varicose veins: compression sclerotherapy, London, 1967, Heinemann Medical.
18. O'Donnell TF Jr et al: Effect of elastic compression on venous hemodynamics in postphlebitic limbs, JAMA 242:2766, 1979.
19. Partsch H: Improvement of venous pumping in chronic venous insufficiency by compression dependent on pressure material, Vasa 13:58, 1984.
20. Yamaguchi K et al: External compression with elastic bandages: its effect on the peripheral blood circulation during skin traction, Arch Phys Med Rehabil 67:326, 1986.
21. Tretbar LL and Pattisson PH: Injection-compression treatment of varicose veins, Am J Surg 120:539, 1970.
22. Callam MJ et al: Arterial disease in chronic leg ulceration: an underestimated hazard, Br Med J 294:929, 1987.
23. Cornwall JV, Dore CJ, and Lewis JD: Leg ulcers: epidemiology and aetiology, Br J Surg 73:693, 1986.
24. Callam MJ et al: Hazards of compression treatment of the leg: an estimate from Scottish surgeons, Br Med J 295:1382, 1987.
25. von Beratung U: Die therapie venoser Beinleiden Kompressionstherapie, medikamentos kombiniert? Der Bayerische Internist 1:46, 1987.
26. Hohlbaum GG: The use of medical compression stockings. In Hohlbaum GG et al, editors: The medical compression stocking New York, 1989, Stuttgart.
27. Reid RG and Rothnie NG: Treatment of varicose veins by compression sclerotherapy, Br J Surg 55:889, 1968.
28. Orbach EJ: The importance of removal of postinjection coagula during the course of sclerotherapy of varicose veins, Vasa 3:475, 1974.
29. Lufkin H and McPheeters HQ: Pathological studies on injected varicose veins, Surg Gynecol Obstet 54:511, 1932.
30. Harridge H: The treatment of primary varicose veins, Surg Clin North Am 40:191, 1960.
31. Goldman MP et al: Sclerosing agents in the treatment of telangiectasia: comparison of the clinical and histologic effects of intravascular polidocanol, sodium tetradecyl sulfate, and hypertonic saline in the dorsal rabbit ear vein model, Arch Dermatol 123:1196, 1987.
32. Fegan WG: Continuing uninterrupted compression technique of injecting varicose veins, Proc R Soc Med 53:837, 1960.
33. Ouvry PA and Davy A: The sclerotherapy of telangiectasia, Phlebologie 35:349, 1982.
34. Goldman MP and Bennett RG: Treatment of telangiectasia: a review, J Am Acad Dermatol 17:167, 1987.
35. Goldman MP, Kaplan RP, and Duffy DM: Postsclerotherapy hyperpigmentation: a histologic evaluation, J Dermatol Surg Oncol 13:547, 1987.
36. Wenner L: Sind endovarikose hamatische Ansammlungen eine Normalerscheinung bei Sklerotherapie? Vasa 10:174, 1981.
37. Struckmann J et al: Venous muscle pump improvement by low compression elastic stockings, Phlebology 1:97, 1986.
38. Louis CE et al: Elastic compression in the prevention of venous stasis: a critical appraisal, Am J Surg 132:739, 1976.
39. Husi EA, Ximenes JOC, and Goyette EM: Elastic support of the lower limbs in hospital patients: a critical study, JAMA 214:1456, 1970.
40. Weber G: Manufacture, characteristics, testing, and care of medical compression hoisery. In Hohlbaum GG: The Medical Compression Stocking New York, 1989, Stuttgart.
41. Somerville JJ et al: The effect of elastic stockings on superficial venous pressures in patients with venous insufficiency, Br J Surg 61:979, 1974.
42. Braverman IM and Keh-Yen A: Ultrastructure of the human dermal microcirculation. IV. Valve containing collecting veins at the dermal-subcutaneous junction, J Invest Dermatol 81:438, 1983.
43. Rooke TW et al: The effect of elastic compression on $TcPO_2$ in limbs with venous stasis, Phlebology 2:23, 1987.
44. Jones NAG et al: A physiological study of elastic compression stockings in venous disorders of the leg, Br J Surg 67:569, 1980.

45. Stoberl Ch, Gabler S, and Partsch H: Indikationsgerechte bestrumpfung — messung der venosen pumpfunktion, Vasa 18:35, 1989.
46. Fentem PH et al: Control of distension of varicose veins achieved by leg bandages, as used after injection sclerotherapy, Br Med J 2:725, 1976.
47. Campion EC, Hoffmann DC, and Jepson RP: The effects of external pneumatic splint pressure on muscle blood flow, Aust N Z J Surg 38:154, 1968.
48. Chant ADB: The effects of posture, exercise, and bandage pressure on the clearance of Na from the subcutaneous tissues of the foot, Br J Surg 59:552, 1972.
49. Lawrence D and Kakkar VV: Graduated, static, external compression of the lower limb: a physiological assessment, Br J Surg 67:119, 1980.
50. Hobbs JT: Surgery and sclerotherapy in the treatment of varicose veins, Arch Surg 109:793, 1974.
51. Doran FSA and White M: A clinical trial designed to discover if the primary treatment of varicose veins should be by Fegan's method or by an operation, Br J Surg 62:72, 1975.
52. Batch AJG et al: Randomized trial of bandaging after sclerotherapy for varicose veins, Br Med J 281:423, 1980.
53. Conrad P: Continuous compression technique of injecting varicose veins, Med J Aust 1:1011, 1967.
54. Orbach J: A new look at sclerotherapy, Folia Angiologica 25:181, 1977.
55. Weissberg D: Treatment of varicose veins by compression sclerotherapy, Surg Gynecol Obstet 151:353, 1980.
56. Tolins SH: Treatment of varicose veins: an update, Am J Surg 145:248, 1983.
57. Sladen JG: Compression sclerotherapy: preparation, technique, complications, and results, Am J Surg 146:228, 1983.
58. Raj TB, Goddard M, and Makin GS: How long do compression bandages maintain their pressure during ambulatory treatment of varicose veins? Br J Surg 67:122, 1980.
59. Coleridge Smith PD, Scurr JH, and Robinson KP: Optimum methods of limb compression following varicose vein surgery, Phlebology 2:165, 1987.
60. Raj TB and Makin GS: A random controlled trial of two forms of compression bandaging in outpatient sclerotherapy of varicose veins, J Surg Res 31:440, 1981.
61. Chou FF et al: The treatment of leg varicose veins with hypertonic saline-Heparin inections, J Formosan Med Assoc 83:206, 1984.
62. Fraser IA et al: Prolonged bandaging is not required following sclerotherapy of varicose veins, Br J Surg 72:488, 1985.
63. Shepard JT: Reflex control of the venous system. In Bergan JJ and Yao JST, editors: Venous problems, Chicago, 1978, Year Book Medical Publishers Inc.
64. Partsch H: Do we need firm compression stockings exerting high pressure? Vasa 13:52, 1984.
65. Chant ADB, Magnussen P, and Kershaw C: Support hose and varicose veins, Br Med J 290:204, 1985.
66. Chant ADB et al: Support stockings in practical management of varicose veins, Phlebology 4:167, 1989.
67. Nabatoff RA: Vulval varicose veins during pregnancy: new support for effective compression, JAMA 173:1932, 1960.
68. Duffy DM: Small vessel sclerotherapy: an overview. In Callen JP et al, editors: Advances in dermatology, vol 3, Chicago, 1988, Year Book Medical Publishers Inc.
69. Bean WB: Vascular spiders and related lesions of the skin, Springfield, 1958, Thomas Publishing Co.
70. Bodian EL: Techniques of sclerotherapy for sunburst venous blemishes, J Dermatol Surg Oncol 11:696, 1985.
71. Faria JLde and Moraes IN: Histopathology of telangiectasias associated with varicose veins, Dermatologica 127:321, 1963.
72. Biegeleisen K: Primary lower extremity telangiectasias — relationship of size to color, Angiology 38:760, 1987.
73. Schalin L: Revaluation of incompetent perforating veins: a review of all the facts and observations interpreted on account of a controversial opinion and our own results. In Tese M and Dormandy JA: Superficial and deep venous diseases of the lower limbs, Torino, Italy, 1984, Edizioni Panminerva Medica.
74. Schroth R: Venose sanerstoffsattigung bei Varicen, Arch Klin Chir 300:419, 1962.
75. Haeger KHM and Bergman I: Skin temperature of normal and varicose legs and some reflections on the etiology of varicose veins, Angiology 14:473, 1963.
76. Gins JA: Arteriovenous anastomoses and varicose veins, Arch Surg 81:299, 1960.
77. Allan JC: The micro-circulation of the skin of the normal leg, in varicose veins and in the post-thromotic syndrome, S African J Surg 10:29, 1972.
78. Dinn E and Henry M: Value of lightweight elastic tights in standing occupations, Phlebology 4:45, 1989.

79. Berg EVD et al: A new method for measuring the effective compression of medical stockings, Vasa 11:117, 1982.
80. Godin MS, Rice JC, and Kerstein MD: Effect of commercially available pantyhose on venous return in the lower extremity, J Vasc Surg 5:844, 1987.
81. Bassi GL and Stemmer R: Traitments mecaniques fonctionnels en phlebologie, Ed Piccin, 1983, Padova.
82. Hohlbaum G: Mass-order Konfektionsstrumpf? Phlebol u Proktol 11:42, 1982.
83. Ashton H: Effect of inflatable plastic splints on blood flow, Br Med J 2:1427, 1966.
84. Cornu-Thenard A: Reduction d'un edeme veineux par bas lastiques, unique ou superposes, Phlebologie 38:159, 1985.
85. Goldman MP et al: Compression in the treatment of leg telangiectasia, J Dermatol Surg Oncol 16:322, 1990.

# 7 | Mechanism of Action of Sclerotherapy

## GENERAL MECHANISM FOR PRODUCING ENDOTHELIAL DAMAGE

Sclerotherapy refers to the introduction of a foreign substance into the lumen of a vessel causing thrombosis and subsequent fibrosis (Fig. 7-1). This procedure, when performed on telangiectasias, is referred to as microsclerotherapy.[1]

The mechanism of action for sclerosing solutions is that of producing endothelial damage (endosclerosis) that eventuates in endofibrosis. The extent of damage to the blood vessel wall determines the effectiveness of the solution. Total endothelial destruction results in the exposure of subendothelial collagen fibers causing platelet aggregation, adherence, and release of platelet-related factors. This series of events initiates the intrinsic pathway of blood coagulation by activating factor XII. Ideally, sclerosing solutions should not otherwise cause activation or release of thromboplastic activity because this would initiate the extrinsic pathway of blood coagulation.

Excessive thrombosis is detrimental to the production of endofibrosis because it may lead to recanalization of the vessel and excessive intravascular and perivascular inflammation and its resulting sequelae (see Chapter 8). This can be prevented or at least minimized with postsclerotherapy compression (see Chapter 6). However, thrombosis usually does occur to some degree as a result of sclerotherapy. If a thrombus is formed, it should be well anchored to the venous wall to ensure against embolization. Wolf[2] in 1920 established that effective sclerosis results in thrombosis that penetrates the full thickness of the adventitia of the vessel wall. Schneider[3] has shown in histologic examinations of sclerosed varices that the strongest fixation of a thrombus occurs in areas where the entire endothelium is destroyed. Therefore, endothelial damage must be complete and should result in minimal thrombus formation with subsequent organization and fibrosis (Fig. 7-2). In addition, Fegan[4] has found on multiple occasions of microscopic examination of varicose veins excised after sclerotherapy that maximal full-thickness fibrosis of the treated segment occurs after 6 weeks of compression. Therefore, in addition to limiting the extent of thrombosis, compression may facilitate endofibrosis (see Chapter 6).

Endothelial damage can be provoked by a number of mechanisms such as changing the surface tension of the plasma membrane or modifying the physical/chemical milieu of the endothelial cell through a change of intravascular pH or osmolarity. The endothelium can be directly destroyed by caustic chemicals or by other physical factors such as heat and cold. For sclerotherapy to be effective without recanalization of the thrombotic vessel occurring, the endothelial damage and resulting vascular necrosis must be extensive enough to destroy the entire blood vessel wall.[5]

## CATEGORIES OF SCLEROSING SOLUTIONS

All sclerosing solutions can be placed into three broad categories based on their mechanisms for producing endothelial injury: detergent, osmotic, or chemical.

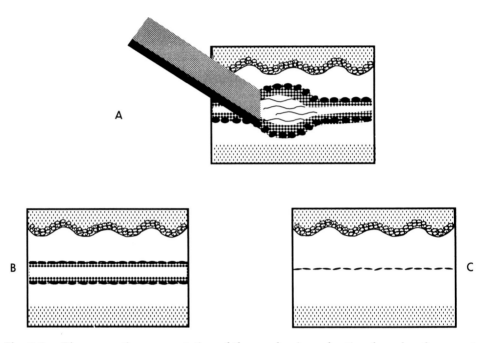

**Fig. 7-1**   Diagrammatic representation of the mechanism of action for sclerotherapy. **A,** Proper placement of needle into the vein and release of sclerosing solution. **B,** Early stage of endothelial destruction and minimal organizing thrombosis. **C,** Late stage demonstrating fibrous cord formation.

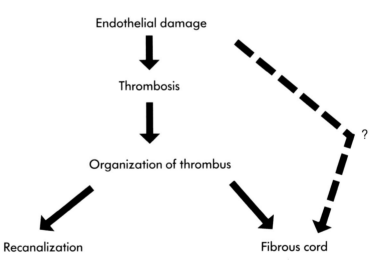

**Fig. 7-2**   Chain of events occurring after sclerotherapy. Ideally, the treated vessel will progress directly from damaged endothelium to a fibrous cord. However, some degree of intravascular thrombosis usually occurs.

## Detergent Solutions

Detergent sclerosing solutions like sodium morrhuate (SM), ethanolamine oleate (EO), sodium tetradecyl sulfate (STS), and polidocanol (POL) produce endothelial damage through interference with the cell surface lipids (Fig. 7-3). Strong detergents such as STS and SM produce maceration of the endothelium within 1 second of exposure.[6] The intercellular "cement" is disrupted resulting in desquamation of endothelial cells in plaques. Because the hydrophilic and hydrophobic poles of the detergent molecule orient themselves so that the polar hydrophilic part is within the water and the hydrophobic part is away from the water, they appear as aggregates in solution or fixed onto the endothelial surface (Fig. 7-4). Because one cannot ensure that the solution is entirely in contact with the endothelial surface, the decrease in surface tension on the endothelial cells may not

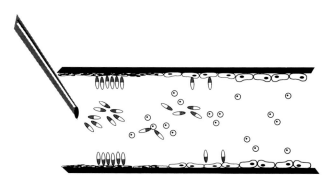

**Fig. 7-3** Diagrammatic representation of the action of a detergent sclerosing solution on the vessel wall, showing formed elements of the blood.

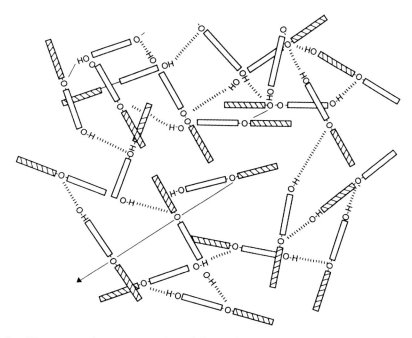

**Fig. 7-4** Diagrammatic representation of the probable molecular orientation of detergent sclerosing solutions into aggregates.

be in direct proportion to the concentration of the solution. Strong detergent sclerosants therefore have a low safety margin.[6]

Detergent sclerosing agents have also been studied regarding their direct toxic effects on the formed elements of blood. One study found that the addition of SM, EO, STS, or POL to citrated plasma did not cause clotting or shorten the prothrombin time or the partial thromboplastin time.[7] However, all of the sclerosing agents examined were directly toxic to both granulocytes and red blood cells at dilutions of up to 1:1000. When tested against cultured endothelial cells, all solutions were toxic to approximately 60% to 80% of endothelial cells at 1:100 dilutions, but only SM and EO were toxic at a further dilution of 1:1000. None of these tested solutions were toxic at 1:10,000 dilutions. Therefore, this study confirms that effective endosclerosis occurs through damage to endothelium and not through thrombosis induced by destruction or damage to red and white blood cells. Another in vitro study, however, found that activated partial thromboplastin time was prolonged in proportion to the fall of factor XII and prekallikrein activity when POL was added to citrated serum.[8] This indicates that in addition to its action on endothelial cells, POL is capable of acting on blood coagulation through activation of the early phase of the intrinsic pathway. The clinical relevance of this finding is unclear.

## Osmotic Solutions

Hypertonic solutions such as hypertonic saline (HS) probably cause dehydration of endothelial cells through osmosis resulting in endothelial destruction[8] (Fig. 7-5). It is speculated that fibrin deposition with thrombus formation on the damaged vessel wall occurs through modification of the electrostatic charge of the endothelial cells.[6] For the vessel wall to be completely destroyed, the osmotic solution must be of sufficient concentration to diffuse throughout the entire vein wall.[9] In contrast to the immediate action of detergent sclerosing solutions, experimental studies have shown that endothelial destruction with HS 22% or glucose 66% occurs only after 3 minutes.[6] The destroyed endothelial cells do not appear to be desquamated as with detergent sclerosing solutions.[6]

Hypertonic solutions have a predictable destructive power that is proportional to their osmotic concentration. This was demonstrated in a comparative study of multiple hypertonic solutions used on the superficial and internal saphenous veins of 27 dogs.[10] The degree of endothelial damage was assessed histologically at multiple times from 30 minutes to 8 weeks after sclerotherapy. The authors ranked the solutions from strongest to weakest as:

Sodium salicylate 40%
Sodium chloride 10% + sodium salicylate 30%
Invert sugar 75%
Saccharose 5%
Phenol 1%
Dextrose 66%
Sodium chloride 20%
Sodium salicylate 30%

The authors concluded that maximal endothelial destruction occurred as early as 30 minutes to 4 days after injection, after which time the injected vessel went through either a reparative or fibrotic process.

## Chemical Solutions

Chemical irritants also act directly on the endothelial cells to produce endosclerosis. Lindemayr and Santler[11] studied the sclerosing effect of 4% polyiodinated

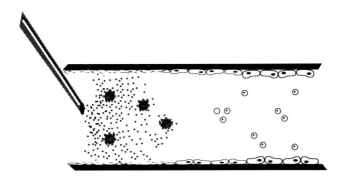

**Fig. 7-5** Diagrammatic representation of the action of a hypertonic sclerosing solution on the vessel wall, showing formed elements of the blood.

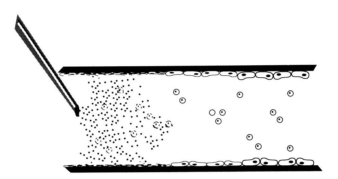

**Fig. 7-6** Diagrammatic representation of the action of a caustic chemical sclerosing solution on the vessel wall, showing formed elements of the blood.

ions (Variglobin) with standard and immunofluorescent microscopy and demonstrated fibrin deposition on the sclerosed veins only. Platelets fixed only to elastin, collagen, basement membrane, and the amorphous material of the subendothelial layer — not to intact endothelial cells. It is also thought that the chemical destruction is in part related to the dissolution of intercellular cement, which has been demonstrated to occur after 30 seconds of exposure.[6] Thus this chemical irritant sclerosing solution produces its end result of vascular fibrosis through the irreversible destruction of endothelial cells with resultant thrombus formation on the subendothelial layer (Fig. 7-6).

The aforementioned mechanism of action has also been visually demonstrated with scanning electron microscopy of sclerosed rabbit veins (agent not noted) by Merlen.[12] He demonstrated intimal cracks and fissures that left intimal connective tissue fibers and elastic lamina exposed. Ultrastructural damage involving stasis of blood and platelet aggregation on intact endothelial intima occurred in 5 minutes in the dorsal rabbit ear vein.

## FACTORS PREDISPOSING TO THROMBOSIS

As discussed previously, optimal clinical results occur when sclerotherapy-induced thrombosis is minimized. Factors predisposing to thrombus formation include decreased velocity of blood flow, hypercoagulability, and endothelial cell damage.[13] The velocity of blood flow is unaffected by the sclerosing agent itself, but flow in general is usually slower in varicose veins and telangiectasias. This relative decrease in blood flow may predispose to thrombus formation in varicose veins and may be a significant contributing factor to the increased incidence of thrombophlebitis and deep vein thrombosis (DVT) in patients with varicose veins (see Chapter 2). However, decreased blood flow probably does not play a significant role in thrombus formation after sclerosing treatment.

Hypercoagulability also predisposes one to thrombus formation. Wuppermann[14] studied fibrinolysis in subjects injected with POL and found a slight, statistically insignificant hyperfibrinolysis in blood drawn from the antecubital vein. He hypothesized that because coagulation factors II, VII, VIII, and IX and platelet function are damaged directly by the sclerosing solution, coagulation at the injection site is delayed. Endosclerosis as measured by fibrinogen gradually occurred over 5 days only at the injection site and did not result in systemic hypercoagulability. Therefore, sclerotherapy should not result in a sudden thrombosis. Earlier work had also demonstrated the lack of effect of POL on coagulation parameters in rabbits.[15] MacGowen et al.[16] combined STS with whole normal blood resulting in a homogeneous red lysate without the formation of thrombin. Therefore, experimental findings do not support the theory of intrinsic hypercoagulability of sclerosing solutions as the mechanism of action for thrombus formation during sclerotherapy.

This lack of hypercoagulability also correlates with clinical experience using POL. When POL is used in patients who are taking systemic anticoagulants, a decrease in its sclerosing action does not occur.[17] Thus it appears that the mechanism of action of POL and STS is to produce endothelial damage[18] and the resultant thrombus formation, but not thrombus formation associated with platelet aggregation. This mode of action is also seen with other (nondetergent) sclerosing agents.

## FACTORS PREDISPOSING TO ENDOFIBROSIS

Whether altered vessels are more susceptible to the action of sclerosing agents than normal vessels is unknown. At times, human varicose and telangiectatic vessels are noted to sclerose focally after the injection of various solutions. The focal nature of endothelial necrosis and thrombus formation may be related to toxic effects of the sclerosing solutions on the surrounding media. Venograms of varicose veins injected with STS demonstrate segmental, intense, and diffuse spasm, both proximally and distally, at the time of injection and 6 minutes after injection.[19] Effective endosclerosis occurs at points of vessel spasm where the entire endothelium is adherent. This agrees with the clinical impression that total compression of the sclerosed vessel is necessary for ideal, long-lasting, and complication-free sclerosis.[20,21]

At one time it was thought that "any solution which will not produce a slough when injected perivenously will generally not be strong enough to obliterate a vein."[22] However, some very effective sclerosing solutions are thought to act selectively on "damaged" varicose endothelium. In fact, experimental studies have documented that effective sclerosing solutions do not have to produce tissue necrosis on intradermal injection (see Chapter 8). The manufacturers of POL state that this agent acts selectively on damaged vessels.*,† In addition, a number of histologic studies of the effect of sclerotherapy on varicose veins have also con-

---

*Dexo SA Pharmaceuticals, France: Product description on hydroxypolyethoxydodecane, May 1985.
†Product insert for aethoxysklerol (1985) from Chemische Fabrik Kreussler & Co GmbH Wiesbaden-Biebrich, West Germany.

cluded that damaged varices are preferentially sclerosed.*[3,6,12] However, experimental injection of sclerosing agents on normal dorsal rabbit ear veins yields effective vessel sclerosis in a concentration-dependent manner.[23,24] Therefore, in addition to the type and concentration of sclerosing solution, other factors including vessel diameter, rate of blood flow, and anatomic site of the vessel may also be important.

Sclerosing solutions affect arteries in a different manner than they do veins. Although thrombosis occurs, intimal damage may not. MacGowen et al.[16] studied the local effects of intraarterial injections of STS. They injected STS 3.0% into the central auricular artery at the base of the rabbit ear and visualized the resulting chain of events through a perplex ear chamber with high-power and oil immersion lenses. Spasm was not noted in any vessels, but within minutes the erythrocytes appeared distorted and broken, with the formation of a central homogeneous thrombus that moved down the arteriole and lodged in a capillary. Intimal damage did not occur. Thus the major effect of STS was on the blood cell mass that it destroyed and converted into an intravascular embolus. Subsequent biopsy of the ears at 1 hour and 5 days demonstrated thrombus only, without evidence of intimal damage. These results are distinctly contrary to the effects of sclerosis on veins.

The reason for this different mechanism of action is unknown but may relate to the difference in velocity of blood flow in arteries and veins. Specifically, STS injected intraarterially may not have enough time to react with endothelium, being both absorbed and inactivated by formed elements in the blood and serum factors and thereby being diluted to a "safe" concentration by the more rapid arterial flow. *Safe* is a relative term since inadvertent intraarterial injections of STS have produced gangrene through thrombosis of vessels downstream of injection (see Chapter 8).

## EXPERIMENTAL EVALUATION OF SCLEROSING SOLUTIONS

Since physicians in the United States are especially limited as to the type of sclerosing solution available, an analysis of the following studies was performed to compare the efficacy of various sclerosing agents.

An important question regarding these studies is whether the experimental animal model is an appropriate system in which to compare the efficacy of various sclerosing solutions. The dorsal marginal rabbit ear vein is similar in size (0.35 to 0.45 mm diameter) to telangiectasias in humans. Reiner[25] found that it was difficult to measure the rate of dilution of sclerosing solutions in the rabbit ear vein because of the great number of collaterals and rapid blood flow caused by the thermoregulatory nature of the ear. Therefore, after injection of the solution, firm pressure for 20 seconds of occlusion on the proximal and distal aspects of the injected vein will help simulate the more sluggish blood flow of human telangiectasias.[23,24] However, study of an animal model may not produce accurate data because one is comparing the action of a sclerosing solution on a normal vessel. In addition, the injected vessels are not compressed in rabbit ear vein studies, thereby resulting in the formation of a larger thrombus, which may allow for a more rapid or increased incidence of recanalization. However, as a model, the rabbit ear vein does allow one to compare the mechanism of action of various

---

*Henschel O: Sclerosing of varicose veins sclerotherapy with aethoxysklerol-Kreussler (product booklet), produced by Chemische Fabrik Kreussler & Co GmbH, Wiesbaden-Biebrich D-6202, Postfach 9105, West Germany.

**Table  7-1**   Clinical use and relative potency of various sclerosing agents

| Relative potency | Clinical use vein diameter | Sclerosing agent | |
|---|---|---|---|
| | | **Brand** | **Percent** |
| I | <0.4 mm | Scleremo | 50 |
| | | POL | 0.25 |
| | | STS | 0.1 |
| | | Scleremo | 100 |
| | | POL | 0.5 |
| | | Variglobin | 0.1 |
| | | HS | 11.7 |
| | | SX | |
| | | EO | 2.0 |
| | | SM | 1.0 |
| II | 0.6-2 mm | STS | 0.25 |
| | | POL | 0.75 |
| | | Variglobin | 1 |
| | | HS | 23.4 |
| | | EO | 5.0 |
| | | SM | 2.5 |
| III | 3-5 mm | POL | 1-2 |
| | | STS | 0.5-1.0 |
| | | Variglobin | 2 |
| | | SM | 5 |
| IV | >5 mm | POL | 3-5 |
| | Perforator veins | STS | 1.5-3 |
| | Saphenopopliteal/ femoral junctions | Variglobin | 3-12 |

sclerosing solutions both clinically and histologically. On the basis of these studies, the physician can achieve a similar therapeutic effect in humans by varying the concentration and type of solution (Table 7-1).

In the 1920s the first studies to elucidate the mechanism of action of sclerosing agents were performed using the dorsal vein of the rabbit ear. Sclerosing agents tested included 1% bichloride of mercury,[26] 30% sodium chloride and 50% grape sugar,[27,28] 30% sodium salicylate,[29] 50% to 60% calorose,[30,31] and SM.[32,33] All of the above solutions achieved venous obliteration through endothelial cell alteration, with inflammation resulting in thrombus formation and eventual production of a fibrous cord.

## Sodium Tetradecyl Sulfate

The mechanism of sclerosis for intravascular sodium tetradecyl sulfate (STS) was elucidated by Schneider[3] and Schneider and Fischer[33] in human varicose veins, by Dietrich and Sinapius[34] in rabbit external jugular veins, and by Imhoff and Stemmer[6] in the dorsal rabbit ear vein. With STS, endothelial damage is concentration dependent and occurs immediately after injection with resulting rapid thrombus formation leading to vascular sclerosis.

In two recent studies, sclerosis with STS produced similar results in a concentration-dependent manner.[23,24] Endothelial damage occurred within 1 hour (Fig. 7-7), followed by the rapid onset of vascular thrombosis with subsequent organization (Fig. 7-8). Histologic recanalization occurred after 30 days with solution concentrations of 0.1% to 0.5% (Fig. 7-9). The histologic findings ex-

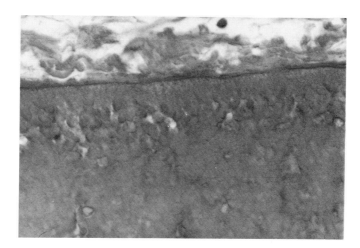

**Fig. 7-7**  Endothelial cells and the vascular wall are entirely destroyed 1 hour after injection with STS 0.5%. Hemolysis of red blood cells and early thrombosis is also present. (Hematoxylin-eosin ×200.)

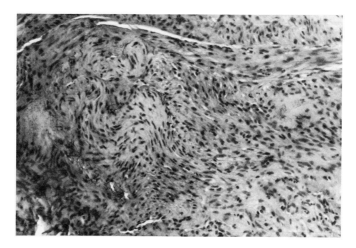

**Fig. 7-8**  Microangiopathic recanalization is apparent 14 days after injection with STS 0.5%. (Hematoxylin-eosin ×100.) (From Goldman MP et al: Arch Dermatol 123:1196, 1987.)

plained the clinical appearance that demonstrated initial thrombosis followed by partial reappearance of the vessel injected with STS 0.1% (Figs. 7-10 to 7-12).

Therefore, there may be a concentration gradient in which an ideal concentration may depend on many factors including vessel diameter, rate of blood flow, animal model, and anatomic region within each animal model.

## Polidocanol

A concentration gradient was also demonstrated in a study of polidocanol (POL) in concentrations of 0.25% to 1.0% (see Fig. 7-9).[23] Only vessels injected with POL 0.5% and 1% were clinically sclerosed, and only the vessels injected with POL 1% maintained sclerosis without revascularization by 60 days (Figs. 7-13 to 7-15; see also Fig. 7-10).

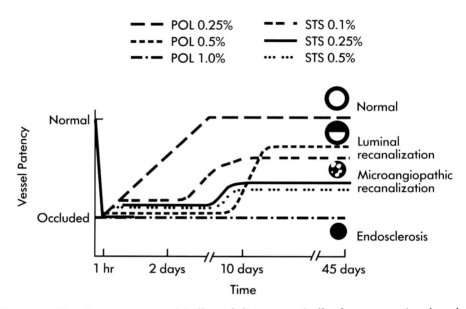

**Fig. 7-9** Vessel patency is graphically and diagrammatically shown over time based on histologic appearance of vessels from which biopsy specimens were taken in time periods previously described.

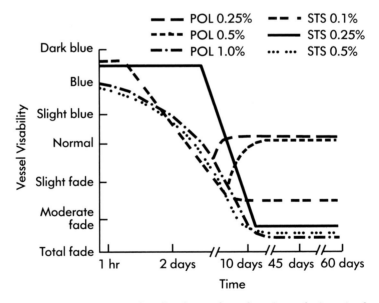

**Fig. 7-10** Vessel visibility is graphically shown for sclerosing solutions in the rabbit ear vein model.

STS 0.5%

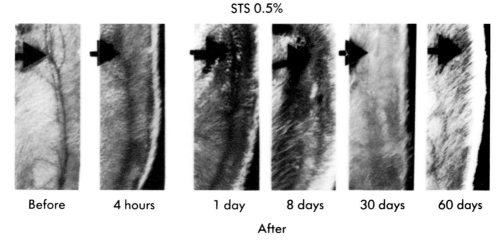

| Before | 4 hours | 1 day | 8 days | 30 days | 60 days |

After

**Fig. 7-11** Photographic composite of the dorsal ear vein injection/biopsy site before injection and 4 hours, 1 day, 8 days, 30 days, and 60 days after injection with STS 0.5%. Arrows indicate injection site. (From Goldman MP et al: Arch Dermatol 123:1196, 1987.)

STS 0.1%

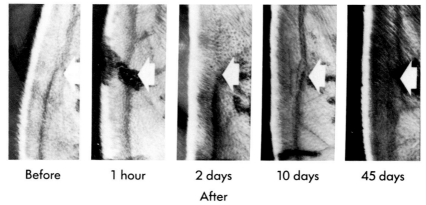

| Before | 1 hour | 2 days | 10 days | 45 days |

After

**Fig. 7-12** Photographic composite of the dorsal ear vein injection/biopsy site before injection and 1 hour, 2 days, 10 days, and 45 days after injection with STS 0.1%. Arrows indicate injection site. (From Martin DE and Goldman MP: J Dermatol Surg Oncol 16:18, 1990.)

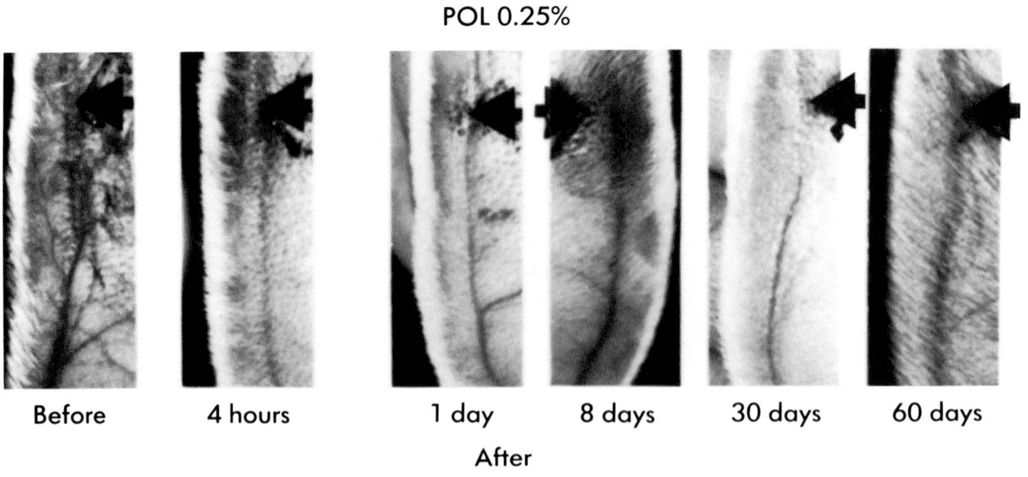

POL 0.25%

| Before | 4 hours | 1 day | 8 days | 30 days | 60 days |

After

**Fig. 7-13** Photographic composite of the dorsal ear vein injection/biopsy site before injection and 4 hours, 1 day, 8 days, 30 days, and 60 days after injection with POL 0.25%. Arrows indicate injection site.

POL 0.5%

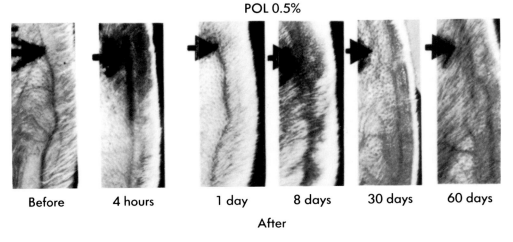

| Before | 4 hours | 1 day | 8 days | 30 days | 60 days |

After

**Fig. 7-14** Photographic composite of the dorsal ear vein injection/biopsy site before injection and 4 hours, 1 day, 8 days, 30 days, and 60 days after injection with POL 0.5%. Arrows indicate injection site.

POL 1.0%

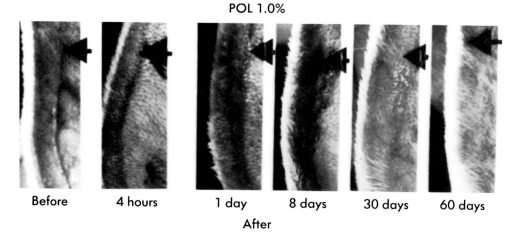

| Before | 4 hours | 1 day | 8 days | 30 days | 60 days |

After

**Fig. 7-15** Photographic composite of the dorsal ear vein injection/biopsy site before injection and 4 hours, 1 day, 8 days, 30 days, and 60 days after injection with POL 1.0%. Arrows indicate injection site.

An examination of the histologic effects of POL on the endothelium specifically between 1 hour and 4 days after injection illustrates the effect of varying the concentration of sclerosing solutions. Endothelial cells exposed to POL 0.25% were at first only partially damaged (Fig. 7-16). Mitotic figures indicating endothelial regeneration were noted 4 days after injection (Fig. 7-17). Likewise, with POL 0.5%, partial luminal recanalization occurred through an initial fibrotic cord in vessels (Fig. 7-18). Only vessels sclerosed with POL 1.0% developed complete endosclerosis (Fig. 7-19). Therefore, POL is probably a weaker detergent type of sclerosing solution than STS, and higher concentrations are necessary to produce complete vascular sclerosis.

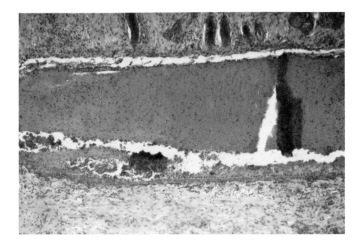

**Fig. 7-16**  Partially damaged endothelial cells with thrombosis is seen 8 hours after injection with POL 0.25% in the rabbit ear vein. (Hematoxylin-eosin ×40.)

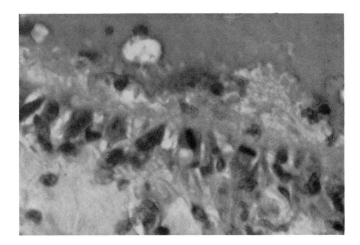

**Fig. 7-17**  Endothelial regeneration is apparent 4 days after injection with POL 0.25% in the rabbit ear vein. (Hematoxylin-eosin ×100.)

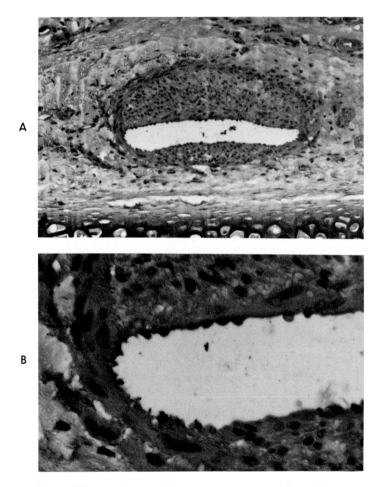

**Fig. 7-18** Advanced luminal recanalization is present 60 days after injection with POL 0.5% as seen in cross section. **A,** ×100; **B,** ×200; note endothelial lining on recanalized lumen. (Hematoxylin-eosin.) (**A** from Goldman MP et al: Arch Dermatol 123:1196, 1987.)

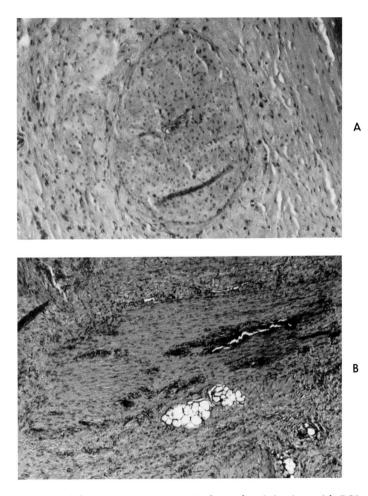

**Fig. 7-19**    Fibrous cord formation is present 30 days after injection with POL 1.0%. The darker areas within the fibrous cord represent hemosiderin-laden macrophages. **A,** Longitudinal section, ×40. **B,** Cross section, ×100. (Hematoxylin-eosin.) (**B** from Goldman MP et al: Arch Dermatol 123:1196, 1987.)

## Hypertonic Saline

The sclerosing effect of hypertonic saline (HS) was histologically examined in the external jugular vein of the dog by Kern and Angle[35] and in human varicose veins by McPheeters and Anderson.[31] These investigators noted endothelial damage with thrombus formation within 1 hour of injection, with ultimate conversion into a fibrous cord within 2 to 4 weeks (Figs. 7-20 and 7-21). This was confirmed in the rabbit ear vein model[23] both clinically (Fig. 7-22) and histologically. Examination of the marginal ear vein 1 hour after exposure to HS 23.4% demonstrated complete endothelial destruction (Fig. 7-23).

However, subsequent evaluation of HS 11.7% in the rabbit ear vein model[35a] demonstrated an immediate thrombosis that only lasted for 48 hours before complete normalization. Endothelial destruction was patchy at 1 hour with perivascular and intraluminal marginization of polymorphonuclear (PMN) cells and eosinophils (EOS). There was no evidence of extravasation of red blood cells (RBCs) in the veins injected with HS 11.7% as opposed to extravasation that was noted in 30% of vessels injected with HS 23.4%. Therefore, the degree of endothelial damage and resulting extravasation of RBCs is proportional to the concentration of HS used.

## Chromated Glycerin

The effect of chemical irritant sclerosing solutions has also been studied in the rabbit ear model.[24] Chromated glycerin (Scleremo [SCL]), 50% and 100%, was injected into the dorsal marginal rabbit ear vein producing clinical and histologic thrombosis that lasted only 2 to 8 days, after which the vessel appeared clinically and histologically normal (Fig. 7-24; see also Fig. 7-21). As noted with POL 0.25% above, the endothelium 1 hour after biopsy was almost undamaged. Therefore, in this experimental model, SCL is a weak solution with a sclerosing effect similar to POL 0.25%. This correlates well with its clinical profile.

## Hypertonic Glucose/Saline

Sclerodex* (SX), a mixture of dextrose, sodium chloride, propylene glycol, and phenethyl alcohol, has recently been studied in the rabbit ear vein model.[35a] Injection produced an immediate thrombosis that lasted for 2 days, after which the vessel recanalized (see Figs. 7-20 and 7-21). At 1 hour, perivascular and intraluminal marginization of PMNs and EOS were present with patchy endothelial destruction. Endothelial mitoses were present at 2 days within a regenerative endothelium. Extravasation of RBCs was not noted. Therefore, SX has a potency similar to HS 11.7%.

## Sodium Morrhuate

Sodium morrhuate† (SM), a mixture of sodium salts of the saturated and unsaturated fatty acids present in cod liver oil, has recently been studied in the rabbit ear vein model (Figs. 7-25 and 7-26).[35a] SM 0.5% produced no clinical evidence of endothelial damage. Temporary histologic evidence of thrombosis was noted at 1 hour only with a mild perivascular mixed cellular infiltrate (MCI). There was no evidence for extravasation of RBCs. Vessels injected with SM 1.0% were throm-

---

*Omega, Montreal, Canada.
†Scleromate, Palisades Pharmaceuticals, Inc, Tenafly, NJ.

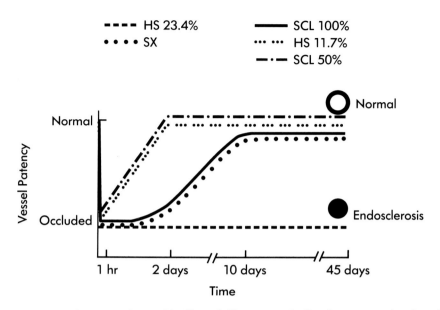

**Fig. 7-20**   Vessel patency is graphically and diagrammatically shown over time based on histologic appearance of vessels from which biopsy specimens were taken in time periods previously described. (From Goldman MP: J Dermatol Surg Oncol 17:354, 1991.)

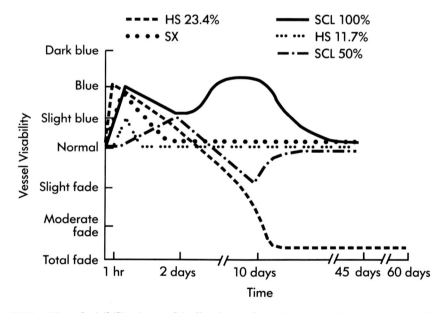

**Fig. 7-21**   Vessel visibility is graphically shown for sclerosing solutions in the rabbit ear vein model. (From Goldman MP: J Dermatol Surg Oncol 17:354, 1991.)

HS 23.4%

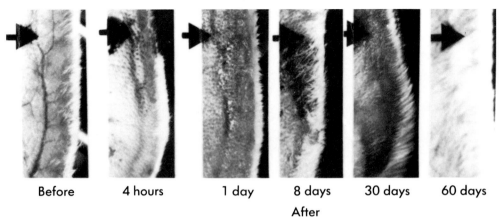

Before    4 hours    1 day    8 days    30 days    60 days

After

**Fig. 7-22**    Photographic composite of the dorsal ear vein injection/biopsy site before injection and 4 hours, 1 day, 8 days, 30 days, and 60 days after injection with HS 23.4%. Arrows indicate injection site.

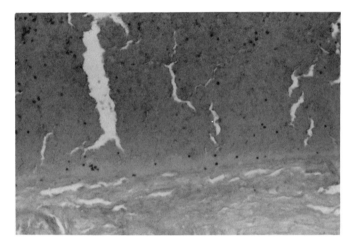

**Fig. 7-23**    The endothelial cells and vascular wall structure is completely homogenized 1 hour after injection of the rabbit ear vein with HS 23.4%. Longitudinal section, ×40. (Hematoxylin-eosin.)

Scleremo (SCL)

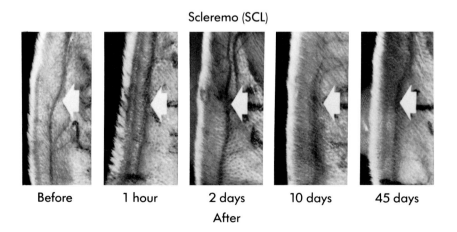

Before    1 hour    2 days    10 days    45 days

After

**Fig. 7-24**    Photographic composite of the dorsal ear vein injection/biopsy site before injection and 1 hour, 2 days, 10 days, and 45 days after injection with Scleremo 100%. Arrows indicate injection site. (From Martin DE and Goldman MP: J Dermatol Surg Oncol 16:18, 1990.)

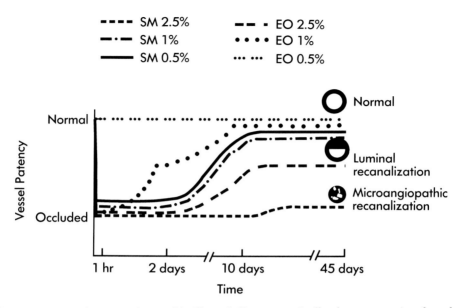

**Fig. 7-25** Vessel patency is graphically and diagrammatically shown over time based on histologic appearance of vessels from which biopsy specimens were taken in time periods previously described. (From Goldman MP: J Dermatol Surg Oncol 17:354, 1991.)

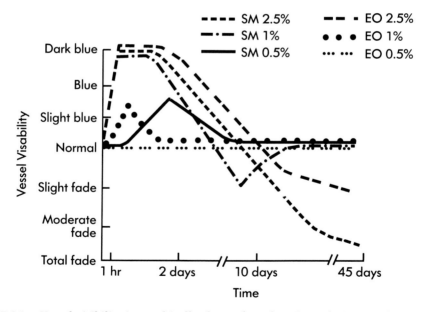

**Fig. 7-26** Vessel visibility is graphically shown for sclerosing solutions in the rabbit ear vein model. (From Goldman MP: J Dermatol Surg Oncol 17:354, 1991.)

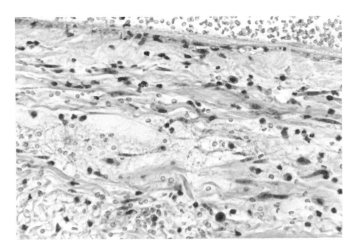

**Fig. 7-27**    Vessel 2 days after injection with SM 1%. Note large numbers of perivascular mast cells. (Hematoxylin-eosin, × 400.)

bosed between 2 and 10 days, after which the vessels normalized. Histologically, the SM 1.0% injected vessel demonstrated a partially destroyed endothelium with extravasation of RBCs. The vessels injected with SM 2.5% demonstrated clinical fibrosis with histologic evidence of microangiopathic recanalization through a fibrotic cord at 45 days after injection. A unique finding noted with injection of SM, both 1.0% and 2.5%, was the presence of large numbers of perivascular mast cells (Fig. 7-27). This finding may correlate with the increased inflammatory nature and allergenicity of SM as compared to other sclerosing solutions (see p. 210).

## Ethanolamine Oleate

Ethanolamine oleate (EO) (Ethamolin*), a synthetic mixture of ethanolamine and oleic acid, is another sclerosing solution that has recently been studied in the rabbit ear vein model (see Figs. 7-25 and 7-26).[35a] No histologic or clinical changes were noted with injection of EO 0.5%. Although an organizing thrombus was produced, complete recanalization occurred in the vessel injected with EO 1% resulting in the returned clinical appearance of the injected vessel. Vessels injected with EO 2.5% had a partially destroyed endothelium followed by luminal recanalization. Evidence of phagocytosis of lipidlike material was noted in a vessel injected with EO 2.5% at 48 hours (Fig. 7-28). This may indicate extravasation of sclerosing solution either during injection or with endothelial destruction. Large numbers of perivascular mast cells were also noted 2 days after injection with EO 1% and 2.5%. Extravasated RBCs occurred in vessels injected with EO 1% and 2.5% at 1 hour and 2 days, but not in vessels injected with EO 0.5%.

A previous study of EO as compared with STS was performed using the rat tail vein model.[35b] In this model EO 5% was compared to STS 3% and 1%. Solution measuring 0.1 ml was injected and the veins were biopsied at 4 weeks. In this study EO 5% was only effective in sclerosing 25% of the treated veins as opposed to a 73% efficacy with STS 1% and a near 100% efficacy with STS 3%. Therefore, results in the rabbit ear vein compare well to those in the rat tail vein.

*Block Drug Company; Piscataway, NJ.

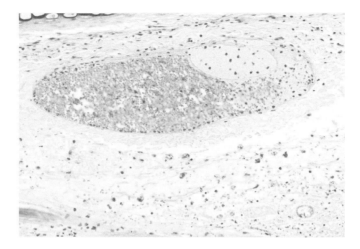

**Fig. 7-28**    Vessel 2 days after injection with EO 2.5%. Note extensive phagocytosis of lipidlike globules. (Hematoxylin-eosin, × 200.)

## Comparative Efficacy in the Animal Model

The mechanism of action for all sclerosing solutions injected into veins in these studies was basically similar, that is, endothelial damage and simultaneous thrombus formation occurred almost immediately after injection. Endothelial damage was less in the vessels injected with SCL, POL 0.25%, SX, and EO 0.5%, which showed early recanalization and a continued normal clinical appearance. POL 0.5%, SM 0.5% and 1%, EO 1%, and HS 11.7% produced endothelial attenuation, not necrosis. Although an organizing thrombus was produced, recanalization occurred resulting in the returned clinical appearance of the injected vessel. Vessels injected with STS 0.5%, SM 2.5% and EO 2.5% also demonstrated recanalization although endothelial necrosis was demonstrated. In contrast to the luminal recanalization that occurred with POL 0.5% and EO 2.5%, recanalization with STS 0.5% and SM 2.5% occurred with multiple minute vascular channels. Vessels sclerosed with STS 0.25% and 0.5% and SM 2.5% never totally reappeared clinically in the 60-day span of this study. The only vessels to histologically demonstrate fibrous cord formation that did not recanalize were sclerosed with HS 23.4% and POL 1.0%.

## Comparative Efficacy in the Human Model

In an effort to assess the effect of sclerosing agents in human leg telangiectasias, I injected 0.1 ml of either POL 0.5% or STS 0.5% into two nearly identical telangiectasias 0.4 mm in diameter over the anterior tibia in a 65-year-old man. This vessel did not have any associated "feeding" reticular veins, and there was no evidence of associated varicose veins or signs of venous insufficiency. The injected vessel was not compressed, and a biopsy of it was taken 48 hours after treatment.

The vessel injected with POL 0.5% demonstrated a blue thrombus (Fig. 7-29) that was histologically confirmed and an endothelium that was relatively intact with extensive cellular vacuolization (Fig. 7-30).

The vessel injected with STS 0.5% demonstrated a deep blue thrombus (Fig. 7-31). Histologically, the endothelium was totally destroyed, showing extensive intravascular thrombosis and early organization (Fig. 7-32). Therefore, this limited human study correlates with the above-mentioned studies on the marginal rabbit ear vein demonstrating that STS is a stronger sclerosing agent than POL.

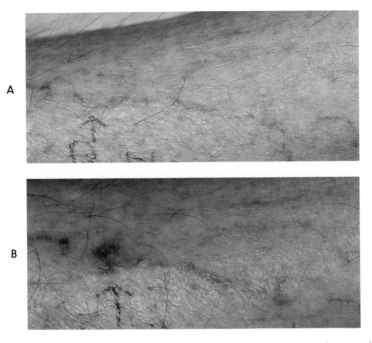

**Fig. 7-29** Anterior tibial telangiectasia. **A**, Before treatment. **B**, 48 hours after injection with POL 0.5%.

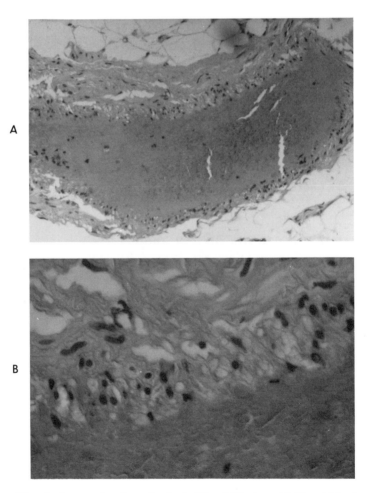

**Fig. 7-30** Histologic examination of vein in Fig. 7-27. **A**, ×40. **B**, ×100; shows endothelial cell vacuolization with thrombosis. (Hematoxylin-eosin.)

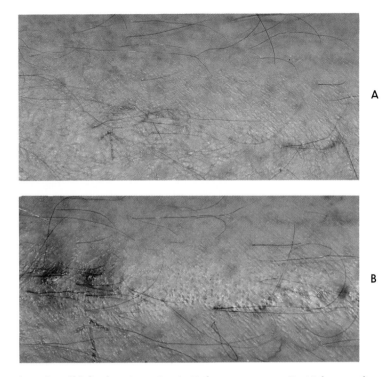

**Fig. 7-31** Anterior tibial telangiectasia. **A,** Before treatment. **B,** 48 hours after injection with STS 0.5%.

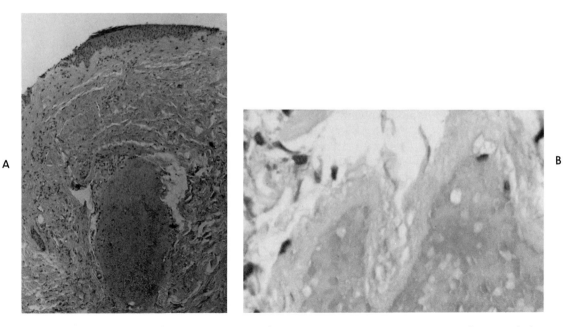

**Fig. 7-32** Histologic examination of vein in Fig. 7-31. **A,** ×40. **B,** ×100; shows endothelial cell homogenization/necrosis with thrombosis. (Hematoxylin-eosin.)

## CLINICAL USE OF SCLEROSING AGENTS

The only sclerosing agents approved for use in the United States by the Food and Drug Administration (FDA) are sodium morrhuate (SM), ethanolamine oleate (EO), and sodium tetradecyl sulfate (STS). All of these agents were approved for use before 1950 and thus have never been subjected to the rigorous toxicity and efficacy studies that would be required by the FDA today. Hypertonic saline (HS) in a 23.4% concentration is available and approved for use as an abortifacient. However, it is commonly used in various concentrations with and without the addition of heparin, procaine, or lidocaine for sclerosis of telangiectasias and superficial varicosities. POL, widely used in the United States today, was introduced in this country by D. Duffy and P. Goldman in 1984. Sclerodex (SX), a solution of dextrose 5% and sodium chloride 10%, is commonly used in Canada for sclerosis of superficial varicosities and telangiectasias. Chromated glycerin (Scleremo [SCL]) is perhaps the most widely used sclerosing agent worldwide for the treatment of leg telangiectasias. It has been popularized in the English literature recently by Ouvry.[36] Polyiodinated iodine (Variglobin) is the most powerful sclerosing agent and is commonly used outside of the United States for sclerotherapy of the saphenofemoral junction. It is not yet approved for use by the FDA in the United States but will be discussed because of its importance in sclerotherapy. Another solution commonly used outside of the United States, sodium salicylate, is not widely used or available here and will not be discussed. The remainder of this chapter reviews the specific advantages and disadvantages of sclerosing agents commonly used in the United States.

## Osmotic Agents

### Hypertonic saline

Hypertonic saline (HS) was first used to sclerose varicose veins by Linser[6] in 1926 and Kern and Angle[35] in 1929. With the advent of more effective synthetic detergent sclerosing solutions in the 1940s, its use declined. Renewed interest in its use occurred in the 1970s, spurred on by numerous publications in the dermatology literature and multiple lectures on its use presented at major meetings.

*Advantage.* Part of the currently experienced popularity stems from the lack of allergenicity of unadulterated HS solution compared with the exaggerated claims of allergenicity associated with all other sclerosing agents. However, HS is not without significant adverse sequelae.

*Disadvantages.* Unlike detergent sclerosing solutions, all hypertonic solutions act nonspecifically to destroy all cells (including red blood cells) within its osmotic gradient. Osmotic agents damage cellular tissues and readily produce ulceration if injected extravascularly or if it diffuses through the vessel extravascularly (see Chapter 8). Therefore, injection technique is critically important when using this sclerosing agent.

Because HS diffuses to some extent through the blood vessel wall, the nerves in the adventitia of the vein may be stimulated causing pain (see Chapter 3). This diffusion may also lead to transient muscle cramping. Hemolysis of red blood cells occurs via hyperosmosis resulting in the release of hemosiderin, which may readily diffuse across the damaged endothelium. This may lead to posttreatment hyperpigmentation. Finally, because osmotic agents are rapidly diluted in the bloodstream, they lose their potency within a short distance of injection. Thus these agents are only rarely effective in treating veins larger than 3 to 4 mm in diameter.

***Modification of the solution and the technique.*** Various modifications of the HS solutions have been made in an effort to increase the efficacy and decrease the pain of injection and other adverse sequelae. In 1975 Foley[37] described the microinjection of "venous blemishes" with a 30-gauge needle using 20% hypertonic saline, 100 U/ml of heparin, and 1% procaine, which he patented as Heparsal. He reported no allergic or anaphylactic reactions and only rare pigmentary problems in over 1000 treatments to more than 100 patients. Foley theorized that the addition of heparin helped to prevent thrombi in larger vessels, and the addition of procaine helped alleviate the pain on injection. Recently, Sadick,[38] in a randomized, blinded 800-patient study, found that the addition of heparin to HS provided no benefit in the treatment of varicose and telangiectatic veins. Bodian,[39,40] because of results of a clinical comparison, also does not believe that the addition of heparin is necessary for effective sclerosis. Finally, it has been demonstrated that the addition of heparin to the culture medium enhances proliferation and increases the life span of endothelial cells.[41] Therefore, its use may be counterproductive.

A number of modifications in injection technique have also been made to limit the unpleasant side effects of HS. Bodian has found that muscle cramps occurring at the site of injection last 3 to 5 minutes and are relieved with gentle massage or ambulation. To limit the risk of extravasation, he recommends injecting a small air bolus before injecting 0.5 to 1 ml of HS to ensure undiluted contact of the HS with the intima to produce maximal irritation of the vessel. He believes that hemolysis caused by the sclerosing solution may lead to or exacerbate hemosiderin staining and thus should be lessened by the prior injection of air, which washes out the red blood cells from the vessel.[42] Finally, regarding the possible exacerbation of hypertension with injection of a large sodium bolus, he states that 1.0 g of sodium chloride injected during a "long treatment session" (5 ml of a 20% HS solution) is well tolerated.

Alderman[43] was the first to advocate dilution of the HS solution to better adjust the osmotic damage to the caliber of the vessel. From his experience with 150 patients with telangiectasias treated over 8 years with 18% to 30% HS, he recommends the following HS concentrations for sclerosis of varicose and telangiectatic veins: 18% to 20% HS for "venous telangiectasias" (blue telangiectasias), 22% to 25% HS for "arterial lesions" (red telangiectasias), and 30% HS for rare large "arterial" lesions. He dilutes the saline with lidocaine to achieve a 0.4% concentration of lidocaine. Tissue necrosis was not noted. The only adverse side effects reported were mild, temporary burning at injection and residual brownish pigmentation that occurred in up to one third of patients. The pigmentation usually resolved, for the most part, over 1 year.

### Hypertonic glucose/saline

Sclerodex* is a mixture of dextrose 250 mg/ml, sodium chloride 100 mg/ml, propylene glycol 100 mg/ml, and phenethyl alcohol 8 mg/ml (as a local anesthetic/preservative) at a pH of 5.9, mainly used in Canada for sclerosis of telangiectasias and small-diameter superficial varicosities.[44] It is essentially a hypertonic solution with a mechanism of action similar to HS. The manufacturer states that the sodium chloride reinforces the sclerosing potency of dextrose.

The manufacturer of Sclerodex recommends that the maximum quantity that should be injected during one visit is 10 ml in divided doses, with a 5-cm interval

*Omega; Montreal, Canada.

between each site of injection.* (The maximum recommended amount to be injected at any one site is 1 ml.) The average dose per treated vein varies between 1 ml in the upper thigh and 0.1 ml in the lower leg. The reason for these recommended doses by the manufacturer is unclear.

*Advantage.* The addition of dextrose allows for a reduction of the concentration of sodium chloride, thereby minimizing the pain and local discomfort that would occur with injection of sodium chloride alone.* However, it is probably the decrease in osmolarity relative to 23.4% HS that allows Sclerodex to produce less pain and muscle cramping.

*Disadvantages.* Despite its lower osmolarity, like HS, it is slightly painful for the patient on injection.[45] Superficial necrosis may occur rarely, with an incidence less than HS.*[44,46] I have noted postsclerosis pigmentation to occur with a frequency similar to that of other sclerosing agents although Mantse[46] notes a decreased incidence of complications with Sclerodex as compared with POL and STS.

Another disadvantage to its use is that the solution becomes sticky in the syringe when blood is withdrawn to ensure an intravenous position. Unfortunately, unlike unadulterated HS, allergic reactions may occur to the phenethyl alcohol component of the solution.* Mantse[44] notes one allergic reaction in 500 patients treated with Sclerodex, for an incidence of 0.2%.

## Chemical Irritants
### Chromated glycerin

Chromated glycerin 72% (Scleremo† [SCL]) is a sclerosing solution that is increasing in popularity in Europe, whereas clinical experience in the United States remains limited. It is distributed in a 5-ml ampule with the maximum recommended amount per injection session being 10 ml of pure solution. Concentrations of 25% to 100% have been used.†[47] Its clinical efficacy has been shown to be dose dependent. SCL, although not approved by the FDA, is the most widely used sclerosing agent for leg telangiectasias in the world; 500,000 vials were sold in 1986.†

The glycerin component of SCL is rapidly absorbed by the intestine and transformed into carbon dioxide or glycogen or is directly used for the synthesis of fatty acids.[48] Therefore, this solution must be used with caution in diabetic patients. One case of reactive hypoglycemia to an infusion of glycogen occurred in a child resulting in a comatose state within 4 minutes of infusion.[49]

The sclerosing quality of glycerin was first studied in 1925 by Jausion, Carrot, and Ervais[50] who found that it induced a mild rapid and complete endosclerosis. Isosmotic glycerol (2.6% m/v) produces 100% hemolysis in 45 minutes.[48,51] However, a review of 500 patients who received glycerol intravenously (at 50 g/500 ml) 6 hours a day for 7 to 10 days demonstrated hemoglobinuria in less than 1% of patients.[52]

The chromium alum component of SCL is a potent coagulating factor that increases the sclerosing power of glycerin. It also prevents somewhat the mild hematuria induced through the use of glycerin alone.[48,53,54]

---

*Correspondence (1986) received from Laboratoire Ondee Ltee; 280 Milice Longueuil; Montreal, Canada.

†Scleremo product information (1987) from Laboratories E. Bouteille; 7 rue des Belges; Limoges 8100, France.

*Advantages.* The relatively weak sclerosing power of SCL corresponds to its promotion as a mild sclerosing solution with more versatile usage and low incidence of side effects. Pigmentation and cutaneous necrosis are exceedingly rare at recommended dosages, and minimal extravascular injection causes only a small temporary ecchymosis without any cutaneous damage.[55,56] Reportedly, the incidence of adverse sequelae is very low.*[24,47]

*Disadvantages.* The disadvantages of SCL include its high viscosity and local pain at injection.[57,58] Both of these drawbacks can be partially overcome by dilution with lidocaine. Hypersensitivity is a very rare complication.[59,60] Hematuria accompanied by ureteral colic can occur transiently after injection of large doses. Ocular manifestations, including blurred vision and a partial visual field loss, have been reported by a single author with resolution in less than 2 hours.[61] These latter two complications may be a result of excessive nonspecific destruction of red blood cells.

### Polyiodinated iodine

Polyiodinated iodine† (Variglobin, Sclerodine) is a stabilized water solution of iodide ions, sodium iodine, and benzyl alcohol. The solution was invented by Imhoff and first used by Sigg in Switzerland in 1958. Others had reported on the use of iodine solutions in sclerotherapy before; however, stabilization of the mixture by Imhoff produced a standardized solution that could be easily obtained. The active sclerosing ingredient is elemental iodine. Sodium and potassium help to make it water soluble. Benzyl alcohol is added as a preservative/stabilizer. Variglobin is available in concentrations of 2%, 4%, 8%, and 12% as a dark-brown solution contained in brown glass vials.

Wenner[62] states that it should only be used in the manufactured concentrations because dilution may allow the chemical effect to propagate away from the injection site. However, others mix it with normal saline or Sclerodex.‡ Raymond-Martimbeu[63] claims that the addition of Sclerodex to the solution potentiates the action and causes a more localized destruction with less risk of diffusion of the sclerosing solution. Mixing with ethanol has been advocated by Wenner[62] to increase the sclerosing potency.[62] Wenner believes that the addition of ethanol delays inactivation of the solution by blood proteins in addition to increasing the potentiating action of ethanol, which directly damages the lipoprotein component of the endothelial surface. He recommends the addition of 50% ethanol to an equal amount of Variglobin 12%. The amount of ethanol injected is likened to a "large glass of wine."

Omega Laboratories recommends that concentrations of 0.15% are optimal to sclerose telangiectasia and recommends 6% to sclerose truncal varicose veins. They recommend injection of 2 ml of a 3% solution into the proximal "internal saphena" and 0.5 ml of a 0.5% solution into the ankle "internal and external saphena." The maximum quantity that can be injected in a single session is 3 ml of a 6% solution.‡ Kreussler Pharma§ recommends the following concentrations: 4%, 8%, or 12% for injection to the saphenofemoral junction, 4% for the saphe-

---

*Sclermo product information (1987) from Laboratories E. Bouteille, 7 rue des Belges, Limoges 8100, France.
†Varigloban (Chemische Fabrik Kreussler & Co, Wiesbaden-Biebrich, West Germany); Variglobin (Globopharm, Switzerland); Sclerodine (Omega, Montreal, Canada).
‡Product information on Sclerodine 6 (1989) from Omega; Montreal, Canada.
§Product information (June 1987) from Kreussler Pharma; Wiesbaden 12, D-6200, West Germany.

nopopliteal junction, 4% to 8% for perforating veins and varicosities greater than 8 mm in diameter, 2% to 4% for varicose veins 4 to 8 mm in diameter, and 2% for varicose veins 2 to 4 mm in diameter. They do not recommend its use in smaller veins.

*Advantage.* The sclerosing effect of Variglobin is based on the direct destruction of the endothelium. It destroys the entire vessel wall through diffusion at the point of injection. It is very short acting because it is neutralized within a few seconds by binding to different blood components, especially proteins.[62] Variglobin is primarily used for large varicosities including the saphenofemoral junction. Sigg[64] performed over 400,000 injections with Variglobin.

*Disadvantage.* Paravenous injections will readily produce tissue necrosis; therefore, its injection should be performed with utmost care. Sigg, Horodegen, and Bernbach[64] and Sigg and Zelikovski[65] never used more than 0.5 ml per injection. Fortunately, Variglobin is painful when injected outside a vein so that improper injection technique is immediately apparent. To prevent nonspecific damage, the concentration, not the volume of solution, is increased to enhance the sclerosing power.

## Detergent Sclerosing Solutions
### Sodium morrhuate

Sodium morrhuate (SM) is a mixture of sodium salts of the saturated and unsaturated fatty acids present in cod-liver oil (see box below). It is prepared by the saponification of selected cod-liver oils. Each milliliter contains morrhuate sodium, 50 mg; benzyl alcohol 2% (as a local anesthetic); water for injection (as much as will suffice); the pH is adjusted to about 9.5 with hydrochloric acid and/or sodium hydroxide. It is available as a 5% concentration that can be diluted with normal saline to the appropriate concentration for the vessel to be treated.

SM was first prepared for injection by Ghosh[66] or Cutting.[67] This sclerosing agent was met with much enthusiasm in the United States by Biegeleisen[32] and others. However, extensive cutaneous necrosis occurs when it is inadvertently injected perivascularly. Many cases of anaphylactic reactions within a few minutes after injection have been reported. More commonly, these reactions occur when therapy is reinstituted after a few weeks. Anaphylaxis has resulted in fatalities,

**FATTY ACID COMPOSITION OF SODIUM MORRHUATE**

| | |
|---|---|
| Linoleic acid | 28.2% |
| Unknown | 20.8% |
| Eicosadienoic acid | 15.5% |
| Palmitoleic acid | 12.1% |
| Arachidonic acid | 8.2% |
| Palmitic acid | 8.1% |
| Myristic acid | 4.2% |
| Oleic acid | 1.8% |
| Stearic acid | 1.1% |

From Monroe P et al: Acute respiratory failure after sodium morrhuate esophageal sclerotherapy, Gastroenterology 85:693, 1983.

albeit rarely (see Chapter 8). SM is approved by the FDA for sclerosis of varicose veins. However, because of its extremely caustic nature, it is not recommended for use as a sclerosing agent for telangiectasias.

### Ethanolamine oleate

Ethanolamine oleate (EO) (Ethamolin) is a synthetic mixture of ethanolamine and oleic acid with an empirical formula of $C_{20}$-$H_{41}$-$NO_3$. It is available as a 5% aqueous solution containing approximately 50 mg ethanolamine oleate per milliliter. Benzyl alcohol, 2% by volume, is used as a preservative. The pH ranges from 8.0 to 9.0. The minimum lethal intravenous dose in rabbits is 130 mg/kg.[68] The oleic acid component is responsible for the inflammatory action. Oleic acid may also activate coagulation in vitro by release of tissue factors and Hageman factor XII.

*Advantage.* EO was first reported to be an ideal sclerosing agent by Biegeleisen[69] in the medical literature in 1937. No toxic effects were noted in 500 injections. EO is thought to have a decreased risk of allergic reactions compared with SM or STS.[70] However, pulmonary toxicity has been associated with this sclerosing agent (see Chapter 8).

The sclerosing action is thought to be related to a dose-dependent extravascular inflammatory reaction caused by diffusion of EO through the venous wall.* Autopsy findings regarding its use in esophageal varix injection demonstrated that variceal obliteration occurred as a result of mural necrosis followed by fibrosis and that thrombosis was a transient phenomenon.[71,72]

*Disadvantage.* Some degree of nonspecific red blood cell hemolysis may also occur with its use. A hemolytic reaction occurred in 5 of 900 patients with injection of over 12 ml of 0.5% EO per patient per treatment session.[73] Acute renal failure with spontaneous recovery followed injection of 15 to 20 ml of Ethamolin in two women.† The patients were described as "feeling generally unwell and shivery, with aching in the loins and passage of red-brown urine. All rapidly recovered with bed-rest and were perfectly normal the next day." Injections of less than 12 ml per treatment session did not result in this reaction.

### Sodium tetradecyl sulfate

Sodium tetradecyl sulfate‡ (STS) is a synthetic, surface-active substance first described by Reiner[25] in 1946. It is composed of sodium 1-isobutyl-4-ethyloctyl sulfate plus benzoyl alcohol 2% (as an anesthetic agent) and phosphate buffered to a pH of 7.6. It is recommended that solutions be protected from light. It is a long-chain fatty acid salt of an alkali metal with properties of a soap. The solution is clear, nonviscid, has a low surface tension, and is readily miscible with blood leading to a uniform distribution after injection.[74] It primarily acts on the endothelium of the vein because if diluted with blood, the molecules attach to the surface of red blood cells causing hemolysis. The recommended maximal dosage suggested by the British manufacturer in a treatment session is 4 ml of a 3% solution.§ The recommended maximum dosage by the United States and Canadian

---

*Product information (1989) from Glaxo Pharmaceuticals; Research Triangle Park, NC. (Ethanolamine now available from Block Drug Company, Piscataway, NJ.)

†Ethanolamin injection, 5%; product information (Dec 1988) from Glaxo Pharmaceuticals Inc.

‡Sotradecol (Elkins Sinn; Cherry Hill, NJ); S.T.D. Injection (S.T.D. Pharmaceuticals; Hereford, England); Tromboject (Omego; Montreal, Canada). Products Ltd.

§S.T.D. Injection product data sheet (1977) from S.T.D. Pharmaceuticals Products Ltd., Hereford, England.

manufacturers is 10 ml of a 3% solution with intervals between treatments of 5 to 7 days.*

It should not be mixed with other anesthetic solutions because it will become turbid and form a new compound.[75] About 60% to 70% of the sclerosing "activity" of this compound is undiluted STS.

It is available as a 1% or 3% solution that can be diluted with sterile water or normal saline to achieve an appropriate therapeutic concentration. The Canadian manufacturer recommends dilution with phosphate-buffered saline to preserve the original pH level.* It is limpid and does not stick to the syringe cylinder when blood is withdrawn to ensure accurate needle placement. Concentrations of 0.1% to 0.3% are commonly used for the treatment of telangiectatic veins 0.2 to 1.0 mm in diameter; 0.5% to 1% for the treatment of uncomplicated varicose veins 2 to 4 mm in diameter; and 1.5% to 3% for the treatment of larger varicose veins, incompetent perforating veins, or an incompetent saphenofemoral junction.

*Advantages.* STS became widely used in the 1950s after its introduction by Reiner.[25] Tretbar[76] in 1978 first reported the injection of a 1% solution into spider angiomata. He noted excellent results in virtually all 144 patients treated. He also noted an unspecified number of episodes of epidermal necrosis without significant sequelae and a 30% incidence of postsclerosis pigmentation that resolved within a few months.

Shields and Jansen[77] in 1982 were first to describe microsclerosis of telangiectasias with STS in the dermatologic literature. They injected STS 1% in 105 patients and reported only 1 episode of necrosis in over 600 treatments in vessels less than 5 mm in diameter. There were no systemic reactions, and the majority of postsclerosis pigmentary changes resolved in 3 to 4 months. However, as more experience with its use in the treatment of leg telangiectasias occurred, even further dilutions (0.1% to 0.3%) were recommended both to achieve clinical efficacy and to limit adverse sequelae (see Chapter 11).

*Disadvantages.* STS, approved for use by the FDA for vein sclerosis, also has a number of disadvantages. Epidermal necrosis frequently occurs with concentrations higher than the above-mentioned recommendations; even when extravasation does not occur, allergic reactions may occur, and postsclerotherapy hyperpigmentation is frequent (see Chapter 8). Therefore, its dilution is critical. The above-mentioned percentages per diameter of treated vein provide only a preliminary guide for effective treatment. In addition, the Canadian manufacturer recommends that as a precaution against anaphylactic shock, 0.3 ml of a 1% solution should be injected into the varicosity, and then the patient should be observed for several hours before proceeding with further injections.* The reason for this recommendation is unclear; it is discussed further in Chapter 8.

### Polidocanol

Polidocanol† (POL) is composed of hydroxypolyethoxydodecane dissolved in distilled water to which ethyl alcohol is added to a concentration of 5% to ensure heat stability. Thus 1 ml of POL contains 50 mg of ethyl alcohol. One brand,

---

*Tromboject product information (rev 10/87) from Omega; Montreal, Canada.
†Brand names: Aetoxisclerol (Laboratories Pharmaceutiques Dexo; Nanterre, France); Aethoxysklerol (Chemische Fabrik Kreussler & Co GmbH; Wiesbaden-Biebrich, West Germany); Sclerovein (Resinag AG; Zurich, Switzerland); Etoxisclerol (Bama; Spain); Sotrauarix (Belg; Switzerland); Laureth 9 (U.S.A.N.).

**Table** 7-2    Maximum daily doses of polidocanol

| Concentration of POL | Dose (ml) according to body weight of patient | | | | |
|---|---|---|---|---|---|
| | **50 kg** | **60 kg** | **70 kg** | **80 kg** | **90 kg** |
| 0.5% | 20 ml | 24 ml | 28 ml | 32 ml | 36 ml |
| 1.0% | 10 ml | 12 ml | 14 ml | 16 ml | 18 ml |
| 2.0% | 5 ml | 6 ml | 7 ml | 8 ml | 9 ml |
| 3.0% | 3.3 ml | 4 ml | 4.6 ml | 5.3 ml | 6 ml |

From Kreussler & Co GmbH: Product insert for Aethoxysklerol, Wiesbaden-Biebrich, West Germany, 1985, Chemische Fabrik.

Aethoxysklerol forte 4% is available in Europe. This product contains 50% ethyl alcohol to increase the sclerosing potency. Therefore, patients taking disulfiram (Antabuse*) should be warned about a possible alcohol-disulfiram reaction. Sclerovein contains chlorobutanolum as a preservative, 0.5 g/100 ml.

POL was synthesized by (BASF) and introduced in 1936 as a local and topical anesthetic under the trade name Sch 600. Unlike the two main groups of local anesthetics, esters (procaine, benzocaine, and tetracaine) and the amides (lidocaine, prilocaine, mepivacaine, procainamide, and dibucaine), POL is a urethane (compounds with an $-NHCO_2-$ linkage). The anesthetic effect is not a direct function of its concentration but is optimum at a concentration of between 3% and 4%.† The maximum daily dose recommended by Kreussler Pharma is found in Table 7-2. Blenkinsopp[78] recommends a maximum daily dosage of 10 ml of a POL 6% solution for an average person based on toxicity experiments extrapolated from rats. However, rats are much less sensitive to POL. Since the lethal dose in 50% of the population ($LD_{50}$) in rabbits and dogs is approximately 11.7 mg/kg, Blenkinsopp's minimal dose is highly toxic.[79]

POL is unique among local anesthetics in its lack of an aromatic ring. The actual active substance is the topical anesthetic agent polidocanol, an aliphatic molecule composed of a hydrophilic chain of polyethylene glycolic ether and a liposoluble radical of dodecylic alcohol. It is used as a topical anesthetic agent in ointments and lotions for mucous membranes including hemorrhoidal treatment.[80] It is also used as a local anesthetic for skin irritation, burns, and insect bites and as an epidural anesthetic.[81-83] The subcutaneous anesthetic effect of a 0.4% solution is equal to a 2% solution of novocaine.[81] The $LD_{50}$ in rabbits at 2 hours is 0.2 g/kg, which is three to six times greater than the $LD_{50}$ for novocaine.[82] The $LD_{50}$ in mice is 1.2 g/kg.[87] The systemic toxicity was similar to procaine and lidocaine.[84] Thus POL was considered an ideal local anesthetic. However, it soon became apparent that intravascular and intradermal instillation produced sclerosis of small diameter blood vessels and "moderate, clinically unimportant reversible damage to healthy tissue."† Therefore, compound Sch 600 was considered for use as a sclerosing agent. The polidocanol preparation Aethoxysklerol was registered at the German health authority, the Burdesgesundheitsaunt, in 1967.[83]

---

*Wyeth-Ayerst Laboratories, New York, NY.

†Henschel O: Sclerosing of varicose veins sclerotherapy with aethoxysklerol-Kreussler (product booklet), Chemische Fabrik Kreussler & Co GmbH, Wiesbaden-Biebrich D-6202, Postfach 9105, West Germany.

Experimental evaluation of absorption, distribution, metabolism, and excretion of POL has been studied in dogs, rats, and humans.[83] POL is rapidly distributed throughout the body within minutes of injection.[83] The compound is rapidly metabolized and eliminated, having a terminal elimination half-life of 1.4 to 1.7 hours. After 72 hours, 97% of the administered compound is excreted (61% in urine, 37% in feces).

In humans the elimination half-life is 4 hours, with 89% of the dose eliminated from the blood within 12 hours. Amounts excreted in the urine and feces are equal, and almost 80% of the injected compound is excreted via respiration through a breakdown into low molecular weight products. POL is completely eliminated from body organs whether patient receives one dose or repeated doses. Therefore, no accumulation takes place. Polidocanol also does not cross the blood-brain barrier.[83]

The capacity of POL to cross the placental barrier was investigated in rats. Of radioactivity from labeled POL, 15% to 87% was recovered from fetal tissue.[83]

POL belongs to the class of detergent sclerosing solutions that are nonionic compounds. It consists of an apolar hydrophobic part, dodecyl alcohol, and a polar hydrophilic part, polyethylene-oxide chain, which is esterified (Fig. 7-33). In solution POL is associated as macromolecules through electrostatic hydrogen bonding between the H− atom of the OH− group in one molecule, and the free electron-pair of an O− atom of a second molecule. This bonding results in the formation of a network (see Fig. 7-4). The sclerotherapeutic activity results from this double hydrophobic and hydrophilic action, and thus POL is a "detergent." The optimal efficacy of the compound coincides with the highest concentration that still permits the existence of nonaggregated molecules, 3%.*

Telangiectasias are treated with concentrations of 0.25% to 0.75%. Recently a randomized study determined that a 0.5% concentration may be ideal for sclerosis of leg telangiectasia.[85] Varicose veins are treated with concentrations of 1% to 5%. Small vessels and telangiectasias respond well. Efficacy is decreased in the treatment of large or medium-sized varicose veins. Kreussler Pharma† recommends the use of POL forte (4%) for treatment of the saphenofemoral and saphenopopliteal junctions, perforating veins, and varicosities greater than 8 mm in diameter. POL 3% is recommended for varicose veins 4 to 8 mm in diameter. Pol 2% is recommended for varicose veins 2 to 4 mm in diameter and 1% solution for veins 1 to 2 mm in diameter. The concentration of solution for telangiectasia ranges from 0.5% to 1%.

***Advantages.*** The safety and efficacy of this agent is such that a derivative of POL, polyoxyethylene dodecanol, was developed by the Vick Chemical Company in the 1950s as a mucolytic wetting agent for use in vaporizers.[86] Toxicity studies on rats demonstrated a lack of sensitization to cutaneous application and no toxicity with oral ingestion or with exposure to steaming electric vaporizers. A clinical study carried out on 168 infants and children treated with this compound in vaporizers showed no harmful effects.[87]

Henschel‡ states that the selective activity on damaged endothelium results from the steric structure of POL. "The macromolecules retard the individual mol-

*Dexo SA Pharmaceuticals, France: Product description on hydroxypolyethoxydodecane. Received with correspondence, May 1985.
†Product information (June 1987) from Kreussler Pharma, Wiesbaden 12, D-6200, West Germany.
‡Henschel O: Sclerosing of varicose veins sclerotherapy with Aethoxysklerol-Kreussler (product booklet), Chemische Fabrik Kreussler & Co GmbH, Wiesbaden-Biebrich D-6202, Postfach 9105, West Germany.

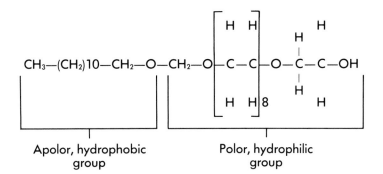

**Fig. 7-33** Structural formula of polidocanol.

ecules and thus shield the tissue from their uninhibited action." This damage is therefore said to be reversible in normal tissue. Henschel goes on to claim that since the surface-active–induced absorption on the varix wall is greatest at the point of injection and falls off rapidly with increasing distance, large quantities can be injected without danger of damage to the deep venous system. He recommends the injection of a maximum of 2 ml of POL 3% at each site with a maximum of 6 ml POL 3% injected in one sclerotherapy session. However, Goldman et al.[23] have demonstrated that POL will sclerose normal vessels (rabbit ear vein) and that the concentration injected is critical to the final outcome of vein sclerosis. POL is a weaker detergent-type sclerosing solution than STS. These experimental studies indicate that its sclerosing power is about 50% of the strength of STS.

POL is unique among sclerosing agents in that it is both painless to inject and will not produce cutaneous ulcerations even with intradermal injection (see Chapter 8). Allergic reactions have only rarely been reported. The degree of pigmentation produced may be less than that of other detergent sclerosing agents (see Chapter 8).

**REFERENCES**

1. Green D: Compression sclerotherapy techniques, Dermatol Clin 7:137, 1989.
2. Wolf E: Die histologischen Veranderungen der venen nach intravenosen sub limatein Spritzungen, Med Klin 16:806, 1920.
3. Schneider W: Contribution to the history of the sclerosing treatment of varices and to its anatomo-pathologic study, Soc Fran Phlebol 18:117, 1965.
4. Fegan WG: Varicose veins: compression sclerotherapy, London, 1967, Heinemann Medical.
5. Hanschell HM: Treatment of varicose veins, Br Med J 2:630, 1947.
6. Imhoff E and Stemmer R: Classification and mechanism of action of sclerosing agents, Soc Fran Phlebol 22:143, 1969.
7. Stroncek DF et al: Sodium morrhuate stimulates granulocytes and damages erythrocytes and endothelial cells: probable mechanism of an adverse reaction during sclerotherapy, J Lab Clin Med 106:498, 1985.
8. Cacciola E et al: Activation of contact phase of blood coagulation can be induced by the sclerosing agent polidocanol: possible additional mechanism of adverse reaction during sclerotherapy, J Lab Clin Med 109:225, 1987.
9. Cooper WM: Clinical evaluation of sotradecol, a sodium alkyl sulfate solution, in the injection therapy of varicose veins, Surg Gynecol Obstet 83:647, 1946.
10. Oscher A and Garside E: Intravenous injection of sclerosing substances: experimental comparative studies of changes in vessels, Ann Surg 96:691, 1932.
11. Lindemayr H and Santler R: The fibrinolytic activity of the vein wall, Phlebologie 30:151, 1977.
12. Merlen JF et al: Histological changes in a sclerosed vein, Phlebologie 31:17, 1978.
13. Virchow R: Gesammelte Abhandlungen zur wissenschaftlichen Medicin, Frankfurt, 1856, Meidingersohn.

14. Wuppermann Th: Study of sclerosis of varicose veins: comparison between the natural fibrinolysis in the blood of the antecubital vein and the test with labelled fibrinogen in the sclerosed leg, Phlebologie 30:145, 1977.
15. Soehring K and Nasemann Th: Beitrage zur Pharmakologie der Alkylpolyathylenoxyderivate. III. Gerinnungszeit bei wiederholtzer Applikation, hamolytische Wirkungen, Arch Int Pharmacodyn 91:96, 1952.
16. MacGowen WAL et al: The local effects of intra-arterial injections of sodium tetra-decyl sulfate (STD) 3%: an experimental study, Br J Surg 59:101, 1972.
17. Dastain JY: Sclerotherapy of varices when the patient is on anticoagulants, with reference to 2 patients on anti-coagulants, Phlebologie 34:73, 1981.
18. Klein-Fein J: What happens during the injection of sclerosant, Phlebologie 30:165, 1977.
19. Williams RA and Wilson E: Sclerosant treatment of varicose veins and deep vein thrombosis, Arch Surg 119:1283, 1984.
20. Wenner L: Sind endovarikose hamatische Ansammlungen eine normalerscheinung bei Sklerotherapie? Vasa 10:174, 1981.
21. Fegan WG: Continuous compression technique of injecting varicose veins, Lancet 2:109, 1963.
22. Schmier AA: Clinical comparison of sclerosing solutions in injection treatment of varicose veins, Am J Surg 36:389, 1937.
23. Goldman MP et al: Sclerosing agents in the treatment of telangiectasia: comparison of the clinical and histologic effects of intravascular polidocanol, sodium tetradecyl sulfate, and hypertonic saline in the dorsal rabbit ear vein model, Arch Dermatol 123:1196, 1987.
24. Martin DE and Goldman MP: A comparison of sclerosing agents: clinical and histologic effects of intravascular sodium tetradecyl sulfate and chromated glycerine in the dorsal rabbit ear vein, J Dermatol Surg Oncol 16:18, 1990.
25. Reiner L: The activity of anionic surface active compounds in producing vascular obliteration, Proc Soc Exp Biol Med 62:49, 1946.
26. Regard GL: The treatment of varicosities by sclerosing injections, Rev Med de la Suisse Rom, Geneve 65:102, 1925.
27. Doerffel J: Klinisches und Experimentelles uber Venenverodung mit Kochsalzlosung und Traubenzucker, Deutsche Med Wohnschr 53:901, 1927.
28. Binet L and Verne J: Evolution histo-physiologie de la veine ala suite de son obliteration experimentale, Presse Med 1:761, 1925.
29. Schwartz E and Ratschow M: Experimentelle und klinische Erfahrungen bei der kunstlichen Verodung von Varicen, Arch Klin Chir 156:720, 1929.
30. Biegeleisen HI: Fatty acid solutions for the injection treatment of varicose veins: an evaluation of 4 new solutions, Ann Surg 105:610, 1937.
31. McPheeters HO and Anderson JK: Injection treatment of varicose veins and hemorrhoids, Philadelphia, 1938, FA Davis and Co.
32. Biegeleisen HI: The evaluation of sodium morrhuate therapy in varicose veins: a critical study, Surg Gynecol Obstet 57:696, 1933.
33. Schneider W and Fischer H: Fixierung und bindegewebige organization artefizieller Thromben bei der Varizenuerodung, Dtsch Med Wschr 89:2410, 1964.
34. Dietrich VHP and Sinapius D: Experimental endothelial damage by varicosclerosation drugs, Arznittel-Forsh 18:116, 1968.
35. Kern HM and Angle LW: The chemical obliteration of varicose veins: a clinical and experimental study, JAMA 93:595, 1929.
35a. Goldman MP: A comparison of sclerosing agents: clinical and histologic effects of intravascular sodium morrhuate, ethanolamine oleate, hypertonic saline (11.7%), and Sclerodex in the dorsal rabbit ear vein, J Dermatol Surg Oncol, 1991 (in press).
35b. Blenkinsopp WK: Comparison of tetradecyl sulfate of sodium with other sclerosants in rats, Br J Exp Pathol 49:197, 1968.
36. Ouvry PA: Telangiectasia and sclerotherapy, J Dermatol Surg Oncol 15:177, 1989.
37. Foley WT: The eradication of venous blemishes, Cutis 15:665, 1975.
38. Sadick N: Treatment of varicose and telangiectatic leg veins with hypertonic saline: a comparative study of heparin and saline, J Dermatol Surg Oncol 16:24, 1990.
39. Bodian EL: Techniques of sclerotherapy for sunburst venous blemishes, J Dermatol Surg Oncol 11:696, 1985.
40. Bodian EL: Sclerotherapy, Sem Dermatol 6:238, 1987.
41. Thornton SC, Mueller SN, and Levine EM: Human endothelial cells: use of heparin in cloning and long-term serial cultivation, Science 222:623, 1983.
42. Bodian E: Sclerotherapy, Dialogues Dermatol 13(3), 1983 (tape recording).
43. Alderman DB: Therapy for essential cutaneous telangiectasias, Postgrad Med 61:91, 1977.

44. Mantse L: A mild sclerosing agent for telangiectasias, J Dermatol Surg Oncol 11:9, 1985.

45. Nguyen VB: Sklerotherapie des varices des membres inferieurs etude de 522 cas, Le Saguenay Medical 23:134, 1976.

46. Mantse L: More on spider veins, J Dermatol Surg Oncol 12:1022, 1986.

47. Ouvry PA: Telangiectasia and sclerotherapy, J Dermatol Surg Oncol 15:177, 1989.

48. Martindale: The extra pharmacopoeia, ed 28, London, 1982, The Pharmaceutical Press.

49. Maclaren NK et al: Glycerol intolerance in a child with intermittent hypoglycemia, J Pediatr 86:43, 1975.

50. Jausion H, Carrot E, and Ervais A: Une methode simple de phlebosclerose: la cure des varices par les injections de glycerine diluee, Bul Soc Fran Dermatol Syph 38:171, 1931.

51. Hammarlund ER and Pedersen-Bjergaard K: Hemolysis of erythrocytes in various iso-osmotic solutions, J Pharm Sci 50:24, 1961.

52. Welch KMA et al: Glycerol-induced hemolysis (letter), Lancet 1:416, 1974.

53. Jausion H: Glycerine chromee et sclerose des ectasies veineuses, La Presse Medicale 53:1061, 1933.

54. Jausion H et al: La sclerose des varices et des hemorroides par le glycerine chromee, Bull Memoires Soc Med Hospitaux Paris, p 587, 1932.

55. Hutinel B: Esthetique dans les scleroses de varices et traitement des varicosites, La Vie Medicale 20:1739, 1978.

56. Nebot F: Quelques points tecniques sur le traitement des varicosites et des telangiectasies, Phlebologie 21:133, 1968.

57. Ducros R and Gruffaz J: Indications, techniques et resultats du traitement sclerosant, La Revue du Praticien 20:2027, 1970.

58. Stemmer R, Kopp C, and Voglet P: Etude physique del injection sclerosante, Phlegologie 22:149, 1969.

59. Ouvry P and Arlaud R: Le traitement sclerosant des telangiectasies des membres inferieurs, Phlebologie 32:365, 1979.

60. Ouvry P and Davy A: Le traitement sclerosant des telangiectasies des membres inferieurs, Phlebologie 35:349, 1982.

61. Wallois P: Incidents et accidents de la sclerose. In Tournay R, editor: La sclerose des varices, ed 4, Paris, 1985, Expansion Scientifique Francaise.

62. Wenner L: Anwendung einer mit Athylalkohol modifizierten Polijodidjonenlosung bei skleroseresistenten Varizen, Vasa 12:190, 1983.

63. Raymond-Martimbeu P: Personal communication, 1990.

64. Sigg K, Horodegen K, and Bernbach H: Varizen-Sklerosierung: Welchos ist das wirUsamste Mittel? Deutsohes Arzteblatt 34/35:2294, 1986.

65. Sigg K and Zelikovski A: Kann die Sklerosierungotherapie der Varizen obne Oparation in jedem Fallwirksam sein? Phlebol Proktol 4:42, 1975.

66. Ghosh S: Chemical investigation in connection with leprosy inquiry, Indian J Med Res 8:211, 1920.

67. Cutting RA: The preparation of sodium morrhuate, J Lab Clin Med 11:842, 1926.

68. Meyer NE: Monoethanolamine oleate: a new chemical for obliteration of varicose veins, Am J Surg 40:628, 1938.

69. Biegeleissen HI: Fatty acid solutions for the injection treatment of varicose veins: evaluation of four new solutions, Ann Surg 105:610, 1937.

70. Hedberg SE, Fowler DL, and Ryan LR: Injection sclerotherapy of esophageal varices using ethanolamine oleate: a pilot study, Am J Surg 143:426, 1982.

71. Ayres SJ et al: Endoscopic sclerotherapy for bleeding esophageal varices: effects and complications, Ann Intern Med 98:900, 1983.

72. Evans DMD et al: Osophageal varices treated by sclerotherapy: a histopathological study, Gut 23:615, 1982.

73. Reid RG and Rothine NG: Treatment of varicose veins by compression sclerotherapy, Br J Surg 55:889, 1968.

74. Nabatoff RA: Recent trends in the diagnosis and treatment of varicose veins, Surg Gynecol Obstet 90:521, 1950.

75. Orbach EJ: Histopathological findings of telangiectasies treated with sodium tetradecyl sulfate-procaine precipitate, Angiopatias (Brasil) 8:103, 1968.

76. Tretbar LL: Spider angiomata: treatment with sclerosant injections, J Kansas Med Soc 79:198, 1978.

77. Shields JL and Jansen GT: Therapy for superficial telangiectasias of the lower extremities, J Dermatol Surg Oncol 8:857, 1982.

78. Blenkinsopp WK: Choice of sclerosant: an experimental study, Angiologica 7:182, 1970.

79. Pfahler B, Kreussler and Co, GMBH: Personal communication, March 29, 1990.

80. Schulz KH: Uber die Verwendung von Alkyl-polathylenoxyd-derivaten als Oberflachenanaesthetica, Dermatol Wochen 126:657, 1952.

81. Soehring K et al: Beitrage zur Pharmakologie der Alkylpolyathylerioxyd derivate. I. Untersuchungen uber die acute und subchronische Toxizitat bein verschiedenen Tierarten, Arch Int Pharmacodyn 87:301, 1951.

82. Siems KJ and Soehring K: Die Ausschaltug sensibler nerven duren peridurale und paravertebrale injektion von alkylpolyathylenoxydathern bei meerschweinchen, Arzneimittelforsche 2:109, 1952.

83. Olesch B: Neuere Erkenntisse zur Pharmakokinetik von Polidocanol (Aethoxysklerol), Vasomed Aktuell 4:22, 1990.

84. Soehring K and Frahm M: Studies on the pharmacology of alkylpolyethyleneoxide derivatives, Arzneimittelforsche 5:655, 1955.

85. Carlin MC and Ratz JL: Treatment of telangiectasia: comparison of sclerosing agents, J Dermatol Surg Oncol 13:1181, 1987.

86. Grubb TC, Dick LC, and Oser M: Studies on the toxicity of polyoxyethylene dodecanol, Toxicol Appl Pharmacol 2:133, 1960.

87. Larkin V De P: Polyethylene dodecanol vaporization in the treatment of respiratory infections of infants and children, NY State J Med 57:2667, 1957.

# 8 Complications and Adverse Sequelae of Sclerotherapy

*Primum non nocere*—above all else do no harm. This has always been a watchword in medicine and should always be considered before embarking on any form of treatment. Rarely in medicine does the physician have the luxury of administering a totally benign therapy, one that has absolutely no chance of harm. Rather, after establishing that the treatment is truly in the best interests of the patient, one should become familiar with the potential hazards of the proposed therapy and be prepared to treat those hazards should they occur. Further, in this era of pervasive medical-legal conflicts, it is advisable to inform the patient of the various potential complications and adverse sequelae of therapy. A cognizant patient can better recognize a problem early and can more willingly participate in the necessary treatment.

Unfortunately, as with any therapeutic technique, sclerotherapy carries with it a number of potential adverse sequelae and complications. Fairly common, and often self-limiting, side effects include perivascular cutaneous pigmentation, edema of the injected extremity, a flare of new perivascular telangiectasias, pain with injection of certain sclerosing solutions, localized urticaria over injected sites, blisters or folliculitis caused by the application of postsclerosis compression, recurrence of previously treated vessels, stress-related problems, and localized hirsutism. Relatively rare complications include localized cutaneous necrosis, systemic allergic reactions, thrombophlebitis of the injected vessel, arterial injection with resultant distal necrosis, deep vein thrombosis (DVT) with pulmonary emboli, nerve damage, and air emboli. This chapter addresses the pathophysiology of these reactions, methods for reducing their incidence, and treatment of their occurrence.

## ADVERSE SEQUELAE
### Postsclerotherapy Hyperpigmentation

Cutaneous pigmentation to some degree is a relatively common occurrence after sclerotherapy of veins varying in size from varicose to capillary (Fig. 8-1). This complication has been reported in up to 30% of patients treated with STS,[1] 30% of patients treated with HS,[2-5] and 10.7%[6] to 30%[3,7] of patients treated with POL. A recent evaluation of patients in one practice found a 1% incidence of pigmentation persisting after 1 year.[8]

#### Etiologic factors

The etiology of this pigmentation is subject to much conjecture. Biegeleisen,[9] Chrisman,[10] and Chatard[11] state (without reported histological evaluation) that this pigmentation results from a *combination* of postinflammatory hyperpigmentation (incontinence of melanin pigment) and hemosiderin deposition. However, Shields and Jansen[12] and Bodian[2] state (again without histological confirmation) that this pigmentation is caused only by hemosiderin staining of the dermis.

Relatively few histologic studies have examined the etiology of postsclero-

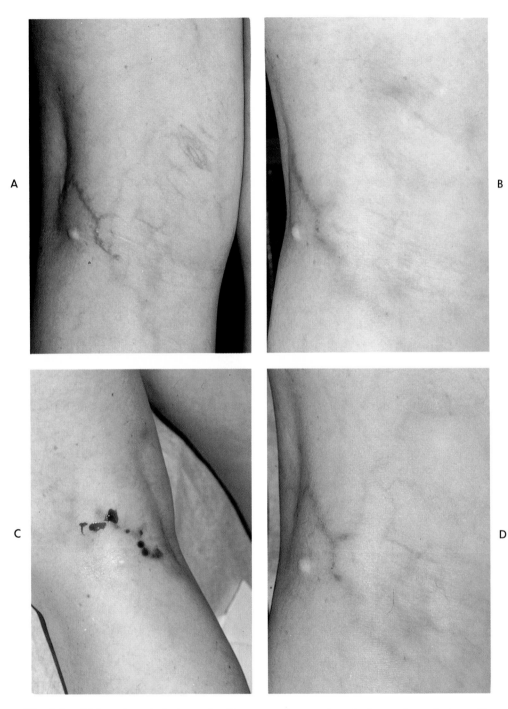

**Fig. 8-1**   This series of photographs illustrates the usual evolution and resolution of hyperpigmentation after sclerotherapy. **A,** Before sclerotherapy appearance of a reticular varicosity not associated with saphenofemoral or saphenopopliteal reflux. **B,** Four weeks after sclerotherapy treatment. Note mild pigmentation at the distal aspect of the treated vein. An obvious thrombotic coagula is present in the main body of the treated vein. **C,** Appearance of coagula after removal (see text for technique). **D,** Three weeks after drainage of coagula showing persistence of some pockets of thrombus within the vessel.

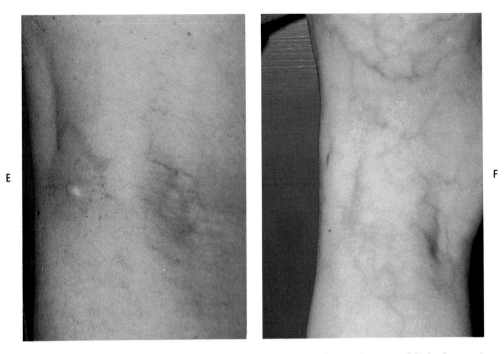

**Fig. 8-1, cont'd.** E, One year after initial treatment with persistence of light hyperpigmentation. F, Two years after initial treatment with complete resolution of the treated vein and hyperpigmentation. Resolution of associated telangiectasia is also apparent.

therapy hyperpigmentation. Biopsy of 14 patients 6 to 54 months after sclerotherapy treatment of varicose veins demonstrated hemosiderin without melanin incontinence.[13] A second histological study performed after injection of varicose veins in patients with spontaneous pigmentation associated with chronic venous insufficiency was reported by Cuttell and Fox.[14] They treated seven patients with STS, using 6 weeks of compression followed by an additional 2 months of wearing elastic stockings. Patients were biopsied both before sclerotherapy and from 10 to 23 months after sclerotherapy. Full-thickness skin biopsies were stained with hematoxylin and eosin, hexamine silver, and Perls' reagent and then blindly reviewed by two histopathologists. All patients demonstrated a decrease in melanin. Dermal hemosiderin was increased in two patients, unchanged in one patient, and curiously decreased in four patients. These authors concluded that "residual pigmentation following sclerotherapy of varicose veins occurs where there has been extravasation of blood at the injection site."

Goldman, Kaplan, and Duffy[15] have microscopically examined this pigmentation in six patients 6 weeks to 6 months after treatment of leg telangiectasias with POL, HS, and STS. Treatment and biopsy characteristics of this study and an additional two patients are listed in Table 8-1. They found that postsclerotherapy pigmentation occurred 6 to 12 weeks after treatment. There were no apparent histologic differences in the degree of pigmentation between the three sclerosing agents. In each biopsy specimen, scattered foci of golden-brown refractile pigment was noted on hematoxylin-eosin stained specimens (Fig. 8-2). Perls' stain revealed iron deposition in the dermis (Fig. 8-3). Fontana's stain demonstrated a normal pattern of melanocytes along the dermal-epidermal junction (Fig. 8-4). Papillary dermal melanophages were not evident in five of six biopsies. Diapedesis of red blood cells was only noted on biopsies taken from the ankle (at 6 and 8

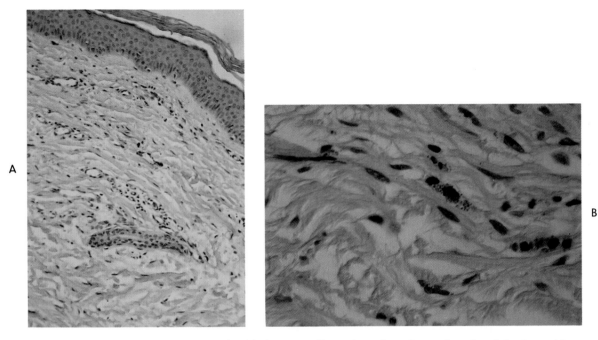

**Fig. 8-2** Section stained with hematoxylin-eosin; taken 6 months after injection with POL 0.75%. Note scattered foci of golden-brown pigment. **A**, Original magnification ×50. **B**, Original magnification ×200. (From Goldman MP, Kaplan RP, and Duffy DM: J Dermatol Surg Oncol 13:547, 1987.)

**Table** | **8-1** | Postsclerotherapy hyperpigmentation treatment characteristics

| Agent | Patient's race | Time of biopsy | Result |
|---|---|---|---|
| POL 0.25% | White | 6 weeks after injection | Heme |
| POL 0.75% | White | 6 weeks after injection | Heme |
| POL 0.75% | Hispanic | 6 months after injection | Heme |
| HS 18% | White | 8 months after injection | Heme |
| HS 20% | White | 2 months after injection | Heme |
| STS 0.5% | White | 5 months after injection | Heme |
| STS 0.25% | Hispanic | 3 months after injection | Heme |
| STS 0.5% | White | 18 months after injection | Heme |

months after injection). Interestingly, periadnexal hemosiderin was prominent in this location and in the popliteal fossae.

Each specimen differed somewhat in the degree of dermal hemosiderin; the more darkly pigmented cutaneous lesions exhibited a greater extent of dermal hemosiderin. In this limited study there appeared to be a greater amount of hemosiderin staining in biopsies taken from the ankle as opposed to the calf or thigh. In addition, darkly pigmented patients did not demonstrate melanin incontinence.

Therefore, three histologic studies on postsclerotherapy pigmentation demonstrated this complication to be caused by hemosiderin only.[13-15] Hemosiderin deposition predominantly occurs in the superficial dermis although it may be present in periadnexal and middermal locations, particularly in the ankle area. This phenomenon probably occurs when red blood cells extravasate into the der-

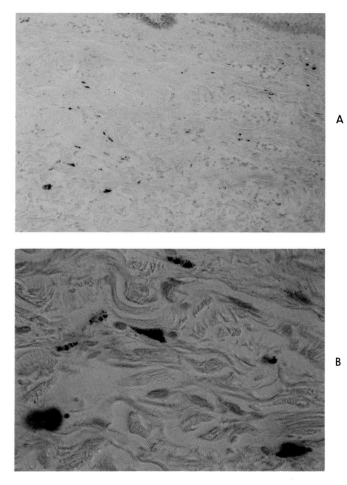

**Fig. 8-3** Perls-stained section from the same patient as in Fig. 8-1. Note scattered foci of green-blue granules within siderophages. **A,** Original magnification ×50. **B,** Original magnification ×200. (From Goldman MP, Kaplan RP, and Duffy DM: J Dermatol Surg Oncol 13:547, 1987.)

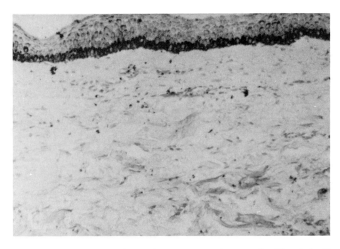

**Fig. 8-4** Fontana-stained section from the same patient as in Fig. 8-1. Note the normal melanocytic pattern of the epidermis. No melanin is present within the dermis (original magnification ×50). (From Goldman MP, Kaplan RP, and Duffy DM: J Dermatol Surg Oncol 13:547, 1987.)

mis after the rupture of treated vessels.[16] Erythrocyte diapedesis is a regular finding in chronic venous insufficiency. Here it is not caused by inflammatory wall alterations, but solely by a pressure rise within the cutaneous vessels[17] (see Chapter 2). Erythrocyte diapedesis may also occur after inflammation of the vessel and is commonly seen after thrombophlebitis.

Perivascular phagocytosis of red blood cells occurs either as intact cells or piecemeal after fragmentation by macrophages.[18,19] The intracellular fragments in the macrophage cytoplasm are further compartmentalized into hemoglobin-containing globules. These are referred to as secondary lysosomes. Since hemosiderin is an indigestible residue of hemoglobin degradation, it may appear as aggregates up to 100 micrometers in diameter.[20] On unstained tissue it appears golden and is 30% iron by weight. Its eventual elimination from the area may take years if it ever occurs.

In addition to its being insoluble, hemoglobin may directly affect cellular function. Recently a histologic examination with x-ray fluorescence analysis on patients with varicose ulceration disclosed an elevation of mean iron levels in periulcerated skin.[21] The authors speculate that free radical formation resulting from local iron accumulation may cause melanocytic stimulation, thereby augmenting brown pigmentation. Indeed, multiple authors have demonstrated melanin incontinence in the presence of venous stasis, complicated by extravascular red blood cells.[22-24] Whether melanocytic stimulation plays a role in the early appearance of postsclerotherapy pigmentation is unlikely. But, this may contribute to the persistence of pigmentation in certain patients.

Irregardless of its etiology, the incidence of pigmentation appears to be related to multiple factors including (1) sclerosing solution type and concentration, (2) sclerotherapy technique, (3) gravitational and other intravascular pressures, (4) innate tendency towards cutaneous pigmentation, and (5) postsclerotherapy treatment.

***Solution type and concentration.*** The type and concentration of the sclerosing solution affect the degree of endothelial destruction. The extent of endothelial destruction with resulting inflammation and extravasation of red blood cells is thought to influence the development of postsclerotherapy hyperpigmentation. Cloutier and Sansoucy[25] and Tournay[1] state that sodium tetradecyl sulfate (STS) has the highest incidence of pigmentation amongst sclerosing solutions. Foley[26] claims that the addition of 100 U/ml of heparin decreases the incidence of pigmentation, but in a large series of patients, Duffy[3] and Sadick[27] have not found this to occur. Sclerosing solutions reported to have the lowest incidence of postsclerotherapy pigmentation are chromated glycerin[8,25,28-30] and sodium salicylate.[8,11] Norris, Carlin, and Ratz[31] have observed an increased incidence of pigmentation (60%) in patients treated with 1% POL compared with those treated with 0.5% POL (20%). Therefore, with excessive endothelial destruction, caused either by high concentrations of sclerosing solutions or the use of extremely caustic agents, perivascular inflammation is increased. This may produce melanoctic changes in the skin or potentiate extravasation of red blood cells.

***Technique.*** To limit the degree of intravascular pressure, larger feeding varices, incompetent varices, and points of high pressure reflux should be treated first. This will minimize the extent of proximal intravascular pressure, which should decrease the risk for extravasation of red blood cells. C. Guarde[32] has found a greater incidence of pigmentation if vessels distal to the saphenofemoral junction are treated before successful closure of the junction. Marley[33] has also reported a decreased incidence of pigmentation in his practice since he began treating legs by injecting veins in order from proximal to distal.

*Gravitational and other intravascular pressures.* Postsclerotherapy pigmentation appears most commonly in vessels treated below the knee[11] but can occur anywhere on the leg. This is probably the result of a combination of increased capillary fragility and increased intravascular pressure by gravitational effects in this location (see Chapter 3). Chatard[11] also has observed an increased incidence of pigmentation when blue venulectases are treated as opposed to the treatment of red telangiectasias. The explanation for this later observation is unknown.

*Predisposition to pigmentation.* The reason that certain individuals appear to be predisposed to the development of pigmentation is unknown. Pigmentation has been reported to be more common and pronounced in patients with dark hair and "dark-toned" skin.[9] This is thought to be caused by an increased incidence of postinflammatory hyperpigmentation in patients with these colorings. However, Chatard[11] reported that pigmentation is unrelated to skin or hair color. I agree with this assessment.

*Postsclerotherapy coagula.* Finally, removal of postsclerotherapy coagula may decrease the incidence of pigmentation. Thrombi, to some degree, are thought to occur after sclerotherapy of all veins, regardless of size. This is because of the inability to completely occlude the vascular lumen with external pressure (see Chapter 6). The persistence of a small vascular lumen even with maximal external pressure has been predicted with experimental models of vein wall.[17] This has also been directly observed with fiber-optic varicography.[34]

Persistent thrombi are thought to produce a subacute "perivenulitis" that can persist for months.[35-37] The perivenulitis favors extravasation of red blood cells through a damaged endothelium or by increasing the permeability of treated endothelium. In addition, intratissue fixation of hemosiderin may occur.[11] This provides a rationale for drainage of all foci of trapped blood between 2 and 4 weeks after sclerotherapy. Sometimes blood can be released even 2 months after sclerotherapy.

Thrombi are best removed by gentle expression of the liquefied clot through a small incision made with a 21-gauge needle, No. 11 blade, or lancet (Fig. 8-5). A rocking action applied around the clot may aid in its expulsion. This should be continued until all dark blood is removed. The art of this procedure is to find the right place to puncture. This is best perceived as a soft, fluctuating spot. If the thrombosis is in the deep dermis, the area should be marked and 1% lidocaine can be infiltrated around the area to facilitate a less painful removal. Compression pads and/or stockings are then worn an additional 3 days to prevent further thrombosis formation and to aid in adherence of the opposing endothelial walls to establish effective endosclerosis.

An alternate technique for extraction of larger segments of thrombotic vein is to remove the thrombus with aspiration through a 16- or 18-gauge needle. This technique usually requires local infiltration with anesthetic along the course of the thrombotic vessel.

Perchuk[38] raises the possibility of infection occurring from stab incisions. This danger was presumed to be caused by the presence of bacteria in varicose veins, which was a commonly held belief by physicians 40 to 50 years ago.[39,40] However, there have been no reports of infections occurring in patients treated with stab incisions into postsclerotherapy clots in the modern medical literature. This problem has not occurred in my practice where this procedure is used routinely.

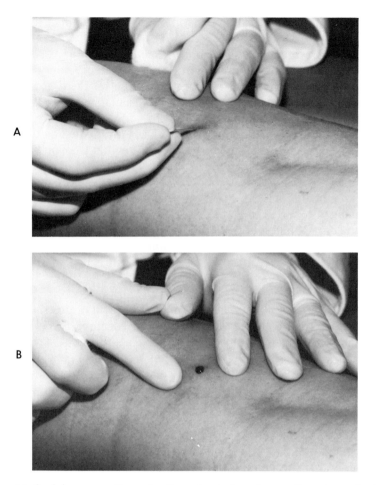

**Fig. 8-5**   Method for evacuation of a thrombosis in a 1-mm diameter reticular varicose vein 2 weeks after sclerotherapy. **A,** Small incision. **B,** Expelling clot (see text for details).

### Duration

Despite therapeutic attempts, pigmentation often lasts from 6 to 12 months.[15] Rarely, pigmentation may last over 1 year. Georgiev[8] estimates that 1% of his patients and Duffy[3] estimates that up to 10% of his patients have pigmentation lasting over 1 year. It is important to recognize that in certain patients this pigmentation may be present over superficial varicosities and telangiectasias before sclerotherapy is performed.[8,11] Hyperpigmentation as a result of "physiologic" diapedesis of red blood cells through fragile vessels is common in venous stasis or over varicose veins (see Chapter 2). Therefore, preoperative documentation, including photographs, may be beneficial during follow-up patient visits.

### Prevention

Although never formally studied, there appears to be a decreased incidence of postsclerosis pigmentation after injection treatment of deeper varicose veins. This may occur because sclerosis of vessels in the deeper dermis results in a more efficient reabsorption of extravasated heme, eventuating in a decreased incidence of overlying pigmentation.

To prevent the development of pigmentation, sclerotherapy should produce limited endothelial necrosis and not total destruction with its resulting diapedesis of red blood cells. This may be achieved by meticulous technique, avoidance of excessive injection pressures, selection of appropriate solution concentration, and treatment of areas of reflux venous return in a proximal to distal manner.

### Treatment

Treatment of pigmentation, once it occurs, is often unsuccessful. Because this pigmentation primarily is caused by hemosiderin deposition and not melanin incontinence, bleaching agents that affect melanocytic function are usually ineffective. Exfoliants (trichloroacetic acid) may hasten the apparent resolution of this pigmentation by decreasing the overlying cutaneous pigmentation, but they carry a risk of scarring, permanent hypopigmentation, and postinflammatory hyperpigmentation. However, some physicians have reported apparent success with this therapeutic modality.[41]

Effective treatments for this pigmentation have only rarely been reported. Chatard[11] has found that light cryotherapy to exfoliate the epidermis and "evict the pigment" is helpful. Cryotherapy has not been found to be useful in my practice.

Terezakis[42] has found that the use of topical retinoic acid enhances resolution of the pigmentation. She speculates that retinoids enhance fibroblastic removal of hemosiderin.

A seemingly logical form of treatment would be chelation of the subcutaneous iron deposition. Myers[42a] reported the use of a 150 mg/ml ointment of disodium ethylenediamine tetraacetic acid (EDTA) in the treatment of 10 patients with pigmentation after sclerotherapy or vein stripping or with pigmentation in chronic postphlebitic legs. He reported a consistent reduction in the shade of the pigmentation in every patient treated. Unfortunately, this was an uncontrolled study, and there has been no further reports of this form of treatment since its presentation in 1965. In my experience, intradermal injections of deferoxamine in an attempt to cause chelation of the hemosiderin has not proven to be beneficial.

The recommended treatment is "flashbulb therapy" or "chronotherapy." Since the majority of patients will have a resolution of pigmentation within 1 year, time and photographic documentation tend to be very satisfactory for the understanding patient (see Fig. 8-1).

# Temporary Swelling
### Etiologic factors

Multiple factors are responsible for swelling of a treated area. These factors include changes in the pressure differential between the intravascular and perivascular space and changes in endothelial permeability. Edema is most common when varicose veins or telangiectasias below the ankle are treated. This relates both to the increase in gravitational intravascular pressure in this area and the relative sparsity of perivascular fascia at the ankle (see Chapters 1 and 3). Riddock[43] speculates that edema is caused by an unduly prolonged reflex spasm spreading to some of the subfascial (deep) veins. Reflex vasospasm is thought to increase proximal intravascular pressures.

The extent of edema is also related to the strength of the sclerosing solutions used. This appears to be correlated with the degree of perivascular inflammation produced by the sclerosing solution. The by-products of inflammation, including release of histamine and various mediators, increase endothelial permeability. Duffy[3] and Goldman[7] estimate the occurrence of pedal edema to be between 2%

and 5%. They do not note a difference in the incidence of pedal edema between HS and POL use.

Edema may also occur if compression is not applied in a graduated manner. Edema may be produced when one tries to apply localized pressure on the thigh over an injected vein with the addition of a tape dressing over or under a graduated compression stocking. If patients are informed of the possibility of a tourniquet effect being produced by the extra compression, they can be advised to remove the dressing at the first sign of edema distal to the dressing.

### Prevention and treatment

There are two techniques that may limit temporary swelling. First, limit perivascular inflammation. Ankle edema occurs much less frequently if one limits the quantity of sclerosing solution to 1 ml per ankle. A second method for limiting the degree of pedal/ankle edema is to routinely apply a graduated pressure stocking after injections in this area. A recent study on the use of 30-to-40 mm Hg compression hosiery in the treatment of leg telangiectasia found a significant decrease in the incidence of ankle edema when a 30-to-40 mm Hg graduated compression stocking was worn for 3 days after sclerotherapy.[44]

## Telangiectatic Matting

The new appearance of previously unnoticed fine red telangiectasias occurs in a number of patients after either sclerotherapy or surgical ligation of varicose veins and leg telangiectasias (Fig. 8-6). This has been termed *distal angioplasia* by Terezakis[45] and *telangiectatic matting* (TM) by Duffy.[3] The reported incidence varies from 5%[7] to 75%.[31] The largest retrospective analysis to date (of 2120 patients with leg telangiectasias) reported a 16% incidence.[46] Duffy[3] has never seen the appearance of TM in male sclerotherapy patients. Other authors do not comment on a sexual predisposition. I have seen the development of TM in one male

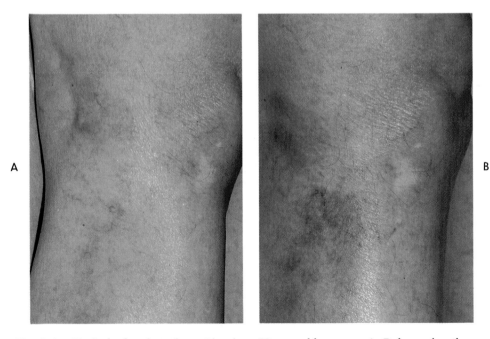

**Fig. 8-6** Typical telangiectatic matting in a 72-year-old woman. **A,** Before sclerotherapy treatment, right lateral knee. **B,** 6 weeks after treatment.

patient with leg telangiectasias. Because of the small number of men seeking treatment, an accurate appraisal of the sexual incidence of TM can not be stated. TM may appear anywhere on the leg but has been reported to occur more frequently on the thighs.[47]

### Etiologic factors

Probable risk factors for the development of TM in patients with leg telangiectasia include obesity, use of estrogen-containing hormones, pregnancy, and a family history of telangiectatic veins. Age and excessive standing do not appear to influence the incidence of TM.[46]

Postsclerosis TM was first described in the 1960s by Ouvry and Davy.[48] They observed that the incidence of matting was proportional to the degree of inflammation and thrombus formation. The etiology of TM is unknown but is thought to be related either to angiogenesis[3,49] or a dilation of existing subclinical blood vessels by the promotion of collateral flow through arteriovenous anastomoses.[49,50] One or both of these mechanisms may occur. Terezakis[45] believes that TM refers to the "survival of the fittest" with new blood vessels developing after occlusion of neighboring vessels. Experimentally, there are a number of etiologic factors that can initiate or contribute to angiogenesis (see box below).

*Angiogenesis.* Angiogenesis is a complex process in which capillary blood vessels grow in an ordered sequence of events. Angiogenic factors either act directly on the endothelium to stimulate locomotion and mitosis or indirectly by mobilization of host helper cells (mast cells and macrophages) and release of endothelial growth factors. When a new capillary sprout grows from the side of a venule, endothelial cells degrade basement membrane, migrate towards an angiogenic source, proliferate, form a lumen, join the tips of two sprouts to generate a capillary loop, and manufacture new basement membrane.[51] Obstruction of outflow from a vessel (which is the end result of successful sclerotherapy) is one of the most important factors contributing to angiogenesis.[52] Initiation of angiogenesis also follows disruption of endothelial continuity or intercellular contact. This results in endothelial cell sprouting and migration.[53] In addition, endothelial damage leads to the release of heparin and other mast cell factors that both promote the dilation of existing blood vessels and stimulate angiogenesis.[54,55] Finally, it is possible that this neovascularization is coming from a platelet-derived endothelial mitogen that is also angiogenic.[56] Thus sclerotherapy provides the mechanisms for new blood vessel formation to occur. Indeed, it is remarkable that one does not see a greater incidence of postsclerosis TM.

Heparin has been demonstrated both to bind to endothelial cells and promote endothelial proliferation in vitro and to produce angiogenesis in vivo through an affinity for growth factors.[54] Heparin potentiates angiogenesis in vivo

---

**ANGIOGENIC FACTORS**

Obstruction of blood flow — thrombosis, anoxia
Disruption of endothelial continuity
Heparin secretion by mast cells
Endothelial leakage of fibrinogen
Inflammation
Estrogen receptors

by stimulating endothelial cell plasminogen activator, endothelial cell chemotaxis, or both.[57] Therefore, it is interesting to speculate that the high incidence of TM reported by Duffy[3] may be related to his use of heparin in the HS sclerotherapy solution. Bodian[47] notes a 10% incidence of TM in his patients with the use of HS saline without the addition of heparin. Weiss and Weiss[5] note an 11% incidence of TM in their patient population treated with HS without heparin.

Sclerotherapy produces some degree of perivascular inflammation.[16] Inflammation may be considered as a hypermetabolic state with new vessel growth occurring as a result of increased metabolic demand.[58] In addition, mast cells are found in increased numbers in inflammatory states such as allergic contact dermatitis or delayed hypersensitivity reactions.[59] Since mast cell heparin is one factor responsible for capillary endothelial cell migration,[54] in an attempt to decrease angiogenic stimuli, one should try to limit the degree of inflammation as much as possible. This is achieved by choosing an appropriate solution concentration for each type of vessel to be treated and limiting the quantity of solution to that amount which will not produce excessive endothelial damage. This was confirmed by Weiss and Weiss[60] who found that in a random sample of 113 sclerotherapy patients, 10 developed TM with injection of POL 1% into vessels less than 1 mm in diameter. When POL 0.5% was used for subsequent treatments in these patients, none developed further areas of TM.

Ouvry and Davy[48] and Mantse[61] note a decreased incidence of TM when the pressure of injection is minimized and the extent of dispersion of sclerosing solution is limited to 1 cm diameter with each injection. These techniques may minimize the degree of perivascular inflammation with sclerotherapy. However, these procedural cautions are discounted by Duffy[3] who advocates the injection of up to 1.5 ml of solution through each injection site and Lary[62] who advocates injection of up to 3 ml per injection site. Duffy[3] has reported that TM occurs in from 20% to 35% of his patients. Lary[62] does not remark on the development of TM in his patients.

Duffy[3] has speculated that estrogen may play a role in the development of TM. Indeed, it appears that there may be an increased incidence of persistent TM among patients who are taking systemic estrogen preparations.[46] Estrogen receptors have been found in a number of tumors including angioma of the nose, soft tissue sarcoma, breast carcinoma, endometrial carcinoma, and unilateral nevoid telangiectasia syndrome. Estrogens have also been noted to play a role in the development of vascular tissues. Spider angiomas have been noted to develop during pregnancy and resolve after delivery.[63,64] Spider nevi are also noted to occur in patients with hepatic cirrhosis associated with elevated serum estradiol.[65] In addition, Davis and Duffy[46] have reported on the virtual disappearance of leg telangiectasia and TM in a 51-year-old woman with estrogen-receptor–positive breast carcinoma after initiation of antiestrogen therapy with tamoxifen citrate (Nolvadex). Thus since estrogen receptors have been implicated in the promotion of angiogenesis,[66] it may be prudent to withhold estrogen therapy during sclerotherapy treatment. However, Sadick[67] could not demonstrate estrogen receptors in a number of biopsies from leg telangiectasias. Therefore, at this time recommending that estrogen preparations be discontinued before sclerosing treatment begins to prevent or minimize the development of TM may be premature.

### Prevention and treatment

Irrespective of the etiology of TM, since patients come for treatment to have leg telangiectasia eliminated, it is most disconcerting for the sclerotherapist to produce new areas of telangiectasia. Therefore, any technique that may limit this side effect, such as limiting the injection blanch to 1 to 2 cm, should be employed. Further recommendations await future studies. Unfortunately, despite one's best efforts, TM will occur in a significant percentage of patients. Fortunately, TM usually resolves spontaneously over 3 to 12 months. Rarely, TM may be permanent. Thus far, except for the pulsed dye laser (see Chapter 12), TM is commonly resistant to treatment.

In the future, modifications of present treatment techniques may minimize this complication. Experimentally, protamine blocks the ability of mast cells and heparin to stimulate migration of capillary endothelial cells.[68] Protamine has also been demonstrated to prevent the neovascularization induced by an inflammatory agent when it is applied locally. It has no effect on established capillaries that are not proliferating.[69] In addition, β-Cyclodextrin tetradeasulfate administered with cortexolone has also been found to be a potent inhibitor of angiogenesis.[70] Thus preventive topical preparations or additives to the sclerosing solution may limit the development of TM.

# Pain

Since a great number of patients who come for treatment of cosmetic leg telangiectasia require a number of separate treatment sessions, each consisting of multiple injections, one should attempt to minimize the unpleasantness of the procedure.

## Prevention

Certain areas are slightly more painful, especially the ankles, upper medial thighs, and medial knees. Two variables of technique that can minimize pain are the type and size of the needle used for injection and the type of sclerosing solution used.

*Type and size of needle.* Using the smallest possible diameter needle for injection is the most obvious way to minimize injection pain (see Chapters 11 and 13). Another factor to consider is the shape of the needle bevel. Needles, even those of the same gauge, are shaped differently and may or may not be coated with a layer of silicone. Acutely tappered needles and those that are silicone coated appear to be perceived by the patient as less painful in my experience. Finally, it appears that with some agents that are inherently painful to inject (for example, hypertonic solutions), pain can be minimized with slow infusion.[5,3] Slow injection will produce a slower distention of tissue. This may decrease nerve stimulation. Therefore, needle type and size are important factors in minimizing the pain of injection.

*Type of sclerosing solution.* The second method for reducing pain is to choose the least painful sclerosing solution. Hypertonic solutions are notorious for causing pain on injection. The cramping pain that may develop after correct intravenous injection usually occurs a few minutes after injection. Weiss and Weiss[5] report that 72% of their patients injected with HS 23.4% experience pain that lasts less than 5 minutes; 4.5% of patients have pain that lasts more than 5 minutes. This pain probably occurs at the time the hypertonic solution reaches the nerve fibers of the adventitia, either through the wall of the vein or through the capillaries. Subsequently, because of stimulation of sympathetic perivenous nerve fibers, an active contraction of the muscle occurs that may also produce a cramping pain.[71] In addition, vascular spasm caused by direct effects of the hypertonic solution itself may occur.

Hypertonic solutions also have the additional effect of producing muscle cramping after injection. With the injection of 5 to 10 ml of Heparsal per injection site into varicose veins, Chou et al.[72] noted that 16% of 310 patients could not tolerate the pain associated with the procedure. Duffy[3] estimates that 82% of his patients treated with HS note moderate cramping or aching. This can be limited somewhat by keeping the volumes injected to 0.1 ml or less per injection site and by massaging the area immediately after injection. Also, adding lidocaine to the sclerosing solution may lessen muscle cramping and allow additional injections into the same area to be done less painfully.[3,4] However, the addition of lidocaine to a hypertonic solution is associated with two problems. First, lidocaine, if acidified (in a multidose bottle), is painful to inject. Therefore, nonacidified lidocaine (found in single dose "cardiac" ampules) should be used as an additive. Second, the addition of lidocaine gives the sclerosing solution the potential to produce an allergic reaction (discussed below).

Chromated glycerin solutions are also painful to inject and may produce a mild muscle cramping if more than 1 ml of solution is injected into a single vein.[30]

Two painless solutions are POL and STS. STS has the advantage of being painful only when it is injected into perivascular tissues, thereby providing a noticeable check on inadvertent perivascular injection. POL is painless with intradermal as well as intravenous injection. Therefore, one does not have the additional sign of pain to ensure accurate placement of the sclerosing solution. In a double-blind comparison of STS, HS, and POL, patients preferred injection with POL.[73] Finally, despite optimal technique and the use of mild sclerosing agents, posttreatment soreness for 1 or 2 weeks after injection has been noted to occur in 20% of patients.[3] With the use of nonosmotic sclerosing solutions and the use of graduated compression stockings after treatment, I have *not* seen soreness in most patients after treatment. If patients do complain of soreness, the cause is usually found to be vessels that are thrombosed and/or inflammed.

## Localized Urticaria

Localized urticaria occurs after injection of all sclerosing solutions (Fig. 8-7). It is usually transient (lasting about 30 minutes) and is probably the result of endothelial irritation. Localized urticaria is not likely an allergic response since it occurs even after injection of 23.4% unadulterated HS. It is probably related to the release of endothelial factors after these cells have been destroyed by the sclerosing solution. Alternatively, it may occur as the earliest manifestation of perivascular inflammation, again through release of endothelial- or platelet-derived factors.

Approximately 40% of patients studied by Norris, Carlin, and Ratz[31] described temporary itching after injections with POL regardless of drug dosage. Duffy[3] reports an almost 100% occurrence of urticaria with injection of either POL or HS-heparin-lidocaine solutions. The urtication is usually more intense when more concentrated solutions are used.[3,7]

### Treatment

In my experience localized urticaria and itching may be diminished by applying topical steroids immediately after injection and by limiting the injection quantity per injection site. This is particularly helpful in patients who are to wear a graduated support stocking after treatment.

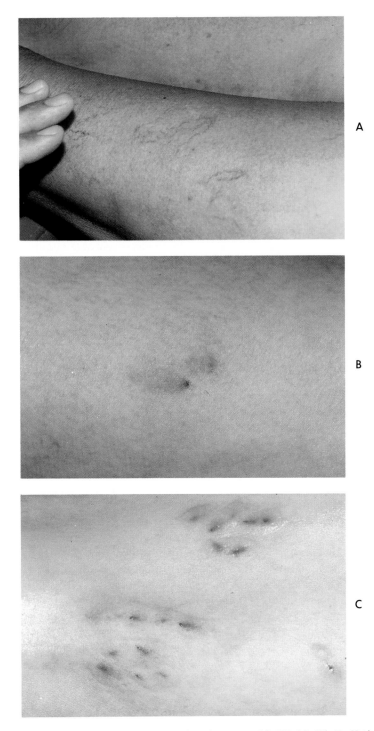

**Fig. 8-7**    **A,** Urtication immediately after sclerotherapy with HS 23.4%. **B,** Urtication immediately after sclerotherapy with STS 0.1%. **C,** Urtication immediately after sclerotherapy with POL 0.5%. Note the relatively increased degree of edema and erythema as compared with urtication with HS and STS.    *Continued.*

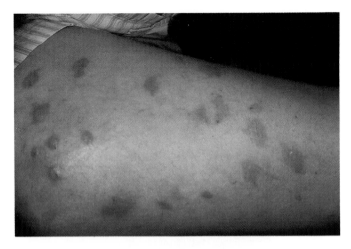

**Fig. 8-7, cont'd.    D,** Urtication immediately after sclerotherapy with Scleremo. Note the blue-green color of the skin, which reflects probable intradermal extravasation of chrome despite injection entirely within the blood vessel.

## Tape Compression Blister

The relatively uncommon cutaneous lesion, tape compression blister, (Fig. 8-8, *A*) occurs when a tape dressing is applied in an area of tissue movement. The blister usually appears as a flacid fluid-filled sack overlying normal-appearing skin. It is usually not associated with induration or erythema of the adjacent skin. Common sites of occurrence are the posterior calf, medial thigh, and popliteal fossae.

Blisters may occur with the use of any tape, but appear more commonly when one uses 3M Microfoam tape* as opposed to hypoallergenic paper tape† over foam pads or cotton balls. This is probably caused by the greater adhesiveness of the Microfoam tape. In addition, Microfoam tape is usually placed over the foam dressing with a slight amount of tension. This increases the tension on either end of the tape. Blistering is also more common in the summer months when the weather is hotter and in elderly patients with thinner, more fragile skin.

The only problem with blistering is that it must be distinguished from early cutaneous necrosis, cutaneous infection, or an allergic reaction. Early cutaneous necrosis may appear as a superficial blister. In this situation, the underlying and adjacent tissue is usually indurated and erythematous. Bullous impetigo can also have a similar physical appearance. Here, the blister is usually overlying warm, erythematous skin. If not warned beforehand, patients may think that the blister is the result of an allergy to the sclerosing solution. A detailed explanation of the cause of the blister is usually required before treatment can continue.

### Prevention

If compression pads are to be used under graduated stockings in a patient susceptible to blistering, a Tubigrip tubular support bandage‡ can be used over the pad to hold it in place while the stocking is being applied (Chapter 6). Al-

*3M Medical Surgical Division, St. Paul, Minn.
†Dermilite II, Johnson & Johnson, New Brunswick, NJ.
‡Seton Products, Inc., Montgomeryville, Penn.

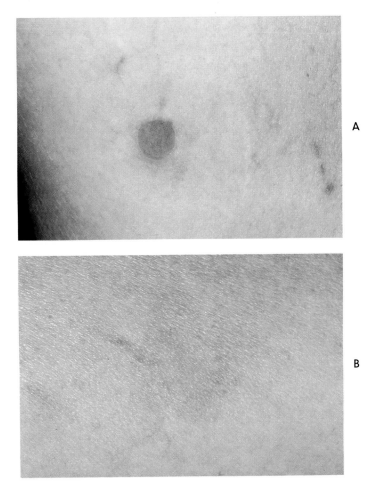

**Fig. 8-8**    A, Superficial blister that developed 1 week after sclerotherapy treatment; compression of the treated area was produced with an STD pad overlaid with 3M Microfoam tape. B, Complete resolution 3 weeks after blister formation.

though somewhat costly, this dressing (similar to a net dressing used in burn patients) will help prevent blister formation. (It can also be used in patients with allergy to tape.)

### Treatment

Fortunately, resolution of the blister occurs within 1 or 2 weeks without any adverse sequelae (Fig. 8-8, *B*). To aid healing and prevent infection of the denuded skin, the use of an occlusive hydroactive dressing such as Duoderm* appears to be helpful. Occlusive dressings may also help alleviate any pain associated with the blister.

## Tape Compression Folliculitis

Occlusion of any hairy area can promote the development of folliculitis (Fig. 8-9). If not associated with secondary alopecia of chronic venous insufficiency, men seeking treatment for varicose veins usually have hairy legs. If a tape dressing is

---

*ConvaTec, Princeton, NJ.

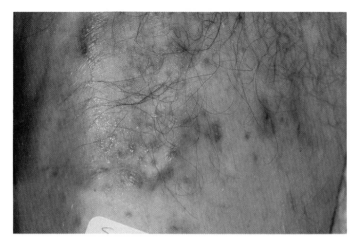

**Fig. 8-9**   Folliculitis apparent 7 days after sclerotherapy; compression of the treated area was produced with STD foam pads overlaid with 3M Microfoam tape.

placed over foam or cotton ball pads under a graduated compression stocking, a follicular inflammation or infection may occur. Folliculitis is more likely to occur in the summer months or when patients are active and perspire under the dressing.

### Treatment

Treatment consists of removal of the occlusive dressing and application of topical treatment with an antibacterial soap such as chlorhexidine gluconate* or a topical antibiotic gel such as erythromycin 2%† or clindamycin phosphate topical solution 1%.‡ The folliculitis usually resolves within a few days. Only rarely will systemic antibiotics be necessary.

## Recurrence

Recurrence of treated vessels has been estimated to occur in from 20% to nearly 100% of leg telangiectasias at 5-year follow-up.[74] Recanalization of initially thrombosed leg veins is procedure dependent. The larger the extent of intravascular thrombosis, the greater the likelihood of recanalization of the thrombosis during organization.[75,76] The recanalization of injected varices without subsequent compression or with inadequate compression is caused by clot contraction and the formation of sinuses that may become lined with endothelium; central clot liquefaction and the formation of vascular tunnels through the thrombosis; formation of vascular organization of the thrombosis and collateral vessel formation of the newly formed capillaries; and formation of peripheral sinuses filled with sludged blood (see Chapter 6) (Figs. 8-10 and 8-11).[76,77] Therefore, the most important factor in preventing recurrence is the limiting of intravascular thrombosis.

### Treatment

Tournay[78] was the first physician to stress the importance of postinjection removal of blood clots in 1938. The importance of draining these postsclerother-

---

*Hibiclens Antimicrobial Skin Cleanser; Stuart Pharmaceuticals, Wilmington, Del.
†Erygel Topical Gel; Herbert Laboratories, Irvine, Calif.
‡Cleocin T; The Upjohn Company, Kalamazoo, Mich.

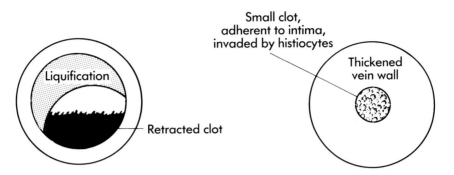

**Fig. 8-10**    Diagrammatic representation of a histologic study from Fegan WG[70] demonstrating the appearance of a varicose vein after sclerotherapy treatment. **A,** Without compression. **B,** With continuous compression for 6 weeks. (After Orbach EJ: Vasa 3:475, 1974.)

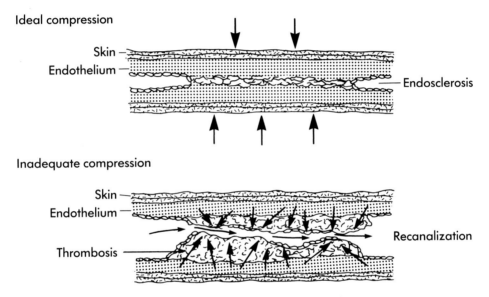

**Fig. 8-11**    Diagrammatic representation of recanalization of a varicose vein through a sclerotherapy-induced thrombosis. (Redrawn from Wenner L: Vasa 15:180, 1986.)

apy thrombi has since been emphasized by Sigg,[79] Pratt,[80] and Hobbs.[81] Orbach[75] advocates the compulsive removal of all postinjection clots, both fluctuating and hard cords. After administration of local anesthesia, he uses a No. 11 blade to make an incision over the vein and a von Graefe cataract knife to dissect the clot completely from the vein wall. This is followed by continuous compression until resolution of the vein occurs.

With proper technique, recurrence of varicose veins only rarely occurs. A biopsy study of 6 patients with "recurrence" of previously treated veins demonstrated that the veins thought to have recurred were in reality new varicose veins.[82] When high recurrence rates are reported, the patients have usually been treated with minimal compression.[75] For example, in one recent study of 310 patients, 83% required reinjection of a treated varicosity. These patients received only 48 hours of compression with elastic bandages.[72]

Unlike recanalization through a varicose vein cord, recanalization is not common through a sclerosed telangiectasia. Posttreatment histologic studies have demonstrated only fibrosis in an area treated with sclerotherapy.[2]

## Stress-Related Symptoms

### Vasovagal reflex

The vasovagal reflex is a common adverse sequellae of any surgical or invasive procedure. It has been estimated to occur in 1% of patients during sclerotherapy[83] and is more frequent when using the technique of Fegan or Sigg.[84] With these later two techniques, 21- to 25-gauge needles are inserted while the patient is sitting or standing, and blood is allowed to flow freely from the punctured vein. Duffy, who performs sclerotherapy with 30-gauge needles in reclining patients, estimates the incidence of vasovagal reactions to be 0.001%.[3] Interestingly, the percentage of men who experience this response far exceeds the percentage of women.

Vasovagal reactions have typical clinical findings. The usual symptoms include light-headedness, nausea, and sweating. The patient may also experience shortness of breath and palpitations. Syncope rarely occurs, but usually provokes the most concern in the physician and staff. Vasovagal reactions are most often preceded by painful injection but may occur just from the patient seeing the needle or smelling the sclerosing solution.

*Prevention.* The main concern in a vasovagal reaction is that the patient will fall and get injured. Therefore, both the nurse and physician should watch the patient closely for signs of restlessness and excessive perspiration. All patients should be warned to sit down if they become dizzy. It is also helpful when needle placement is performed on a standing patient for the patient to hold on to an arm rail or other support. All such reactions are easily reversible when the patient assumes the supine or Trendelenburg position. Preventative measures consist of recommending that the patient eat a light meal before the appointment, maintaining good ventilation in the treatment room, and maintaining constant communication with the patient during the procedure.

It is important that the physician recognize the vasovagal response in a patient and not assume that an allergic reaction is occurring. If subcutaneous epinephrine is given in the mistaken belief that an anaphylactic reaction is occurring, the symptoms will both become exaggerated and obscured. This only further confuses the clinical situation and adds to patient apprehension regarding further treatment sessions.

### Underlying medical disease

More serious stress-induced problems include exacerbation of certain underlying medical diseases. Patients with a history of asthma may experience wheezing, which can be treated with a bronchodilator such as metaproterenol sulfate,* albuterol,† or over-the-counter epinephrine bitartrate‡ metered dose inhalers. Patients with coronary artery disease may develop angina, treatable with sublingual nitroglycerin tablets. Urticaria is easily treated with an oral antihistamine but may be a sign of systemic allergy. Therefore, one should carefully evaluate use of the sclerosing agent in future treatment sessions. It is intriguing that urticaria and periorbital edema have occurred even with injection of unadulterated HS.[85] This may be related to histamine release from irritated perivascular mast cells. Finally, triggering of frequent migraine headaches has also been noted to occur after sclerotherapy.[3]

---

*Alupent; Boehringer Ingelheim Pharmaceuticals, Inc., Ridgefield, Conn.
†Proventil; Schering Corporation, Kenilworth, NJ.
‡Primatene; Whitehall Laboratories Inc., NY.

## Localized Hirsutism

Localized hypertrichosis developing after sclerotherapy with the use of multiple sclerosing agents has been described in the literature several times.

The etiology is thought to be the result of an improved cutaneous oxygen content with localized increase in hair growth or the result of a long-standing low-grade inflammatory reaction involving stimulation of new hair growth. In this regard, two patients have been reported to have developed localized hair growth after surgical treatment of venous insufficiency with cutaneous inflammation.[86]

Hair growth at the site of injection has been described in three patients treated with STS.[87] All patients were given injections of between 1 to 6 ml of STS over 5 to 10 sessions. Localized hair growth developed 4 to 7 months after the last injection. The site of hair growth was related to the area of skin most damaged by venous incompetence. Weissberg[88] has also reported on the development of localized hirsutism in 1 of 62 patients. The hair growth occurred at the site of injection 1 month after treatment. It lasted 4 months and then subsided. Sclerotherapy with polyiodinated iodine has also been associated with hypertrichosis at the injection site in three cases.[82]

## COMPLICATIONS
### Cutaneous Necrosis
#### Etiology

Cutaneous necrosis may occur with the injection of any sclerosing agent (Figs. 8-12 to 8-14). Its cause may be the result of (1) extravasation of a sclerosing solution into the perivascular tissues, (2) injection into a dermal arteriole or an arteriole feeding into a telangiectatic or varicose vein, (3) a reactive vasospasm of the vessel, or (4) excessive cutaneous pressure created by compression techniques.

*Extravasation.* Extravasation of caustic sclerosing solutions may directly destroy tissue. The solutions are not always deposited entirely within the vessel lumen (Fig. 8-15). During the injection of an abnormal vein or telangiectasia, even the most adept physician may inadvertently inject a small quantity of sclerosing

**Fig. 8-12**  Superficial cutaneous necrosis. Photograph shows healing 8 weeks after injection with HS 20%.

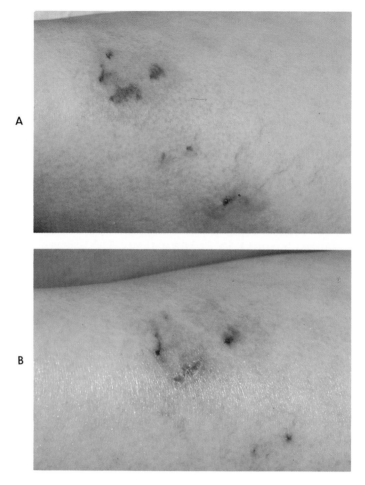

**Fig. 8-13**  Cutaneous necrosis after injection with STS 0.5%. **A,** Immediately after injection. **B,** Necrotic epidermis apparent 2 weeks after injection.

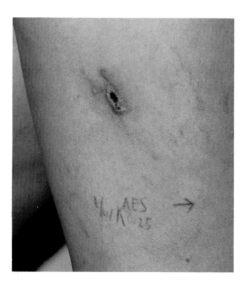

**Fig. 8-14**  Cutaneous necrosis 6 weeks after sclerotherapy with POL 0.25%. Note that 2 ml of solution was injected into a feeder vein approximately 10 cm distal to the necrotic area.

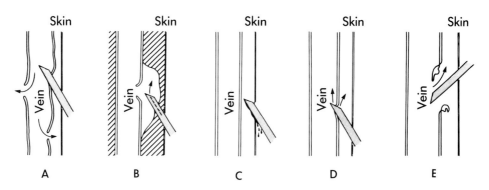

**Fig. 8-15** Mechanism for extravasation of sclerosing solution. **A,** Extravasation through multiple needle puncture holes. **B,** Extravasation from injection of sclerosing solution after slight withdrawal of the needle. **C,** Extravasation of sclerosing solution along needle shaft. **D,** Extravasation from injection with needle bevel both in and out of the vein. **E,** Extravasation through excessive destruction of the vein wall. (Redrawn from Biegeleisen HI: Varicose veins, related diseases, and sclerotherapy: a guide for practitioners, Montreal, 1984, Eden Press.)

solution into the perivascular tissue. Also, a tiny amount of sclerosing solution may be left in the tissue when the needle is withdrawn, and sclerosing solution may leak out of the injected vessel, which has been traumatized by multiple or through-and-through needle punctures. Rarely, the injection of a strong sclerosing solution into a fragile vessel may lead to endothelial necrosis and rupture producing a "blow-out" of the vessel and perivascular extravasation of sclerosing solution. Therefore, injection technique is an important, but not a foolproof, factor in avoiding this complication, even under optimal circumstances.

Sclerosing solutions vary in the degree of cellular necrosis they produce. If minimal tissue necrosis is caused by a sclerosing agent, it may even be suitable for perivascular injection in the treatment of telangiectatic mats whose vessels cannot be cannulated even with a 33-gauge needle.

HS 23.4% is a caustic sclerosing agent as demonstrated in intradermal injection experiments. Clinically, small punctate spots of superficial epidermal damage occur at points of injection, especially when a small bleb of the solution escapes from the vein. However, subcutaneous injection of up to 1 ml of HS 23.4% (by mistake) in lieu of lidocaine into the neck or cheek has been reported to result in no adverse sequellae.[89,90] In this situation, cutaneous necrosis was most likely avoided by rapid physiologic dilution of HS. Alternatively, dermal tissue may be more resistent to the caustic effects of hypertonic solutions.

POL appears experimentally to be the least toxic to subcutaneous tissue. Jaquier and Loretan[91] and Hoffer[92] advocate the use of intradermal POL 0.5% to treat telangiectatic leg veins smaller than the diameter of a 30-gauge needle and report no evidence of cutaneous necrosis. However, POL in sufficient concentration has been reported to cause cutaneous necrosis. Solutions of POL over 1.0% may produce superficial necrosis with intradermal injection in patients.[91] This unfortunately occurred with the mistaken injection of 0.1 ml POL 5% solution into a leg telangiectasia 0.2 mm in diameter in my practice. This injection resulted in extensive overlying cutaneous necrosis that took 8 weeks to heal (Fig. 8-16). Therefore, POL is not without the risk of cutaneous necrosis if a strong enough concentration is injected.

However, even when sclerotherapy is performed with expert technique, us-

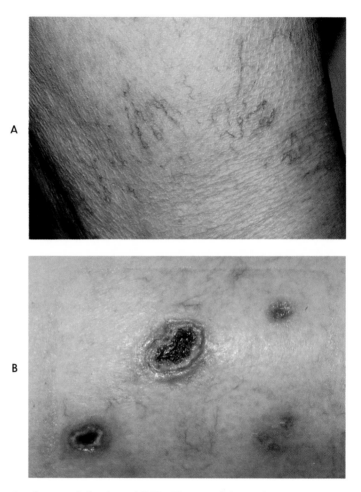

**Fig. 8-16** Inadvertent injection of POL 5%, 0.1 ml into telangiectatic veins on the thigh. A, Immediately before injection. B, Four weeks after injection.

ing the safest sclerosing solutions and concentrations, cutaneous ulceration may occur (see Fig. 8-14). Therefore, it appears that extravasation of caustic sclerosing solutions alone is not totally responsible for this complication.

*Arteriolar injection.* De Faria and Moraes[94] have observed that 1 in 26 leg telangiectasias are associated with a dermal arteriole. It is my opinion that inadvertent injection into or near this communication is the most common cause of cutaneous ulcerations.

POL has been injected intradermally to effect sclerosis of TM in my practice without the development of cutaneous ulceration, even with the injection of 0.5 ml of a 0.75% solution. However, I have noted the development of 3-to-6 mm diameter ulcerations in approximately 0.0001% of injections with POL 0.5%.

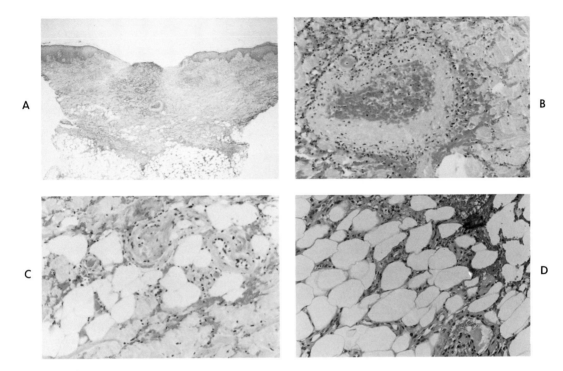

**Fig. 8-17** **A,** Low-power view showing skin ulceration and focal inflammation extending into the subcutaneous fat. A thrombosed vessel, most likely an artery, is present directly under the area of necrosis. (Hematoxylin-eosin ×25.) **B,** Higher magnification of same area as in **A** showing the thrombosed vessel that caused the infarct. The lumen is completely occluded by a fresh thrombus; there is also red cell extravasation in the adjacent dermis (Hematoxylin-eosin ×200). **C,** View of adjacent dermis-fat interface showing thrombi in the luminae of small vessels (Hematoxylin-eosin ×200). **D,** Mononuclear cell inflammation and fresh hemorrhage is present focally in the subcutaneous tissue (Hematoxylin-eosin ×200).

Three consecutive ulcerations that appeared over the course of 6 months were excised. In these patients each cutaneous ulceration developed as the result of the occlusion of the feeding dermal arteriole. This produced a classic wedge-shaped arterial ulceration (Fig. 8-17). Therefore, it appears that this complication may be unavoidable to some extent.

*Vasospasm.* Rarely, after injection of the sclerosing solution, one notes an immediate porcelain-white appearance to the skin at the site of injection (Fig. 8-18). A hemorrhagic bullae usually forms over this area within 2 to 48 hours, which progresses to an ulcer (Figs. 8-19 and 8-20).[35] This cutaneous reaction might represent an arterial spasm. In an attempt to reverse the spasm, vigorous massage when the white macule appears has been shown in my practice to sometimes avert ulceration. However, the prevention of the ulceration is not always successful. Arterial spasm may also explain the development of cutaneous ulceration upstream from the injection site (see Fig. 8-14). In this later case, 2 ml of POL 0.25% was injected into a feeding reticular vein as shown by the *arrow*. That was the only injection given to the patient in that sclerotherapy session.

*Lymphatic injection.* Injection into a lymphatic vessel may also lead to cutaneous necrosis. Histologic studies have disclosed evidence of lymphovenous

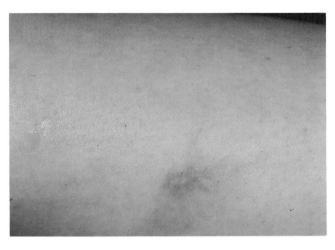

**Fig. 8-18**    Porcelain-white cutaneous reaction immediately after injection with POL 0.25%. This area healed within 4 weeks without any complication.

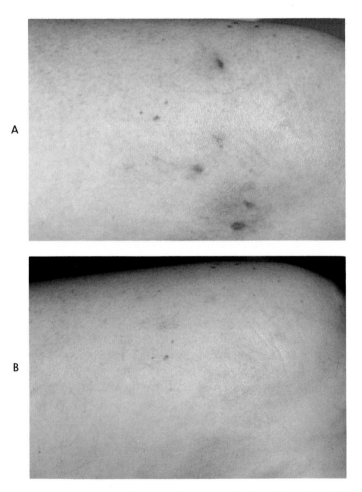

**Fig. 8-19**    A, Hemorragic macular reaction 1 week after injection with POL 0.5%. B, Complete resolution without treatment occurred after 2 months.

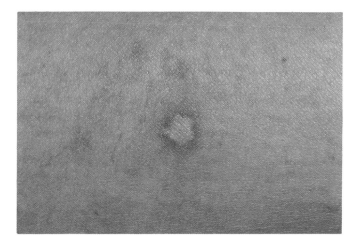

**Fig. 8-20**   Porcelain-white cutaneous reaction immediately after injection with POL 0.5% in the upper lateral thigh. This area progressed into a frank cutaneous ulceration.

anastomoses in humans.[95] It is possible that injection into such an anastomosis could result in necrosis of the associated lymphatic vessel and infiltration of the sclerosing solution extravascularly. If the sclerosing solution is caustic to extravascular tissues, this may result in tissue necrosis.

*Excessive compression.* Finally, excessive compression of the skin overlying the treated vein may produce tissue anoxia with the development of localized cutaneous ulceration (see Chapter 6). Subcutaneous tissue flow in the leg is decreased when cutaneous pressure exceeds 20 mm Hg.[96] In addition, external pressure above 30 mm Hg reduces muscle blood flow in some patients.[97] Therefore, excessive compression may produce tissue ischemia. However, both of the above-mentioned studies employed indirect measurements of subcutaneous tissue flow and calf muscle blood flow and thus need to be viewed with caution. A more physiologic method for measuring the effect of compression on blood flow was recently performed through determination of femoral blood flow.[98] These authors demonstrated that in the recumbent patient, static, graduated, external compression of approximately 20 mm Hg at the ankle, reduced to about 10 mm Hg in the upper thigh, produces an increase in femoral flow of up to 75%. However, if calf pressures exceed 30 mm Hg when the patient is recumbent, a progressive fall in subcutaneous tissue flow and deep venous velocity occurs. Therefore, it is recommended that patients not wear a graduated compression stocking of over 30 to 40 mm Hg when lying down for prolonged periods of time.

One method for applying compression to treated veins that could be varied with patient position is that of using a double layer of graduated compression stockings. This would ensure that maximal pressure over the vein is maintained while the patient is ambulatory. When the patient is recumbent, the outer stocking is removed, thereby decreasing the cutaneous pressure to 20 to 30 mm Hg at the ankle, which should prevent a reduction in cutaneous and subcutaneous blood flow.

### Treatment

Whatever the cause of the ulceration, it must be dealt with when it occurs. Fortunately, ulcerations, when they do occur, are usually fairly small, averaging

4 mm in diameter in my practice. At this size, primary healing usually leaves an acceptable scar (Fig. 8-21). Bodian,[47] who uses 23.4% HS, notes that ulceration usually takes 3½ months to heal even when judicious wound care is given. He advocates treatment with daily application of 20% benzoyl peroxide powder* under moist dressings cut to fit snugly over the ulcer. The use of a number of occlusive or hydrocolloid dressings has been found by myself to result in an apparent decrease in wound healing time. More importantly, occlusive dressings decrease the pain associated with an open ulcer. However, because an ulcer may take 4 to 6 weeks to completely heal, even under ideal conditions, if possible, excision and closure of these lesions are recommended at the earliest possible time. This affords the patient the fastest healing and an acceptable scar.

## Systemic Allergic Reaction/Toxicity

Systemic reactions caused by sclerotherapy treatment occur very rarely.

### Minor reactions

Minor reactions like urticaria are easily treated with an oral antihistamine such as diphenhydramine† 25 to 50 mg by mouth, or hydroxyzine‡ 10 to 25 mg by mouth. Rarely, one would need to add corticosteroids if the reaction did not subside readily. A short course of prednisone, 40 to 60 mg per day for 1 week, in conjunction with systemic antihistamine every 6 to 8 hours, would be helpful. Suppression of the adrenal axis is not a problem with this short course, so a tapering schedule is not necessary.

---

*Vanoxide Acne Lotion; Dermik Labs, Fort Washington, Penn.
†Benadryl; Parke-Davis, Morris Plains, New Jersey.
‡Atarax; Roerig, New York.

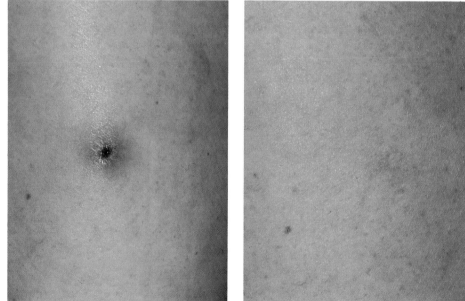

A        B

**Fig. 8-21**   Cutaneous ulceration on the posterolateral thigh. **A,** Three weeks after treatment with POL 0.5%. **B,** After 6 months. Treatment consisted of a duoderm dressing that was changed every 4 days until complete healing occurred in 5 weeks. Note the cosmetically acceptable stellate scar.

Because of the possibility of angioedema or bronchospasm, each patient with evidence of an allergic reaction should be examined for stridor and wheezing by auscultating over the neck and chest while the patient breathes normally. Supine and sitting blood pressure and pulse should be checked to rule out orthostatic changes, hypotension, or tachycardia that might result from the vasodilation that precedes anaphylactic shock.

Minor degrees of angioedema can, again, be treated with oral antihistamines; however, if stridor is present, an intramuscular (IM) injection of diphenhydramine and intravenous (IV) corticosteroids should be administered, and a laryngoscope and endotracheal tube should be available.

Bronchospasm is estimated to occur after sclerotherapy in 0.001% of patients.[3] It usually responds to the addition of an inhaled bronchodilator or IV aminophylline, 6 mg/kg over 20 minutes, to the antihistamine/corticosteroid regimen already noted.

### Major reactions

Four types of potentially serious systemic reactions specific to the type of sclerosing agent have been noted: anaphylaxis, pulmonary toxicity, cardiac toxicity, and renal toxicity. These reactions will be discussed both in general and separately for each sclerosing solution.

Anaphylaxis is a systemic hypersensitivity response caused by exposure or more commonly reexposure to a sensitizing substance. Anaphylaxis is usually an IgE-mediated, mast cell–activated reaction that occurs most often within minutes of antigen exposure. Other classes of immunoglobin such as IgG may also produce anaphylaxis.[99] Since the risk of anaphylaxis increases with repeated exposures to the antigen, one should always be prepared for this reaction in every patient.[100]

The principal manifestations of anaphylaxis occur in areas where mast cell concentrations are highest: skin, lungs, and gastrointestinal tract. Histamine release is responsible for the clinical manifestations of this reaction. Although urticaria and abdominal pain are common, the three principal manifestations of anaphylaxis are airway edema, bronchospasm, and vascular collapse. Urticaria alone does not constitute anaphylaxis and should not be treated as such because of the potential side effects of treatment with epinephrine, especially in the older patient.

The signs and symptoms of anaphylaxis may initially be subtle and often include anxiety, itching, sneezing, coughing, urticaria, and angioedema. Wheezing may be accompanied by hoarseness of the voice and vomiting. Shortly after these presenting signs, breathing becomes more difficult, and the patient usually collapses from cardiovascular failure resulting from systemic vasodilation.

The recommended treatment is to give epinephrine 0.2 to 0.5 ml 1:1000 subcutaneously. This can be repeated three to four times at 5-to-15 minute intervals to maintain a systolic blood pressure above 90 to 100 mm Hg. This should be followed with establishment of an intravenous line of 0.9% sodium chloride. Diphenhydramine hydrochloride 50 mg is next given along with cimetidine 300 mg; both IV and oxygen are given at 4 to 6 L/minute. An endotracheal tube or tracheostomy is necessary for laryngeal obstruction. For asthma or wheezing, IV theophylline 4 to 6 mg/kg is infused over 15 minutes. At this point it is appropriate to transfer the patient to the hospital. Methylprednisolone sodium succinate 60 mg is given IV and repeated every 6 hours for four doses. Corticosteroids are not an emergency medication since their effect only appears after 1 to 3 hours. They are given to prevent the recurrence of symptoms 3 to 8 hours after the initial event. The patient should be hospitalized overnight for observation.

## Allergic Reactions to Sclerosing Agents
### Sodium morrhuate

Although touted by the manufacturer as "the natural sclerosing agent," sodium morrhuate (SM) causes a variety of allergic reactions ranging from mild erythema with pruritus[101-103] to generalized urticaria[103-105] to gastrointestinal disturbances with abdominal pain and diarrhea[101,102] to anaphylaxis. It has been estimated that "unfavorable reactions" occur in 3% of patients.[106] The reason for the high number of allergic reactions with this product may be related to the inability to remove all the fish proteins that are present in SM. In fact, 20.8% of the fatty acid composition of the solution is unknown.[107]

Many cases of anaphylaxis have occurred within a few minutes after the drug is injected or more commonly when therapy is reinstituted after a few weeks.[103,108-110] Most of these cases occurred before 1950. Rarely, anaphylaxis has resulted in fatalities,[105,106,111] many of which have not been reported in the medical literature.[101]

Pleural effusions with pulmonary edema and acute respiratory failure appearing as *adult respiratory distress syndrome* are common with esophageal injection.[107] It has been estimated that pleural effusions occur in 46% of patients with esophageal injection.[112] With injection into esophageal varices, the sclerosing solution rapidly enters the pulmonary circulation causing increased permeability of the pulmonary microvasculature.[107] There have been no reports of pleural effusions with injection into varicose veins of the legs.

Prolonged dysrhythmia requiring permanent pacemaker has been reported in two cases.[113] This complication has been attributed to a direct cardiotoxic effect of SM.

### Ethanolamine oleate

Ethanolamine oleate* (EO) is a synthetic mixture of ethanolamine and oleic acid with an empirical formula of $C_{20}H_{41}NO_3$. The minimal lethal intravenous dose in rabbits is 130 mg/kg.[104] The oleic acid component is responsible for the inflammatory action. Oleic acid may also activate coagulation in vitro by release of tissue factor and Hageman factor. This agent was first reported in the medical literature to be an ideal sclerosing agent by Biegeleisen[114] in 1937. He observed no toxic effects in 500 injections. Ethanolamine is thought to have a decreased risk of allergic reactions compared with SM or STS.[115] However, pulmonary toxicity and allergic reactions have been associated with this sclerosing agent.

Pleural effusion, edema, and infiltration and pneumonitis have been demonstrated in human trials with the injection of esophageal varices. Pleural effusion or infiltration has been estimated to occur in 2.1% of patients and pneumonia in 1.2% of patients by the product manufacturer.† One study of 75 patients treated for esophageal varices disclosed abnormal chest x-ray films showing infiltration or effusion in 45 patients for an incidence of 60%.[116] These conditions usually resolve spontaneously within 48 hours.[116]

Anaphylactic shock has been reported by the product manufacturer after injection in three cases.† Another case of a nearly fatal anaphylactic reaction during the fourth treatment of varicose leg veins with 1 ml of solution has also been reported.[117] In one additional case a fatal reaction occurred in a man with a known allergic disposition.† Another episode of a fatal anaphylactic reaction occurred in a woman having her third series of injections.[101] This represented one

---

*Ethamolin; Block Drug Company, Piscataway, NJ.
†Product information (1989) from Glaxo Pharmaceuticals, Research Triangle Park, NC.

reaction in 200 patients from that author's practice. Generalized urticaria occurred in about 1 in 400 patients; this symptom responded rapidly to an antihistamine.[118]

Acute renal failure with spontaneous recovery occurred after injection of 15 to 20 ml of Ethamolin in two women.* A hemolytic reaction occurred in 5 patients in a series of over 900 patients, with injection of over 12 ml of 0.5% EO per patient per treatment session.[118] The patients were described as "feeling generally unwell and shivery, with aching in the loins and passage of red-brown urine. All rapidly recovered with bed rest and were perfectly normal the next day." Injections of less than 12 ml per treatment session have not resulted in this reaction.

Transient chest pain has also been reported in 13 of 23 patients treated for esophageal varices.[119] However, pyrexia and substernal chest pain are said to be common sequelae of esophageal varicosis injection with any sclerosing agent.[115]

### Sodium tetradecyl sulfate

A synthetic detergent developed in the 1940s, sodium tetradecyl sulfate (STS) has been used throughout the world as a sclerosing solution. Although some outspoken dermatologists have claimed that it is hazardous to use because of the risk of fatal allergic reactions, in reality the risk is very small. A comprehensive review of the medical literature (in multiple specialties and languages) disclosed a total of 47 cases of nonfatal allergic reactions in a review of 14,404 treated patients. This included six case reports.[120] A separate review of treatment in 187 patients with 2249 injections disclosed no evidence of allergic or systemic reactions.[121] An additional report of 5341 injections given to an unknown number of patients found "no unfavorable reaction."[122] If one were to combine only those reviews of over 1000 patients, the incidence of nonfatal allergic reactions would be about 0.3%.[4,118,123-125]

Fegan[126] has reviewed his experience with STS in 16,000 patients. He reported 15 cases of "serum sickness, with hot stinging pain in the skin, and an erythematous rash developing 30 to 90 minutes after injection." These patients subsequently underwent additional uneventful treatment with STS after premedication with antihistamines. Ten additional patients developed "mild anaphylaxis" that required treatment with epinephrine.

The product manufacturer notes two fatalities associated with the use of STS.† One fatality occurred in a patient who was receiving an antiovulatory agent. Another death (fatal pulmonary embolism) was reported in a 36-year-old woman who was not taking oral contraceptives. MacGowan et al.[127] note only one fatality recorded in a series of over one million patients injected. This fatality was attributed to the injection of over 5 ml of a 3% solution in one sitting.

Since all reported cases of allergic reactions are of the IgE-mediated immediate hypersensitivity type, it is recommended that patients remain in or near the office for 30 minutes after sclerotherapy when STS is used. However, patients may also develop allergic reactions hours or days after the procedure.[125,128] For example, urticaria occurred 8 hours after treatment in one patient,[128] and 2 weeks after treatment in two other patients.[125] Therefore, patients should be warned about the possibility of allergic reactions and how to obtain care should a reaction occur.

Recently, in a review of 2300 patients treated over 16 years, four cases of

*Product information (1989) from Glaxo Pharmaceuticals, Research Triangle Park, NC.
†Product information (1976) from Elkins-Sinn, Inc.

allergic reactions were reported (0.17% incidence).[128] Reactions in this study were described as periorbital swelling in one patient and *urticaria* in three. All reactions were easily treated with oral antihistamines. It is of interest that French phlebologists advocate a 3-days-before and 3-days-after treatment course with an antihistamine. P. Flurie[129] noted no episodes of allergic reactions in 500 patients treated in this manner.

As of January 1990, a total of 37 reports of adverse reactions have been reported to the FDA's Drug Experience Monitoring Program. However, this information cannot be used to estimate the incidence of adverse drug reactions since there was no central reporting agency before August 1985. A review of these adverse reactions was remarkable in that five cases of suspected anaphylaxis and two cases of asthma induced by injection were reported. One of the cases of anaphylaxis resulted in death (see below). Numerous reports of cutaneous necrosis were also reported along with a number of other nonspecific "complications." A review of the available notes on the complications were remarkable for the poor technique and inexperience on the part of the treating physician. In addition, on review it was unclear to me whether anaphylaxis indeed occurred in every reported case.

In short, anaphylaxis has been reported only rarely.[130] The most common systemic reaction consists of transient low-grade fever and chills lasting up to 24 hours after treatment.[131] This has also been noted in one of my patients. Of note is that three patients with allergic systemic reactions to monoethanolamine oleate had no evidence of allergy to STS.[131]

A fatality was recently reported[132] that occurred after a test dose of 0.5 ml of STS 0.5% was given to a 64-year-old woman. An autopsy performed by the Hennipin County coroner's office revealed no obvious cause of death. Subsequently, mast cell tryptase studies were performed on blood collected approximately 1 hour after the reaction while the patient was on life-support systems. A normal tryptase level is less than 5 ng/ml; in experimental anaphylactic reactions induced in the laboratory, levels up to 80 ng/ml have been seen. In this patient the levels were extremely high at 6000 ng/ml, suggesting that an anaphylactoid reaction had caused her death. Unfortunately, tryptase levels are experimental at this time, and it is unclear how such a high level could be obtained. Therefore, it is also unclear whether fatal anaphylaxis is a significant possibility with STS.

A hemolytic reaction occurred in 5 patients in a series of over 900 patients with injection of over 8 ml of STS 3%.[118] Like a similar reaction that occurred with EO, patients were described as "feeling generally unwell and shivery, with aching in the loins and passage of red-brown urine. All rapidly recovered with bed rest and were perfectly normal the next day." Injections of less than 8 ml per treatment session did not result in this reaction. Intravascular hemolysis was also reported to the FDA after injection of STS into an hepatic artery feeding a hepatic tumor.

The intravenous $LD_{50}$ in mice is 90 mg/kg.[133] The lethal volume after IV injection in the rat is about four to six times as high for STS as for POL in equivalent concentrations.[93]

### Polidocanol

Allergic reactions to polidocanol (POL) have been reported in only four patients in a recent review of the world's literature with an estimated incidence of 0.01%.[120] Amblard[134] reported no allergic reactions in over 250 patients, no allergic reactions even in two patients who were intolerant to STS. Hoffer[92] reported no allergic reactions in over 19,000 cases. In addition, patients who are allergic to STS or iodine have no allergic manifestations to injections of POL.[134-136] However, rare allergic reactions have been reported, including a case of nonfatal anaphylactic shock to 1 ml of POL 2% injected into a varicose vein during the fourth treatment session.[128,137-139] Also, Ouvry, Chandet, and Guillerot[140] reported a patient who developed generalized urticaria with cough and dyspnea after receiving 2 ml of POL 2%; the condition resolved in 30 minutes with IV corticosteroids.

Jaquier and Loretan[91] believe that the decrease in antigenicity is the result of the absence of a benzene nucleus and a paramine group and the presence of a lone free alcohol group. Dexo SA Pharmaceuticals, the product manufacturer in France, recommends that this substance not be used in subjects with an allergic diathesis (asthma, etc.).* But Kreussler and Co., the product manufacturer in Germany, states that there are no contraindications that arise from the product itself.† Thus allergic reactions to POL are much rarer than those reported with STS.

Like EO and SM, POL has demonstrated a dose-dependent cardiac toxicity when injected into esophageal varices. POL has a negative inotropic effect and reduces atrioventricular and intraventricular conduction. Animal studies demonstrate a reversible, dose-dependent decrease in myocardial contractility, blood pressure, and pulse rate and a prolongation of the P-Q interval.[141] This effect may explain the etiology of heart failure in three elderly patients with severe liver failure, who were given massive quantities of POL during esophageal sclerotherapy (760 mg in a 74-year-old woman; 600 mg in a 70-year-old woman; 750 mg in a 76-year-old woman).[142,143]

The $LD_{50}$ in rabbits at 2 hours is 0.2 g/kg, which is three to six times greater than the $LD_{50}$ for procaine hydrochloride.[144] The $LD_{50}$ in mice is 1.2 g/kg.[145] The systemic toxicity is similar to lidocaine and procaine.[146]

### Chromated glycerin

Chromated glycerin 72% (Scleremo [SCL]) is a sclerosing solution whose incidence of side effects is very low.‡[12,17,147] Hypersensitivity is a very rare complication.[148,149] Hematuria accompanied by ureteral colic can occur transiently after injection of large doses. Ocular manifestations, including blurred vision and a partial visual field loss, have been reported by a single author with resolution in less than 2 hours.[150]

An additional case was recently reported of transient hypertension and visual disturbance after the injection of 12 ml of 50% SCL into spider and "feeder" leg veins in a fourth treatment session. These symptoms occurred 2½ hours after treatment and lasted over a 3-hour period without treatment. This may have represented a retinal spasm or an ophthalmic migraine.[151]

### Polyiodide iodine

Polyiodide iodine§ (Variglobin, Sclerodine) is a stabilized water solution of iodide ions, sodium iodine, and benzyl alcohol. Sigg et al.[152] reported on his experience in over 400,000 injections with Variglobin. Paravenous injections

---

*Product description of hydroxypolyethoxydodecane (May 1985) received with correspondence from Dexo SA Pharmaceuticals, France.
†Product insert for Aethoxysklerol from Chemische Fabrik Kreussler & Co GmbH, West Germany.
‡Scleremo product information (1987) from Laboratories E. Bouteille, 7 rue des Belges, Limoges 8100, France.
§Varigloban (Chemische Fabrik Kreussler & Co GmbH, Wiesbaden-Biebrich, West Germany); Variglobin (Globopharm, Zurich, Switzerland); Sclerodine 6 (Omega; Montreal, Canada).

readily produced tissue necrosis. In 1975 he reported an incidence of side effects of 1.25 per 1000 injections, 0.13 per 1000 allergic cutaneous reactions, 0.04 per 1000 instances of localized necrosis, and 1 per 1000 instances of varicophlebitis. No systemic allergic reactions were observed.[153] Obvious contraindications to the use of variglobin are hyperthyroidism and allergies to iodine and benzyl alcohol.

Iodine solutions may also produce bronchiomucosal lesions if used in high concentration. Therefore, Wenner[154] recommends that a maximum of 5 ml of 12% solution be used in a single sclerosing session.

### Hypertonic saline

Alone, hypertonic saline (HS) shows no evidence of allergenicity or toxicity. The only complication from its specific use is hypertension that may be exacerbated in predisposed patients when an excessive sodium load is given. In addition, Dodd[154a] has reported painless hematuria in five patients injected with HS. Sometimes blood appears in the urine after one to two acts of micturition, sometimes at additional times throughout the day. There are usually no other ill effects, and the hematuria resolves spontaneously. Hematuria probably occurs because of hemolysis of red blood cells during sclerotherapy.

Recently, Coverman[155] described two patients injected with up to 6 ml of HS 23.4% who developed "peculiar visual symptoms in just one eye." This was described as either blurred vision or an aura. There were no other symptoms, and each incidence passed quickly and spontaneously. Coverman speculates that this may be caused by the addition of lidocaine to the HS solution.

### Heparin in hypertonic saline

Whereas many authors use hypertonic saline solutions in concentrations from 15% to 30% for the treatment of varicose and telangiectatic leg veins, some advocate the addition of heparin to the solution to prevent the theoretical risk of embolization associated with sclerotherapy.[13] Although the necessity for heparin has been discounted in a well-controlled 800-patient randomized study,[14] Foley's solution, "Heparsal," consisting of HS 20% with heparin 100 U/ml and procaine 1%, is commonly used in the treatment of telangiectatic leg veins. Therefore, the risk of adverse reactions to heparin should be mentioned.

Commercial preparations of heparin consist of straight-chain anionic polysaccharides of variable molecular weight (usually 7000 to 40,000). Heparin prepared from different tissues also appears to vary: more protamine is required to neutralize a unit of beef lung heparin than porcine mucosal heparin. Plasma lipolytic activity, antifactor $X_a$ activity, and activated partial thromboplastin time ratios are significantly different.[156]

Fever, urticaria, and anaphylaxis occur occasionally after administration of heparin.[156-160] Necrosis has been reported in patients receiving subcutaneous heparin.[152,161-164] Necrosis usually occurred 3 to 10 days after multiple subcutaneous injections. Pruritus, local tenderness, and burning sensations associated with large, indurated, erythematous plaques were also reported to occur in six patients 10 to 20 days after beginning prophylactic doses of heparin.[165] Therefore, there is a measurable risk of toxicity to heparin.

Although heparin is not a totally benign substance, there have been no reports by those who use Heparsal of any adverse reactions that could be attributed to the heparin component.[3,13,14,72] The lack of side effects has even been reported when volumes of 10 to 20 ml have been injected into varicose veins in one series of 310 patients.[72] Therefore, in the doses used, heparin in Heparsal may be without significant side effects, but one must be aware of the potential dangers associated with its use.

### Lidocaine in hypertonic saline

Alderman[4] and Duffy[3] advocate the addition of lidocaine (to achieve a 0.4% final concentration) to minimize patient discomfort during injection of HS. This addition means that this sclerosing mixture has the potential to be allergenic. Although the most common etiologies of previous allergic reaction in a patient to lidocaine are psychogenic or vasovagal reactions,[166] allergic reactions may occur.

The amide class of anesthetics has a very low risk of allergic reaction.[167-172] Allergy is most likely caused by the methylparabens or sodium metabisulfite that is used as a preservative in the anesthetic solutions.[167,168,173-175] Therefore, to keep the allergic risk as low as possible, one should use single-dose vials of lidocaine without preservatives.

Despite the low risk of allergenicity to lidocaine, multiple allergic reactions, including anaphylaxis have been reported.[176-183] Therefore, HS, when adulterated with lidocaine, may place the patient at risk for allergic reactions.

## Superficial Thrombophlebitis

Before the advent of modern day sclerotherapy, which employs graduated compression to limit thrombosis, thrombophlebitis, both superficial and deep, occurred in a significant number of sclerotherapy patients.[184] In fact, it was commonly thought that the incidence of phlebitis was so common a sequelae of sclerotherapy that there was doubt over whether this form of therapy was legitimate.[185] With the use of compression and the realization that many adverse effects resulted from thrombus formation in treated veins, the incidence of thrombophlebitis greatly decreased.

Certain patients may be predisposed to the development of thrombophlebitis. Fegan[186] states that this complication occurs more commonly if perforator veins in the region of treatment are undiagnosed and not treated.

### Etiology

Superficial thrombophlebitis appears 1 to 3 weeks after injection as a tender erythematous induation over the injected vein (Fig. 8-22). Duffy[3] estimates that it occurs in 0.5% of his patients. Mantse[125] reported an incidence of 1% in the treatment of varicose (nontelangiectatic) veins despite the use of a tensor bandage for 6 weeks. Mantse notes that the patients who developed superficial thrombophlebitis found the bandage to be too tight and reapplied it too loosely at home. In my experience, this complication occurs in some degree in approximately 0.01% of patients. Severe cases requiring treatment with compression and antiinflammatory agents occur very rarely (less than 0.001% of patients comprising over 10,000 separate injections).

### Prevention and treatment

The decreased incidence in my practice may be the result of the greater degree and length of compression used in treating all injected veins. Indeed, the cause of thrombophlebitis is related in part to treatment technique. An inadequate degree or length of compression results in excessive intravascular thrombosis. Sigg[187] notes that perivenous inflammation is observed only at those parts of the limb not covered by a compression dressing. Thus to avoid this complication, one should prevent and/or minimize the development of postsclerosis thrombosis. This is accomplished with compression pads and hosiery.

However, even when appropriate compression is used over treated varicose veins, thrombosis and perivascular inflammation may occur. Ascending phlebitis in the LSV or its long tributaries starting at the upper edge of the compression stocking is relatively common. Here the sclerosing action continues up the abnor-

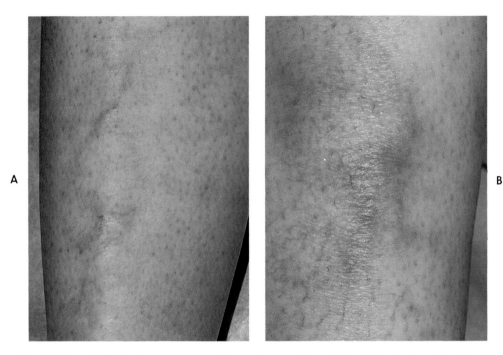

**Fig. 8-22** A, Clinical appearance of the vein over the anterior tibia before injection. B, Acute thrombophlebitis developed 10 days after sclerotherapy with POL 0.5%.

mal vessel (even beyond what appears to be the extent of the abnormality). It is thought that the sclerosing solution destroys damaged endothelium to a greater extent than normal endothelium.*,† Therefore, the placement of a sorbo pad extending above the compression stocking or bandage to create a gradual transition of pressure from compressed to noncompressed vein may provide a safety margin. Also, this may prevent damage to the vein by the otherwise abrupt cut-off of the pressure stocking.

In addition to adequate compression, drainage of thrombi after liquification occurs in 2 weeks will hasten resolution of the otherwise slow painful resorption process.[187]

Thrombophlebitis is not a complication that should be taken lightly (see Chapter 2). If untreated the inflammation and clot may spread to perforating veins and the deep venous system, which leads to valvular damage and possible pulmonary embolic events. Therefore, when thrombophlebitis occurs, the thrombus should be evacuated, and adequate compression and frequent ambulation should be maintained until the pain and inflammation resolves. Aspirin or other nonsteroidal antiinflammatory agents may be helpful in limiting both the inflammation and pain.

## Arterial Injection

The most feared complication in sclerotherapy is inadvertent injection into an artery. Fortunately, this complication is very rare.[188-190] Five examples of this complication had been reported to the Medical Defense Union in Great Britain by 1985.[191] The mechanism of action for the development of an embolus when a

---

*Product description on Hydroxypolyethoxydodecane received with correspondence, May 1985.
†Product insert (1985) for Aethoxysklerol from Chemische Fabrik Kreussler and Co. GMBH.

sclerosing solution is injected into an artery has been examined in the dog femoral artery.[127] The results of these experiments indicated that there is little effect on the major vessel (artery) with injection. Spasm does not occur. The sclerosing solution acts to denature blood in smaller arteries and produce a sludge embolus, which obstructs the microcirculation causing stagnation, secondary thrombosis, and necrosis.

### Etiology

The most common location for arterial injection to occur is in the posterior or medial malleolar region, specifically in the posterior tibial artery.[186,190,192] The patient will usually, but not always, note immediate pain. Cutaneous blanching of the injected area usually occurs in an arterial pattern associated with a loss of pulse and progressive cyanosis of the injected area.

Another area where the artery and veins are in close proximity is the junction of the femoral and superficial saphenous veins. A review of one sclerotherapy practice over 20 years disclosed two cases of accidental arterial injection in this area requiring thigh amputations.[193] In this location the external pudendal artery bifurcates and may surround the LSV shortly after the location of its connection with the femoral vein (see Chapter 1). Because of anatomical variation of these collateral arteries in this location, duplex scanning is important before injection of sclerosing solution.

### Prevention and treatment

Arterial injection is a true sclerotherapy emergency. The extent of cutaneous necrosis usually is related to the amount of solution injected. Therapeutic efforts to treat this complication are usually unsatisfactory but should be attempted.[190] Browse[84] recommends that on realization of arterial injection, blood and sclerosing solution should be aspirated back into the syringe to empty the needle of solution. In addition, aspiration of the injected artery as rapidly and completely as possible may help remove the injected sclerosing solution if performed immediately. The needle should not be withdrawn, but the syringe should be replaced with one containing 10,000 U of heparin, which should be injected slowly into the artery. Periarterial infiltration with procaine 3%, 1 ml, will complex with STS and render it inactive.[186,192] The foot should be cooled with ice packs to minimize tissue anoxia. Immediate heparinization to be continued for 6 days and administration of IV dextran 10%, 500 ml per dose, for 3 days is recommended. IV streptokinase also may be considered if there are no other contraindications for its use. Finally, use of oral prazosin, hydralazine or nifedipine for 30 days should be considered.

Recently, a favorable resolution of arterial injection occurred with injection of tissue-type plasminogen activater.[194] In this patient promazine was injected into an artery. Heparin, axillary plexus blockade, and IV sodium nitroprusside were not successful. Brachial artery injection of tissue-type plasminogen activater (Actilyse, 50 mg over 8 hours) resulted in therapeutic efficacy. Therefore, local fibrinolytic therapy should be considered if conservative treatments prove ineffective.

Given the known relationship of injection site to the development of this problem, one must consider the necessity for injecting vessels in the vicinity of the medial malleolus. In this regard, there is an interesting report in the *British Medical Journal*,[188] of a legal case brought against a physician for performing such an injection, which resulted in a transmetatarsal amputation. The case was found in favor of the physician after several renowned sclerotherapists stated that if the patient would benefit from the injection it should be attempted, since the risks are infrequent and the benefits significant.

Prevention of this dreaded complication is best accomplished by visualization of the blood emanating from the needle. If it is pulsatile and continues to flow after the leg is horizontal, injection should not be attempted at this site. Mantse[125] advises that the placement of the sclerosing needle should be performed while the patient is standing so the varix is bulged and the distance between the artery and vein is increased.

## Pulmonary Embolism/Deep Venous Thrombosis

Pulmonary emboli only very rarely occur. In the 1930s and 1940s pulmonary emboli after sclerotherapy of varicose veins occurred in, at most, 0.14% of patients.[195,196] In a series of 45,000 injections given to 7500 patients, only one episode of pulmonary embolism was reported.[197] Sicard, in 1928, reported 325,000 injections without a pulmonary infarction.[198] Linser[199] reported four cases of pulmonary embolism after 75,000 injections, only one of which was fatal. More recently, with the onset of compression techniques in combination with sclerotherapy, this complication has become even less common. Sigg[200] has reported pulmonary emboli occurring only once in 42,000 injections. A French vascular surgeon who treats about 75 sclerotherapy patients a week, amounting to 25,000 yearly injections, reported only one case of pulmonary embolism in 20 years.[189] And Fegan[126] reported that he has never seen conclusive evidence of DVT after injection treatment of 16,000 patients in his clinic.

### Cause

The cause of DVT with pulmonary embolism development after sclerotherapy is unclear. The chemical endophlebitis produced by sclerotherapy should anchor the thrombus to the site of injection. Histologic examination of treated varicose veins has demonstrated that a firm thrombosis occurs only on the abnormal endothelium. Nonadherent thrombosis occurs on normal endothelium.[201] Therefore, the most logical explanation for the development of emboli is damage to the deep venous system by migration of sclerosing solution or a partly attached thrombosis into deep veins from superficial veins as a result of either injection of large quantities or physical inactivity after injection.[202] Also, tributary communicating veins, if not compressed, may force early clots into the deep circulation with muscle contraction.

*Amount of injection per site.* The circulation and direction of blood flow in varicose veins has been determined radiographically to be stagnant or reversed (away from the heart) so that the chemically induced thrombus is forced distally towards the smaller branching veins.[203] However, recent cinematographic studies documented that a small amount of sclerosing solution entered the deep circulation after injection of between 0.5 and 1.0 ml of solution into a superficial varicosity during 7 of 15 injections in nine subjects (see Chapter 9).[204] Fortunately, no adverse effects were noted in these patients treated with a relatively mild agent, POL 2%. The lack of adverse effects was probably related to rapid compression and ambulation of treated individuals and the resulting rapid dilution of the sclerosing agent within the deep venous system. Therefore, one must both limit the quantity of sclerosing solution per injection site to assure that the agent will remain within the superficial system and also rapidly stimulate blood flow in the deep venous system after sclerotherapy with compression and muscle movement.

Recently, impedance plethysmography and Doppler ultrasonic examination was performed before and after sclerotherapy treatment by the classic Fegan technique in 67 legs.[205] This study confirmed that there were no alterations in deep venous blood flow at 1 and 2 weeks after injection treatment. This confirmed the clinical experience that sclerotherapy using the Fegan technique is highly unlikely to be complicated by the development of DVT.

DVT and embolic episodes usually occur 4 to 28 days after the sclerotherapy treatment session.[195] Most cases have been reported to occur with injection of large quantities of sclerosing solution (12 ml) in a single site.[206] However, two case reports of these complications occurring with injection of less than 0.5 ml of POL 1% have been published.[207] In the latter case, the veins injected were leg telangiectasias. In addition, the injection of 0.5 to 1 ml of sclerosing solution above the midthigh resulted in a presumed thrombus at the saphenofemoral junction with resulting pulmonary emboli.[118] This prompted Reid and Rothine[118] to recommend that injections not be given above the midthigh.

*Inappropriate compression.* The inappropriate tourniquet effect of an excessively tight wrap in the thigh is a rare cause for the development of DVT.[208] In this case, the occlusion of deep venous flow resulted in thrombosis of the popliteal vein. This resolved with conservative treatment. The adverse effects of nongraduated compression again emphasizes the importance of properly fitted graduated support stockings in sclerotherapy treatment.

*Excessive thrombosis.* The mechanism for thromboembolic disease in women who use oral contraceptives is multifactorial. It has been estimated that oral contraceptives are responsible for one case of superficial or DVT per 500 women users per year.[209] Oral contraceptive users as a group have numerous alterations in their coagulation system including hyperaggregable platelets, decreased endothelial fibrinolysis, elevated levels of procoagulants, and decreased levels of antithrombin III.[210] Any of these factors, alone or in combination, may predominate in women taking oral contraceptives. The extent of this derangement in the hemostatic system will determine whether thrombosis will occur. When one then initiates endothelial damage with sclerotherapy in this population, an increased incidence of thrombosis may occur.

The most important factors preventing clot propagation are antithrombin III and vascular stores of tissue-type plasminogen activator (t-PA).[210-213] Antithrombin III levels have been demonstrated to be 20% lower in some women taking oral contraceptive agents.[211] Of women using oral contraceptive agents who have thromboembolic events, 90% have a twenty-fivefold decrease in releasable t-PA;[210-212] 51.6% have an abnormally low plasminogen activator content in the vein walls.[213] Therefore, a certain subgroup of women taking birth control pills are at particular risk for thromboembolic disease. Since it is practically impossible and also impractical at this time to determine which women are at risk, it would appear prudent to recommend that patients consider discontinuing this medication before sclerotherapy treatment.

Another subgroup of patients is also at an increased risk for DVT. Protein C and protein S are two vitamin K–dependent proteins that are important anticoagulant factors that prevent thrombosis. It has been estimated that the prevalence of heterozygous protein C deficiency may occur in 1:300 persons in the United States.[214] Over 95% of these subjects are asymptomatic and without a history of thrombotic disease. It has been speculated that damaged endothelium in combination with this deficiency may be necessary for symptomatic thrombosis to occur.[215] Therefore, patients who exhibit excessive thrombosis with sclerotherapy as well as patients who have a family history of thrombotic disease should be screened for deficiencies of protein C and protein S before treatment.

### Prevention and treatment

Because of the potentially lethal nature of excessive thrombosis, all attempts should be made to minimize its occurrence. The sclerosing solution quantity should be limited to 0.5 to 1 ml per injection site to prevent leakage of the solution into the deep venous system.[192] Other techniques that will minimize damage to the deep venous system include rapid compression of the injected vein with a 30 to 40 mm Hg pressure stocking followed by immediate ambulation or calf movement of the injected extremity and frequent ambulation thereafter to promote rapid dilution of the solution from the injected area. Using these recommendations, Fegan[216] reported no cases of DVT or pulmonary emboli in 13,352 patients when the sclerosing solution quantity was limited to 0.5 ml and rapid compression was used.

Foley[26] advocates the addition of heparin, 100 U/ml, to HS to prevent the theoretical possibility of embolization associated with "microthrombus formation" in sclerotherapy. However, a well-controlled, randomized study of 800 patients treated with and without heparin in the sclerosing solution found no evidence for embolization and no difference in the incidence of thrombophlebitis or microthrombosis requiring puncture evacuation.[27]

Fegan[186] states that STS is rapidly inactivated by the blood and is, in fact, a hemolytic and not a thrombotic agent. Therefore, he states that this complication is extremely rare with use of this sclerosing agent. However, he does recommend against treating women who are taking oral contraceptive agents because of a theoretical increase of thromboembolic events.

## Nerve Damage

Because of close proximity, the saphenous and sural nerves may be injected with solution during sclerotherapy (see Chapter 1). Injection into a nerve is reported to be very painful and, if continued, may cause anesthesia and sometimes a permanent interruption of nerve function.[84]

Occasionally, a patient may complain of an area of paresthesia in the treated leg. This is probably caused by perivascular inflammation extending from the sclerosed vein to adjacent superficial nerves. Steps to limit inflammation, including nonsteroidal antiinflammatory medications and high-potency topical steroids, may hasten resolution of this minor annoyance. However, this complication may take 3 to 6 months to resolve.[126]

## Air Embolism

When one uses the air block[217,218] or foam techniques to inject sclerosing solutions, the theoretical possibility of air embolism is raised. The danger would be that if enough air entered the heart at one time, it might lead to vascular collapse. In addition, if air enters a cerebral vascular artery, a cerebral vascular infarction may occur. More likely, transient ischemic symptoms might occur with this injection technique.

Introduction of air in small amounts into the venous system does not lead to clinical air embolism.[217,218] It appears that small amounts of air are absorbed into the blood stream before it enters the pulmonic circulation. It has been estimated that 480 ml of air would have to be put into the venous system within 20 to 30 seconds to cause death in a person weighing 60 kg.[219] This has never been

**Table** 8-2  Sclerosing agents for telangiectasias

| Agent | Active ingredient | Allergic reaction | Necrosis | Pain |
|---|---|---|---|---|
| Sodium morrhuate* | Fatty acids in cod-liver oil | Occasional | Occasional‡ | Mild |
| Sotradecol* | Sodium tetradecyl sulfate | Rare | Occasional‡ | Mild |
| Ethamolin* | Ethanolamine oleate | Occasional | Rare‡ | Mild |
| Hypertonic saline | 18%-30% saline | None | Occasional‡ | Moderate |
| Polidocanol† | Hydroxypolyethoxy-dodecane | Very rare | Very rare‡ | None |
| Sclerodex† | 10% saline + 5% dextrose | Very rare | Occasional | Mild |
| Scleremo† | 1.11% chromated glycerin | Very rare | Very rare | Moderate |
| Variglobin† | Iodide, sodium iodine | Very rare | Frequent‡ | Moderate |

Modified from Goldman MP and Bennett RG: Treatment of telangiectasia: a review, J Am Acad Dermatol 17:167, 1987.
*Approved for use by the Food and Drug Administration.
†Not approved for use in the United States.
‡Concentration dependent, especially with extravasation.

reported in the medical literature and has not occurred in a series of 297 cases with the air block technique.[217]

## Summary

In summary, sclerotherapy of varicose and telangiectatic leg veins may be associated with a number of adverse sequelae, which may occur despite optimal treatment and complications. Some adverse sequelae may be preventable to a limited degree, but given a large enough number of procedures, these adverse sequelae will occur in any practice. Complications may also be avoidable to some extent. As with any invasive procedure, however, sclerotherapy has inherent risks. Therefore, each patient should be evaluated and cautioned accordingly before initiating treatment. A summary of the common complications that can occur with the commonly used sclerosing agents is presented in Table 8-2.

**REFERENCES**

1. Tournay PR: Traitment sclerosant des tres fines varicosites intra ou saous-dermiques, Soc Fran Phlebol 19:235, 1966.
2. Bodian EL: Techniques of sclerotherapy for sunburst venous blemishes, J Dermatol Surg Oncol 11:696, 1985.
3. Duffy DM: Small vessel sclerotherapy: an overview. In Callen JP et al, editors: Advances in dermatology, vol 3, Chicago, 1988, Year Book Medical Publishers, Inc.
4. Alderman DB: Surgery and sclerotherapy in the treatment of varicose veins, Conn Med 39:467, 1975.
5. Weiss R and Weiss M: Resolution of pain associated with varicose and telangiectatic leg veins after compression sclerotherapy, J Dermatol Surg Oncol 16:333, 1990.
6. Cacciatore E: Experience of sclerotherapy with aethoxysklerol, Minn Cardioang 27:255, 1979.
7. Goldman P: Sclerotherapy of superficial venules and telangiectasias of the lower extremities, Dermatol Clin 5:369, 1987.
8. Georgiev M: Postsclerotherapy hyperpigmentations: a one-year follow-up, J Dermatol Surg Oncol 16:608, 1990.
9. Biegeleisen HI and Biegeleisen RM: The current status of sclerotherapy for varicose veins, Clin Med 83:24, 1976.

10. Chrisman BB: Treatment of venous ectasias with hypertonic saline, Hawaii Med J 41:406, 1982.
11. Chatard H: Discussion de la question de J-C Allart: pigmentations post-sclotherapiques, Phlebologie 29:211, 1976.
12. Shields JL and Jansen GT: Therapy for superficial telangiectasias of the lower extremities, J Dermatol Surg Oncol 8:857, 1982.
13. Barner FR, Holzegel K, and Voigt K: Über Hyperpigmentation nach Krampfaderverödung, Phebol u Proktol 6:54, 1977.
14. Cuttell PJ and Fox JA: The etiology and treatment of varicose pigmentation, Phlebologie 35:387, 1982.
15. Goldman MP, Kaplan RP, and Duffy DM: Postsclerotherapy hyperpigmentation: a histologic evaluation, J Dermatol Surg Oncol 13:547, 1987.
16. Goldman MP et al: Sclerosing agents in the treatment of telangiectasia: comparison of the clinical and histologic effects of intravascular polidocanol, sodium tetradecyl sulfate, and hypertonic saline in the dorsal rabbit ear vein model, Arch Dermatol 123:1196, 1987.
17. Moreno AH et al: Mechanics of distention of dog veins and other thin-walled tubular structures, Circ Res 27:1069, 1970.
18. Bessis M: Living blood cells and their ultrastructure, Berlin, 1973, Springer-Verlag.
19. Leu HJ et al: Veranderungen der transendothelialen Permeabilitat als Ursache des Odems bei der chronisch-venosen Insuffizienz, Med Welt 31:781, 1980.
20. Bessis M, Lessin LS, and Beutler E: Morphology of the erythron. In Williams WJ et al, editors: Hematology, ed 3, New York, 1983, McGraw-Hill Book Co.
21. Ackerman Z et al: Overload of iron in the skin of patients with varicose ulcers, Arch Dermatol 124:1376, 1988.
22. Chatarel H and Dufour H: Note sur la nature mixtre, hématique et mélanique, des pigmentations en phlébologie, Phlébologie 36:303, 1983.
23. Merlen JF, Coget J, and Sarteel AM: Pigmentation et stase veinëuse, Phlébologie 36:307, 1983.
24. Klüken N and Zabel M: La pigmentation est-elle un signe caractéristique de L'insuffisance veineuse chronique? Phlébologie 36:315, 1983.
25. Cloutier G and Sansoucy H: Le traitment des varices des membres inferieurs par les injections sclerosantes, L'Union Medicale du Canada 104:1854, 1975.
26. Foley WT: The eradication of venous blemishes, Cutis 15:665, 1975.
27. Sadick N: Treatment of varicose and telangiectatic leg veins with hypertonic saline: a comparative study of heparin and saline, J Dermatol Surg Oncol 16:24, 1990.
28. Hutinel B: Esthetique dans les scleroses de varices et traitement des varicosites, La Vie Medicale 20:1739, 1978.
29. Nebot F: Quelques points tecniques sur le traitement des varicosites et des telangiectasies, Phlebologie 21:133, 1968.
30. Landart J: Traitment medical des varices des membres inferieurs, La Revue du Practician 26:2491, 1976.
31. Norris MJ, Carlin MC, and Ratz JL: Treatment of essential telangiectasia: effects of increasing concentrations of polidocanol, J Am Acad Dermatol 20:643, 1989.
32. Guarde C: Personal communication, 1989.
33. Marley W: Low-dose sotradecol for small vessel sclerotherapy, Newsletter of North Am Soc Phlebol 3(2):3, 1989.
34. Muntlak H: Personal communication, (Paris) 1989.
35. Wenner L: Sind endovarikose hamatische ansammlungen eine normalerscheinung bei sklerotherapie? Vasa 10:174, 1981.
36. Leu HJ, Wenner A, and Spycher MA: Erythrocyte diapedesis in venous stasis syndrome, Vasa 10:17, 1981.
37. Orbach EJ: Hazards of sclerotherapy of varicose veins — their prevention and treatment of complications, Vasa 8:170, 1979.
38. Perchuk E: Injection therapy of varicose veins: a method of obliterating huge varicosities with small doses of sclerosing agent, Angiology 25:393, 1974.
39. De Takats G: Problems in the treatment of varicose veins, Am J Surg 18:26, 1932.
40. Biegeleisen HI: Sclerotherapy: clinical significance, Clin Med Surg 47:140, 1940.
41. Bernier EC and Escher E: Treatment of postsclerotherapy hyperpigmentation with trichloracetic acid, a mild and effective procedure. Proceedings of the second annual International Congress of the North American Society of Phlebology, New Orleans, La, February 25, 1989.
42. Terezakis N: Personal communication, 1989.
42a. Myers HL: Topical chelation therapy for varicose pigmentation, Angiology 17:66, 1966.
43. Riddock J: Treatment of varicose veins, Br J Med 2:671, 1947.
44. Goldman MP et al: Compression in the treatment of leg telangiectasia, J Dermatol Surg Oncol 16:322, 1990.

45. Terezakis N: Sclerotherapy treatment of leg veins. Presented at the summer session of the American Academy of Dermatology, San Diego, Calif, June 17, 1989.

46. Davis LT and Duffy DM: Determination of incidence and risk factors for post-sclerotherapy telangiectatic matting of the lower extremity: a retrospective analysis, J Dermatol Surg Oncol 16:327, 1990.

47. Bodian EL: Sclerotherapy, Semin Dermatol 6(3):238, 1987.

48. Ouvry P and Davy A: Le traitement sclerosant des telangiectasies des membres inferieurs, Phlebologie 35:349, 1982.

49. Merlen JF: Telangiectasies rouges, telangiectasies bleues, Phlebologie 23:167, 1970.

50. Biegeleisen K: Primary lower extremity telangiectasias, relationship of size to color, Angiology 38:760, 1987.

51. Shing Y et al: Angiogenesis is stimulated by tumor-derived endothelial cell growth factor, J Cell Biochem 29:275, 1985.

52. Ashton N: Corneal vascularization. In Duke-Elder S and Perkins ES, editors: The transparency of the cornea, Oxford, 1960, Blackwell Scientific Publications Inc.

53. Haudenschild CC: Growth control of endothelial cells in atherogenesis and tumor angiogenesis. In Altura BM, editor: Advances in microcirculation, vol 9, Basel, 1980, Karger.

54. Folkman J and Klagsbrun M: Angiogenic factors, Science 235:442, 1987.

55. Ryan TJ: Factors influencing the growth of vascular endothelium in the skin, Br J Dermatol 82(suppl 5):99, 1970.

56. Miyazono K et al: Purification and properties of an endothelial cell growth factor from human platelets, J Biol Chem 262:4098, 1987.

57. Castellot JJ Jr et al: Heparin potentiation of $3T_3$-adipocyte stimulated angiogenesis: mechanisms of action on endothelial cells, J Cell Physiol 127:323, 1986.

58. Barnhill RL and Wolf JE Jr: Angiogenesis and the skin, J Am Acad Dermatol 16:1226, 1987.

59. Dvorak AM, Mihm MC Jr, and Dvorak HF: Morphology of delayed-type hypersensitivity reactions in man. II. Ultrastructural alterations affecting the microvasculature and the tissue mast cells, Lab Invest 34:179, 1976.

60. Weiss RA and Weiss MA: Incidence of side effects in the treatment of telangiectasias by compression sclerotherapy: hypertonic saline vs polidocanol, J Dermatol Surg Oncol 16:800, 1990.

61. Mantse L: More on spider veins, J Dermatol Surg Oncol 12:1022, 1986.

62. Lary BG: Varicose veins and intracutaneous telangiectasia: combined treatment in 1500 cases, South Med J 80:1105, 1987.

63. Corbett DA: Discussion, Br J Dermatol 26:200, 1914.

64. Bean WB: The vascular spider in pregnancy. In Bean WB, editor: Vascular spiders and related lesions of the skin, Springfield, Ill, 1958, Charles C Thomas, Publisher.

65. Pirovino M et al: Cutaneous spider nevi in liver cirrhosis: capillary microscopical and hormonal investigation, Klin Wochenschr 66:298, 1988.

66. Saski GH, Pang CY, and Wittcliff JL: Pathogenesis and treatment of infant skin strawberry hemangiomas: clinical and in vitro studies of normal effects, Plast Reconstr Surg 73:359, 1984.

67. Sadick NS and Niedt GW: A study of estrogen and progesterone receptors in spider telangiectasias of the lower extermities, J Dermatol Surg Oncol 16:620, 1990.

68. Azizkhan RG et al: Mast cell heparin stimulates migration of capillary endothelial cells in vitro, J Exp Med 152:931, 1980.

69. Taylor S and Folkman J: Protamine is an inhibitor of angiogenesis, Nature 297:307, 1982.

70. Folkman J et al: Control of angiogenisis with synthetic heparin substitutes, Science 243:1490, 1989.

71. De Takats G and Quint H: The injection treatment of varicose veins, Surg Gynecol Obstet 50:545, 1930.

72. Chou F-F et al: The treatment of leg varicose veins with hypertonic saline–heparin injections, J Formosan Med Assoc 83:206, 1984.

73. Carlin MC and Ratz JL: Treatment of telangiectasia: comparison of sclerosing agents, J Dermatol Surg Oncol 13:1181, 1987.

74. Alderman DB: Therapy for essential cutaneous telangiectasias, Postgrad Med 61:91, 1977.

75. Orbach EJ: The importance of removal of postinjection coagula during the coarse of sclerotherapy of varicose veins, Vasa 3:475, 1974.

76. Orbach EJ: A new approach to the sclerotherapy of varicose veins, Angiology 1:302, 1950.

77. Fegan WG: Sound film: varicose veins — compression sclerotherapy. Produced by Pharmaceutical Research Limited, 6-7 Broad St, Hereford HR 4 9 AE, England.

78. Tournay R: Collections hematiques intra ou extra-veineuses dans les phlebites superficielles ou apres injections sclerosantes de varicies a quel moment la thrombectomie? Soc Fran Phlebol 19:339, 1966.

79. Sigg K: Varizenverodung am hochgelgerten Bein. Deutsches Arzteblatt — Arztliche Mitteilungen. 69. Jahrang, Heft 14, S. 809-818. 6. April 1972. Postverlagsort Koln.

80. Pratt D: The technique of injection and compression. Stoke Mandeveille Hospital Symposium: The treatment of varicose veins by injection and compression, Oct 15, 1971.

81. Hobbs JT: The Management of recurrent and residual veins. Stoke Mandeville Hospital Symposium: The treatment of varicose veins by injection and compression, Oct 15, 1971.

82. Holzegel VK: Uber Krampfaderverodugen, Dermatol Wocheuschr 153:137, 1967.

83. Winstone N. In The treatment of varicose veins by injection and compression. Proceedings of the Stoke Mandeville Symposium, Hereford, England, 1971, Pharmaceutical Research STD Ltd.

84. Browse NL, Burnard KG, and Thomas ML: Diseases of the veins: pathology, diagnosis, and treatment, London, 1988, Edward Arnold.

85. Duffy DM: Personal communication, 1989.

86. Schraibman IG: Localized hirsuties, Postgrad Med J 43:545, 1967.

87. Marks G: Localized hirsuties following compression sclerotherapy with sodium tetradecyl sulphate, Br J Surg 61:127, 1974.

88. Weissberg D: Treatment of varicose veins by compression sclerotherapy, Surg Gynecol Obstet 151:353, 1980.

89. Coverman M: Personal communication, 1989.

90. Eaglstein W: Personal communication, 1990.

91. Jaquier JJ and Loretan RM: Clinical trials of a new sclerosing agent, aethoxysklerol, Soc Fran Phlebol 22:383, 1969.

92. Hoffer AE: Aethoxysklerol (Kreussler) in the treatment of varices, Minn Cardioang 20:601, 1972.

93. Blenkinsopp WK: Choice of sclerosant: an experimental study. Angiologica 7:182, 1970.

94. de Faria JL and Moraes IN: Histopathology of the telangiectasias associated with varicose veins, Dermatologia 127:321, 1963.

95. Chavez CM: The clinical significance of lymphatico-venous anastomoses, Vasc Dis 5:35, 1968.

96. Chant ADB: The effects of posture, exercise, and bandage pressure on the clearance of 24Na from the subcutaneous tissues of the foot, Br J Surg 59:552, 1972.

97. Campion EC, Hoffman DC, and Jepson RP: The effects of external pneumatic splint pressure on muscle blood flow, Aust N Z J Surg 38:154, 1968.

98. Lawrence D and Kakkar V: Graduated, static, external compression of the lower limb: a physiological assessment, Br J Surg 67:119, 1980.

99. Beall GN, Casaburi R, and Singer A: Anaphylaxis — everyone's problem (Specialty Conference), West J Med 144:329, 1986.

100. Wasserman SI: Anaphylaxis. In Middleton E, Reed CE, and Ellis EF, editors: Allergy: principles and practice, ed 2, St Louis, 1983, The CV Mosby Co.

101. Shelley J: Allergic manifestations with injection treatment of varicose veins: death following injection of monoethanolamine oleate, JAMA 112:1792, 1939.

102. Schmier AA: Clinical comparison of sclerosing solutions in injection treatment of varicose veins, Am J Surg 36:389, 1937.

103. Zimmerman LM: Allergic-like reactions from sodium morrhuate in obliteration of varicose veins, JAMA 102:1216, 1934.

104. Meyer NE: Monoethanolamine oleate: a new chemical for obliteration of varicose veins, Am J Surg 40:628, 1938.

105. Lewis KM: Anaphylaxis due to sodium morrhuate, JAMA 107:1298, 1936.

106. Dick ET: The treatment of varicose veins, N Z Med J 65:310, 1966.

107. Monroe P et al: Acute respiratory failure after sodium morrhuate esophageal sclerotherapy, Gastroenterology 85:693, 1983.

108. Dale ML: Reaction due to injection of sodium morrhuate, JAMA 108:718, 1937.

109. Ritchie A: The treatment of varicose veins during pregnancy, Edinburgh Med J 40:157, 1933.

110. Probstein JG: Major complications of intravenous therapy of varicose veins, J Missouri Med Assoc 33:349, 1936.

111. Dodd H and Oldham JB: Surgical treatment of varicose veins, Lancet 1:8, 1940.

112. Kilby A et al: Abnormal chest roentgenograms following endoscopic injection sclerosis of esophageal varices, Hepatology 2:709, 1982.

113. Perakos PG, Cirbus JJ, and Camara S: Persistent bradyarrhythmia after sclerotherapy for esophageal varices, South Med J 77:531, 1984.

114. Biegeleisen HI: Fatty acid solutions for the injection treatment of varicose veins: evaluation of four new solutions, Ann Surg 105:610, 1937.

115. Hedberg SE, Fowler DL, and Ryan LR: Injection sclerotherapy of esophageal varices using ethanolamine oleate: a pilot study, Am J Surg 143:426, 1982.

116. Hughes RW Jr et al: Endoscopic variceal sclerosis: a one-year experience, Gastrointest Endosc 28:62, 1982.
117. Foote RR: Severe reaction to monoethanolamine oleate, Lancet 2:390, 1944.
118. Reid RG and Rothine NG: Treatment of varicose veins by compression sclerotherapy, Br J Surg 55:889, 1968.
119. Harris OD, Dickey JD, and Stephenson PM: Simple endoscopic injection sclerotherapy of esophageal varices, Aust N Z J Med 12:131, 1982.
120. Goldman MP and Bennett RG: Treatment of telangiectasia: a review, J Am Acad Dermatol 17:167, 1987.
121. Steinberg MH: Evaluation of sotradecol in sclerotherapy of varicose veins, Angiology 6:519, 1955.
122. Nabatoff RA: Recent trends in the diagnosis and treatment of varicose veins, Surg Gynecol Obstet 90:521, 1950.
123. Wallois P: Incidents et accidents au cours du traitement sclerosant des varices et leur prevention, Phlebologie 24:217, 1971.
124. Mantse L: A mild sclerosing agent for telangiectasias, J Dermatol Surg Oncol 11:855, 1985.
125. Mantse L: The treatment of varicose veins with compression sclerotherapy: technique, contraindications, complications, Am J Cosmetic Surg 3:47, 1986.
126. Fegan G: Varicose veins: compression sclerotherapy, London, 1967, Heinemann Medical.
127. MacGowan WAL et al: The local effects of intra-arterial injections of sodium tetradecyl sulphate (S.T.D.) 3%, Br J Surg 59:101, 1972.
128. Fronek H, Fronek A, and Saltzbarg G: Allergic reactions to sotradecol, J Dermatol Surg Oncol 15:684, 1989.
129. Passas H: One case of tetradecyl-sodium sulfate allergy with general symptoms, Soc Fran Phlebol 25:19, 1972.
130. Schneider W: Contribution al'historique du traitement sclerosant des varices et a son etude anatomo-pathologique, Soc Fran Phlebol 18:117, 1965.
131. Dingwall JA, Lin W, and Lyon JA: The use of sodium tetradecyl sulfate in the sclerosing treatments of varicose veins, Surgery 23:599, 1948.
132. Clinical Case 1. Presented at the third annual meeting of the North American Society of Phlebology, Phoenix, Ariz, Feb 21, 1990.
133. Cooper WM: Clinical evaluation of sotradechol, a sodium tetradecyl sulfate solution, in the injection therapy of varicose veins, Surg Gynecol Obstet 83:647, 1946.
134. Amblard P: Our experience with Aethoxysklerol, Phlebologie 30:213, 1977.
135. Hartel S: Complications and side effects of sclerotherapy, Zarztl Furtbild (Jena) 78:331, 1984.
136. Heberova V: Treatment of telangiectasias of the lower extremities by sclerotization: results and evaluation, Cs Dermatol 51:232, 1976.
137. Eichenberger H: Results of phlebosclerosation with hydroxypolyethoxydodecane, Zentralbl Phlebol 8:181, 1969.
138. Jacobesen BH: Aethoxysklerol: a new sclerosing agent for varicose veins, Ugeskr Laeg 136:532, 1974.
139. Feuerstein W: Anaphylactic reaction to hydroxypolyaethoxydodecon, Vasa 2:292, 1973.
140. Ouvry P, Chandet A, and Guillerot E: First impressions of Aethoxysklerol, Phlebologie 31:75, 1978.
141. Thies E, Lange V, and Iven H: Cardiac effects of polidocanol, a sclerotherapeutic drug — experimental evaluations, Chirurgisches Forum 192:313, 1982.
142. Imperiali G et al: Heart failure as a side effect of polidocanol given for esophageal variceal sclerosis, Endoscopy 18:207, 1986.
143. Paterlini A et al: Heart failure and endoscopic sclerotherapy of variceal bleeding, Lancet 2:1241, 1984.
144. Siems KJ and Soehring K: Die Ausschaltug sensibler nerven duren peridurale und paravertebrale injektion von alkylpolyathylenoxydathern bei meerschweinchen, Arzneimittelforsche 2:109, 1952.
145. Soehring K et al: Beitrage zur pharmakologie der alkylpolyathylenoxyd-derivate I: Untersuchungen uber die acute und subchronische toxizitat bei verschiedenen tierarten, Arch Int Pharmacodyn 87:301, 1951.
146. Soehring K and Frahm M: Studies on the pharmacology of alkylpolyethyleneoxide derivatives, Arzneimittel Forsch 5:655, 1955.
147. Nguyen VB: Sclerotherapie des varices des membres inferieurs etude de 522 cas, Le Saguency Medical 23:134, 1976.
148. Ouvry P and Arlaud R: Le traitement sclerosant des telangiectasies des membres inferieurs, Phlebologie 32:365, 1979.

149. Ouvry P and Davy A: Le traitement sclerosant des telangiectasies des membres inferieurs, Phlebologie 35:349, 1982.

150. Wallois P: Incidents et accidents de la sclerose. In Tournay R, editor: La sclerose des varices, ed 4, Paris, 1985, Expansion Scientifique Francaise.

151. Zimmet SE: Letter to the editor, J Dermatol Surg Oncol 16:1063, 1990.

152. Sigg K, Horodegen K, and Bernbach H: Varizen-Sklerosierung: Welchos ist das wirUsamste Mittel? Deutsohes Arzteblatt 34/35:2294, 1986.

153. Sigg K and Zelikovski A: Kann die Sklerosierungotherapie der Varizen obne Oparation in jedem Fallwirksam sein? Phlebol Proktol 4:42, 1975.

154. Wenner L: Anwendurg einer mit Athylalkahol modifizierten Polijodidjonenlosung bei skleroseresistenten Varizen, Vasa 12:190, 1983.

154a. Dodd H: The operation for varicose veins, Br Med J 2:510, 1945.

155. Coverman M: Personal communication, 1989.

156. Anticoagulants. In Bennett R, editor: AMA drug evaluations, ed 5, Chicago, 1983, American Medical Association.

157. Zinn WJ: Side reactions of heparin in clinical practice, Am Cardiol 14:36, 1964.

158. Gervin AS: Complications of heparin therapy, Surg Gynecol Obstet 140:789, 1975.

159. White PW, Sadd JR, and Nensel RE: Thrombotic complications of heparin therapy, including six cases of heparin-induced skin necrosis, Ann Surg 190:595, 1979.

160. Dukes MNG, editor: Meyler's side effects of drugs: an encyclopaedia of adverse reactions and interactions, ed 9, Amsterdam, 1980, Excerpta Medica Foundation.

161. O'Toole RD: Heparin: adverse reaction, Ann Int Med 79:759, 1973.

162. Hume M, Smith-Petersen M, and Fremont-Smith P: Sensitivity to intrafat heparin, Lancet 1:261, 1974.

163. Hall JC, McConahay D, and Gibson D: Heparin necrosis: an anticoagulation syndrome, JAMA 244:1831, 1980.

164. Shelley WB and Ayen JJ: Heparin necrosis: an anticoagulant-induced cutaneous infarct, J Am Acad Dermatol 7:674, 1982.

165. Tuneu A, Moreno A, and de Moragas JM: Cutaneous reactions secondary to heparin injections, J Am Acad Dermatol 12:1072, 1985.

166. DeShago RD and Nelson HS: An approach to the patient with a history of local anesthia hypersensitivity: experience with 90 patients, J Allergy Clin Immunol 63:387, 1979.

167. de Jong RH: Local anesthetics, ed 2, Springfield, Ill, 1977, Charles C Thomas, Publisher.

168. Swanson JG: Assessment of allergy to local anesthetic, Ann Emerg Med 12(5):316, 1983.

169. de Jong RH: Toxic effects of local anesthetics, JAMA 239(12):1166, 1978.

170. Incaudo G et al: Administration of local anesthesia to patients with a history of adverse reaction, J Allergy Clin Immunol 61:339, 1978.

171. Thomas RM: Local anesthetic agents and regional anesthesia of the face, J Assoc Military Dermatol 8:28, 1982.

172. Fregert S, Tegner E, and Thelin I: Contact allergy to lidocaine, Contact Dermatitis 5:185, 1979.

173. Covino BG and Vassallo HG: Local anesthetics: mechanisms of action and clinical use, New York, 1976, Grune & Stratton.

174. Eriksson E: Illustrated handbook of local anesthesia, ed 2, Philadelphia 1980, WB Saunders Co.

175. Baker JD and Blackmon BB: Local anesthesia, Clin Plast Surg 12:25, 1985.

176. Kennedy KS and Cave RH: Anaphylactic reaction to lidocaine, Arch Otolaryngol Head Neck Surg 112:671, 1986.

177. Promisloff RA and Dupont DC: Death from ARDS and cardiovascular collapse following lidocaine administration, Chest 83:585, 1983.

178. Aldrete JA: Sensitivity to lidocaine, Anesth Intensive Care 7:73, 1979.

179. Gill C and Michaelides PL: Dental drugs and anaphylactic reactions: report of a case, Oral Surg 50:30, 1980.

180. Chin TM and Fellner MJ: Allergic hypersensitivity to lidocaine hydrochloride, Int J Dermatol 19:147, 1980.

181. Ravindranathan N: Allergic reaction to lidocaine: a case report, Br Dent J 111:101, 1975.

182. Lehner T: Lidocaine hypersensitivity, Lancet 1:1245, 1971.

183. Fischer MM and Pennington JC: Allergy to local anaesthesia, Br J Anaesth 54:893, 1982.

184. Garber N: A criticism of present-day methods in the treatment of varicose veins, S Afr Med J 21:338, 1947.

185. Ogilvie WH: Some applications of the surgical lessons of war to civil practice, Br Med J 1:619, 1945.

186. Fegan WG: The complications of compression sclerotherapy, The Practitioner 207:797, 1971.

187. Sigg K: The treatment of varicosities and accompanying complications, Angiology 3:355, 1952.

188. From our Legal Correspondent: Hazards of compression sclerotherapy, Br Med J 3:714, 1975.

189. Goldstein M: Les complications de la sclerotherapie, Phlebologie 32:221, 1979.

190. Oesch A, Stirnemann P, and Mahler F: Das akute ischamiesyndrom des Fusses nach Varizen-verodung, Schweiz Med Wschr 114:1155, 1984.

191. MacGowan WAL: Sclerotherapy: prevention of accidents: a review, J R Soc Med 78:136, 1985.

192. Orbach J: A new look at sclerotherapy, Folia Angiologica 25:181, 1977.

193. Benhamou AC and Natali J: Les accidents des traitements sclerosant et chirurgical des varices des membres inferieurs: a propos de 90 cas, Phlebologie 34:41, 1981.

194. Bounumeaux H et al: Severe ischemia of the hand following intra-arterial promazine injection: effects of vasodilatation, anticoagulation, and local thrombolysis with tissue type plasminogen activator, Vasa 19:68, 1990.

195. Smith L and Johnson MA: Incidence of pulmonary embolism after venous sclerosing therapy, Minn Med 31:270, 1948.

196. Natali J and Marmasse J: Enquete sur le traitement chirugical des varices, Phlebologie 15:232, 1962.

197. Barber THT: Modern treatment of varicose veins, Br Med J 1:219, 1930.

198. Kern MM and Angle LW: The chemical obliteration of varicose veins: a clinical and experimental study, JAMA 93:595, 1929.

199. Linser P and Vohwinkel H: Moderne Therapie der Varizen, Hamorrhoiden und Varicocele, Stuttgart, 1942, Ferdinand Enke.

200. Sigg K: Zur Behandlung der Varicen der Phlebitis und ihrer Komplikationen, Hautarzt 1-2:443, 1950.

201. Schneider W and Fischer H: Fixierung und bindegewebige Organisation artefizieller Thromben bei der Varizenverodung, Dtsch Med Wschr 89:2410, 1964.

202. Atlas LN: Hazards connected with the treatment of varicose veins, Surg Gynecol Obstet 77:136, 1943.

203. McPheeters HO and Rice CO: Varicose veins — the circulation and direction of venous flow, Surg Gynecol Obstet 49:29, 1929.

204. Muller JHA, Petter O, and Kostler H: Kinematographische Untersuchugen bei der Varizenverodungstherapie, Z arztl Fortbild 78:345, 1984.

205. Williams RA and Wilson SE: Sclerosant treatment of varicose veins and deep vein thrombosis, Arch Surg 119:1283, 1984.

206. D'addato M: Gangrene of a limb with complete thrombosis of the venous system, J Cardiovasc Surg 7:434, 1966.

207. Goor W, Leu HJ, and Mahler F: Thrombosen in tiefen Venen und in Arterian nach Varizensklerosierung, Vasa 16:124, 1987.

208. Tretbar LL and Pattisson PH: Injection-compression treatment of varicose veins, Am J Surg 120:539, 1970.

209. Stadel BV: Oral contraceptives and cardiovascular disease, N Engl J Med 305:612, 1981.

210. Dreyer NA and Pizzo SV: Blood coagulation and idiopathic thromboembolism among fertile women, Contraception 22:123, 1980.

211. Pizzo SV: Venous thrombosis. In Koepke JA, editor: Laboratory hematology, vol 2, New York, 1984, Churchill Livingstone.

212. Miller KE and Pizzo SV: Venous and arterial thromboembolic disease in women using oral contraceptives, Am J Obstet Gynecol 144:824, 1982.

213. Astedt B et al: Thrombosis and oral contraceptives: possible predisposition, Br Med J 4:631, 1973.

214. Miletich J, Sherman L, and Broze G Jr: Absence of thrombosis in subjects with heterozygous protein C deficiency, N Engl J Med 317:991, 1987.

215. Rick ME: Protein C and protein S: vitamin K–dependent inhibitors of blood coagulation, JAMA 263:701, 1990.

216. Fegan WG: Continuous compression technique of injecting varicose veins, Lancet 2:109, 1963.

217. Orbach EJ: Sclerotherapy of varicose veins: utilization of intravenous air block, Am J Surg 66:362, 1944.

218. Orbach EJ: Clinical evaluation of a new technic in the sclerotherapy of varicose veins, J Inter Coll Surg 11:396, 1948.

219. Richardson HF, Coles BC, and Hall GE: Experimental air embolism, Can Med J 36:584, 1937.

# 9 Clinical Methods for Sclerotherapy of Varicose Veins

Varicose veins represent tortuous dilations of existing superficial veins. They arise because of multiple factors but are always associated with a relatively elevated venous pressure.[1] Therefore, initially, treatment consists of cutting off the point of high pressure inflow to the veins (either through surgical or sclerotherapeutic methods) before treating the varicose veins themselves.[2,3]

## HISTORICAL REVIEW OF TECHNIQUES
### Tournay (French) Technique

This procedure encompasses the basic principle of "French phlebology" developed by Tournay[4]: treating varicose veins "from high to low" ("de haut en bas").[3] Treating from proximal to distal sites also serves to eliminate the weight of the column of blood on the sclerosed point. This has the advantage of minimizing thrombosis and extravasation of red blood cells from a sclerosed vein segment. Interestingly, this same philosophy towards treatment was also reported from the Mayo Clinic in 1941 by Heyerdale and Stalker.[5] The principle of eliminating reflux from the saphenofemoral junction was espoused even earlier in 1927 by Moszkowicz[6] in Germany and de Takats and Quint[7] in the United States in 1930.

In addition to developing a treatment regimen with this tenet in mind, it is critical to accurately obliterate the saphenofemoral junction because its location and anatomy is so variable (see Chapter 1). To determine the origin of high pressure in the varicose vein, a noninvasive diagnostic evaluation of the patient should first be performed (see Chapter 5). The hand-held Doppler will help detect points of reflux from the deep to the superficial veins either through incompetent saphenofemoral or saphenopopliteal junctions and communicating and perforating veins. In certain circumstances additional testing may be required. If any points of reflux are detected, they should be treated first. After the high pressure flow has been eliminated, treatment should proceed first with injection of the largest varicose veins, then injection of the reticular feeding veins, and finally, treatment of the remaining "spider" veins.

In defense of the logic of the "French" technique, de Groot[3] pointed out that any vein in the leg belongs to either the long saphenous "system" or the short saphenous "system" (Fig. 9-1). This concept implies that a vein within the defined area of the long saphenous vein (LSV) eventually drains into the LSV. Therefore, reflux in that vein is derived from reflux at the saphenofemoral junction. This concept directs treatment toward the reflux point. Unfortunately, clinical examination regarding location of a vein does not always correctly determine the point of reflux. Therefore, the clinical examination must be correlated with a noninvasive examination to establish the optimal order of therapy.

### Sigg (Swiss) Technique

In contrast to the French technique, the Swiss technique of Sigg[8] and the modification by Dodd and Cockett[9] advocate total sclerosation of the entire varicose vein without any apparent pathophysiologic orientation. Whereas this method

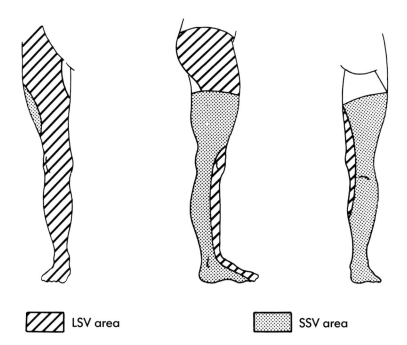

LSV area          SSV area

**Fig. 9-1**   Diagram of the long and short saphenous vein "systems." (Redrawn from de Groot WP: J Dermatol Surg Oncol 15:191, 1989.)

guarantees destruction of the treated vein, theoretical disadvantages to it include a higher incidence of recanalization, hyperpigmentation, and telangiectatic matting. These complications are thought to be partially related to the failure to eliminate the high pressure reflux at the junctions and/or perforators. This technique has also been adopted by some physicians who modify Fegan's technique of sclerotherapy of the incompetent perforating veins (described below). Included in this school are Reid and Rothnie[10] who treated 1358 legs of 974 patients and found that selective injection of perforating veins was ineffective, requiring multiple additional treatments of the entire vein. They therefore evolved a technique of placing multiple injections at intervals along the varicose veins to produce a diffuse sclerosis and have reported very favorable results. This latter technique will be referred to as the *total-vein sclerotherapy technique.*

## Fegan Technique

Fegan[11] proposes a view opposite the one mentioned above, namely that saphenofemoral incompetence could occur as a result of perforator incompetence alone. He reached this conclusion by demonstrating that the calf muscle pump is more powerful than the abdominal or femoral muscles in regard to venous flow in the leg. Therefore, he proposes that sclerotherapy of the incompetent perforating veins should be performed first to restore normal function. Fegan's examination of the saphenofemoral junction and LSV with phlebography after sclerotherapy of incompetent perforating veins showed a narrowing of the vessel lumen in 9 of 11 patients.[12] However, surgical exploration of clinically diagnosed areas of perforating vein incompetence has found at best a 60% incidence of perforating veins being correctly identified clinically.[13] In addition, phlebography examination performed on 112 patients with clinically suspected incompetent perforators showed that the clinical examination correctly identified only 38% of perforating veins below the knee and only 17% of thigh perforators.[14]

Despite the lack of accuracy of clinical diagnosis of incompetent perforating veins, many authors have found Fegan's technique to give excellent results. Tolins[15] reported favorable results using Fegan's technique; he injected areas of fascial defects with 0.5 ml of STS at up to 23 sites per leg. Three quarters of the patients had 2 to 5 injections. Doran and White[16] concluded after 2 years of follow-up that there was no difference between Fegan's technique and ligation and stripping procedures for varicose veins. Hobbs[17] concluded from his comparative study of sclerotherapy with Fegan's technique versus traditional surgery that the best treatment of nontruncal varicose veins and incompetent perforating veins of the lower leg is sclerotherapy. Tretbar and Pattisson[18] have found in their follow-up examinations of 264 patients treated with Fegan's technique that treatment failures usually occurred in patients with very large or fat legs with varicosities originating above the knee. This failure was thought to be caused by the difficulty of accurately placing injections within the veins of these patients and maintaining adequate compression. Sladen[19] analyzed 263 limbs with up to 7 years of follow-up and found that over 95% of his patients were satisfied with treatment and said they would have it repeated. He estimated a retreatment rate of about 5% per year. His patients average 3.6 to 5.25 injections per treatment session and 46% to 74% required one treatment session only. In agreement with Hobbs, Sladen found that all patients with saphenofemoral reflux all eventually required surgery. Therefore, although varicose veins treated with Fegan's technique respond well to treatment, the supposition of Fegan's technique, that sclerosis of the incompetent perforating veins is of primary importance and may reverse the remaining pathology in the LSV system, may not be correct.

Hobbs[20] has also provided evidence that when saphenofemoral and perforator incompetence occur together, both abnormalities should be corrected. Kerner and Schultz-Ehrenburg[21,22] studied the functional effects of sclerotherapy with photoplethysmography and concluded that the greatest functional improvement occurred with obliteration of the saphenofemoral junction. Obliteration of the incompetent perforating veins of the lower legs was of variable importance. Treatment of perforating veins of the upper leg was found to have no functional significance.

## Treatment of Reflux from the Saphenofemoral Junction

There are at least three schools of thought regarding which type of therapy is appropriate for initial treatment of the junctional points of reflux: surgical ligation (with or without limited stripping) of the saphenofemoral junction versus sclerotherapy of the saphenofemoral junction versus sclerotherapy of incompetent perforating veins alone. Bergan (see Chapter 10), Goldman,[23] de Groot,[3] Hobbs,[17] and others argue that surgical treatment of the junctions is the most appropriate and successful mode of treatment. This opinion is not new. As far back as 1934, Cooper,[24] in a series of over 85,000 injections in over 3000 patients, documented that the number of sclerosing injections required to produce obliteration of the varicose vein was markedly decreased after ligation of the saphenofemoral junction. In addition, Butie[25] has shown that sclerotherapy of the saphenofemoral junction is difficult and unreliable with the use of STS 3%, which is the strongest sclerosing agent approved for use by the United States Food and Drug Administration (FDA). Also, there is a risk of damaging the deep venous system and the femoral vein when sclerosing solution is injected in the upper thigh region. This has been demonstrated by radiologic examination showing the rapid flow of contrast media from a varicose LSV into the femoral vein when injections are performed in the upper thigh.[26] Therefore, these authors reserve sclerotherapy for treatment of residual varicosities after surgery.

**Table 9-1** Summary of "schools" of sclerotherapy

| School | Injection site | Compression | Instructions prescribed after procedure |
|---|---|---|---|
| Tournay | Proximal to distal | No | None |
| Sigg | Entire varicosity | Yes | None |
| Fegan | Perforating vein | Yes (6-week minimum) | Walking |

Raymond-Martimbeau,[27] Schultz-Ehrenburg,[28] and others, however, argue that the junctions can be successfully closed with sclerotherapy alone. In fact, a 6-year follow-up study has demonstrated a nearly 90% success rate with sclerotherapy.[27] By whatever method, closure of the saphenofemoral junction has been shown in pressure studies to prevent retrograde flow in the saphenous and perforator systems.[29] This suggests that incompetence of the perforating veins occurs as a result of a primary development of saphenofemoral reflux. Therefore, when the LSV or its tributaries are involved, the saphenofemoral junction, when incompetent, should be the first area treated.

In summary, long-term comparative studies of the various techniques is lacking. The literature consists mainly of anecdotal reports and studies with short follow-up periods. It is my opinion that no one "school" is absolute, but that the correct order of treatment should be individualized for each patient. Some patients may have only perforator incompetence and a normal saphenofemoral junction, thus Fegan's technique would be adequate. Other patients with saphenofemoral incompetence require treatment of that junction before initiating treatment elsewhere. Still other patients may have no obvious hemodynamic etiology for the origin of their varicose veins, thus directing treatment towards the entire varicosity as described by Sigg. Obviously, a careful work-up of all patients is necessary before beginning therapy. Besides deciding on the sequence of treatment, to be considered are various modifications of the injection procedure that some physicians profess have various benefits. Again, comparative studies of these treatment modifications have not been reported. Therefore, this chapter discusses sclerotherapy treatment of varicose veins, perforating veins, and the saphenofemoral junction with a review of the available literature. Variations in treatment are addressed and illustrative cases presented. A summary of the three schools of sclerotherapy is found in Table 9-1.

## INJECTION TECHNIQUE
## Patient Position

**Standing.** Although the above description of the treatment of varicose veins appears simplistic, the actual treatment methods for achieving effective sclerotherapy are numerous. Until the 1950s or so, sclerotherapy was performed with the patient standing throughout the procedure. The purpose was both to distend the varicose vein allowing easier needle insertion and also to produce firm thrombosis of the treated vein.[30] Multiple disadvantages of varicose thrombosis were realized (see Chapter 8), and various methods were devised to limit postsclerotherapy thrombosis. In addition, injecting sclerosing solution while the patient is standing forces the injection to occur against the hydrostatic pressure of a large column of blood. This may cause the sclerosing solution to seep along the needle into the perivenous tissues, which may lead to a chemical phlebitis or tissue necrosis.[31]

One of the earliest methods used to limit thrombosis was that of isolating the injected vein segment with pressure placed above and below the needle insertion site after first milking the blood out of the vein.[32] The importance of these "empty vein" injections was emphasized in a histologic evaluation of treated veins by Lufkin and McPheeters[33] in 1932, and the significance of compressing the vein to minimize thrombosis has been stressed by Orbach since 1943.[34] Therefore, these modifications are not new. They have been shown to result both in improved efficacy and in decreased incidence of complications when treatment is directed at the saphenofemoral junction.[16] The improved efficacy may be the result of a longer length of sclerosis of the varicose vein caused by gravitational flow of the sclerosing solution. However, recent evaluations comparing standing and reclining methods of treating varicose veins below the saphenofemoral junction have not been performed.

**Standing/reclining.** A modification of the standing technique, the standing/reclining technique, was described in 1926 by Meisen.[35] In the standing position, the needle was inserted while the vein was distended. Then with the needle still in the vein, the patient reclined on a table and the leg was elevated. This produced a relative emptying of blood from the vein. The sclerosing solution was then injected into an "empty" vein that was immediately compressed to prevent or minimize thrombosis.

In addition to excessive thrombosis at the injection site, another disadvantage of the total standing technique is that the sclerosing solution may escape through a perforating vein and damage the deep veins.[36] One radiographic study[37] has shown that an injection of 0.5 ml of contrast media travels rapidly (in 5 seconds) 8 cm distal to the injection site. Also, this amount of contrast did not completely fill the vein. Another radiographic study of the standing position, using Amipaque 150 as the contrast media (diluted to an isomolarity and specific gravity similar to polidocanol), showed that the injection of 1.5 ml remained in contact with a convoluted varicosity for about 10 seconds before flowing rapidly into the deep venous system through a presumed perforating vein (Fig. 9-2, *A* and *B*).[38] In contrast, when the patient was supine, the contrast media extended proximally along the varicosity and remained relatively undiluted for over 18 seconds (Fig. 9-2, *C* and *D*).[38] However, injections in some patients, when using the latter technique, also resulted in the contrast media remaining in contact with the varicosity for a longer period with the patient in the standing position (Fig. 9-3). Therefore, multiple variables, including the type of varicosity, its location, the location of associated perforator veins, and the movements of the patient (with associated calf and foot muscle contraction) while standing may all affect the distribution of the sclerosing solution.

**Leg elevated (Fegan).** Another obvious disadvantage of the standing technique is the vasovagal reaction (see Chapter 8). To prevent the sequelae of a vasovagal reaction, Fegan[39] recommends that patients sit at the end of the examining table with their legs hanging down while the physician, sitting in front on a low stool, inserts the needle. The leg is then raised while the patient fully reclines for 1 to 2 minutes. The physician stands to support the raised leg on the shoulder or against the chest, and the varicose veins are injected. With this or any technique that moves the patient after the needle is inserted, it is important to ensure that the needle is not displaced from the vein, either by fixing it to the skin with tape (if butterfly catheters or needles attached to syringes are used) or by holding the needle while the leg is raised. Since the varicose veins will collapse when the leg is raised, it is important to check for blood withdrawal as soon as possible

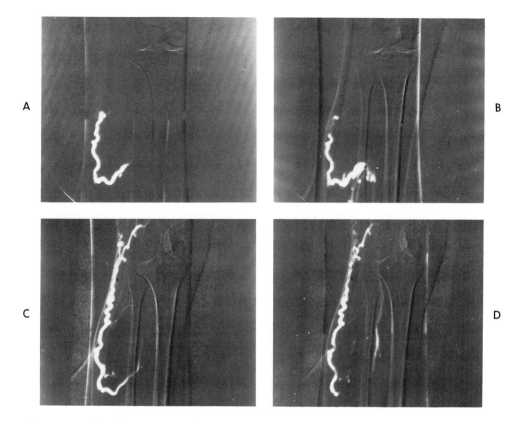

**Fig. 9-2**    Injected contrast media, 1.5 ml, shown 9.5 seconds, **A,** and 18.5 seconds, **B,** after injection into a varicose vein while the patient was standing. Injected contrast media, 1.5 ml, shown 9.5 seconds, **C,** and 18.0 seconds, **D,** after injection into a varicose vein while the patient was supine. (Courtesy George Heyn, M.D., Dept. of Vascular Surgery, DDR-Berlin.)

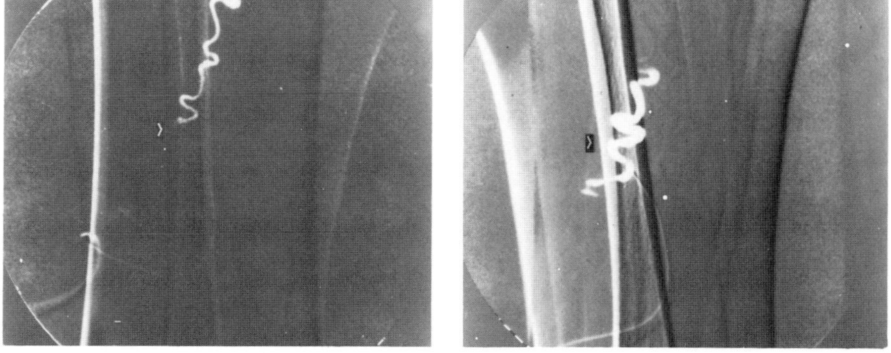

**Fig. 9-3**    **A,** Contrast media, 1.5 ml, shown 10 seconds after injection into a varicose vein while the patient was supine. Note the distribution of the contrast media proximally within the varicose vein. **B,** Contrast media, 1.5 ml, shown 10 seconds after injection into a varicose vein while the patient was standing. Note the contrast media remains for a relatively long time within the venous convolution. (Courtesy George Heyn, M.D., Dept. of Vascular Surgery, DDR-Berlin.)

after the leg is raised to ensure that the needle has not slipped out of the vein. The ease of blood withdrawal and the lack of spontaneous pulsatile flow from the needle without an attached syringe is proof of nonarterial placement of the needle.

To ensure that the sclerosing solution acts on the intended vein segment during injection, Fegan[39] applies pressure with his fingers a few centimeters proximal and distal to the injection point. Finger pressure is maintained for 30 to 60 seconds, and the leg is then bandaged from the toes to the injection site. With this method one injects only at the points of fascial defects (which are thought to represent sites of incompetent perforating veins as previously discussed). Injections proceed from distal to proximal sites with each vein segment/fascial defect being treated.

After injecting varicose veins in the elevated leg, compression should be applied immediately to prevent the vein from filling up with blood. This can be easily performed using the following method. Before inserting the needle, a compression stocking is placed over the foot and heel and allowed to bunch up at the ankle. After the needle is inserted into the varicosity, the leg is raised. Proper placement is then confirmed through blood withdrawal, and the sclerosing solution is injected. A foam pad is then placed over the injection site and secured in place with foam or elastic tape. The compression bandage can then be advanced over the injection site and foam pad in a distal to proximal manner (Fig. 9-4). With this technique, radiographic studies after injection of 0.5 ml of contrast medium show that when the leg is raised above the horizontal plane, the contrast medium travels rapidly for 30 cm before reaching the deep venous system.[37] Therefore, the sclerosing solution is diluted and probably inactivated by the time it reaches the deep venous system (see Chapter 7). In addition, with this technique it may not be necessary to repeat injections every few cm in the varicose vein.

With the leg-raising technique one assumes that the varicose vein is empty of blood; however, Perchuk[40] found otherwise. In "huge" varicosities as much as 18 ml of blood could be withdrawn. Therefore, he developed a method for ensuring an "empty" vein. His method consists of inserting the needle into the varicose vein, elevating the leg 45 degrees and then withdrawing blood through that needle into a syringe until further blood withdrawal is impossible. Then a syringe with sclerosing solution is attached to the needle and the injection is made, followed by application of local pressure for 5 minutes. The use of compression bandages or stockings after treatment was not mentioned. A two-way stop-cock may also be employed for this technique. Perchuk, in an evaluation of 84 patients, found that this technique produced excellent results and limited all complications. Pigmentation, thrombophlebitis, and recurrence were very rare. Fegan, however, disagrees with Perchuk's conclusions and states that the vein would empty of blood if raised for a longer time and at a more acute angle.[41]

**Two-phase (Sigg).** A variation on the method described above is the two-phase technique of Sigg.[8] The variation involves the way in which the needle is inserted into the vein. Sigg recommends that the needle be passed through the vein with the syringe unattached or with a finger placed over the hub and then slowly drawn back until the escape of blood indicates proper placement. The needle is left open and unobstructed while an assistant places a basin beneath it to catch the dripping blood. The leg is then raised above the horizontal plane and bleeding stops. A syringe is then attached and blood is withdrawn. After proper placement is confirmed by withdrawl of venous blood and the vein is emptied of

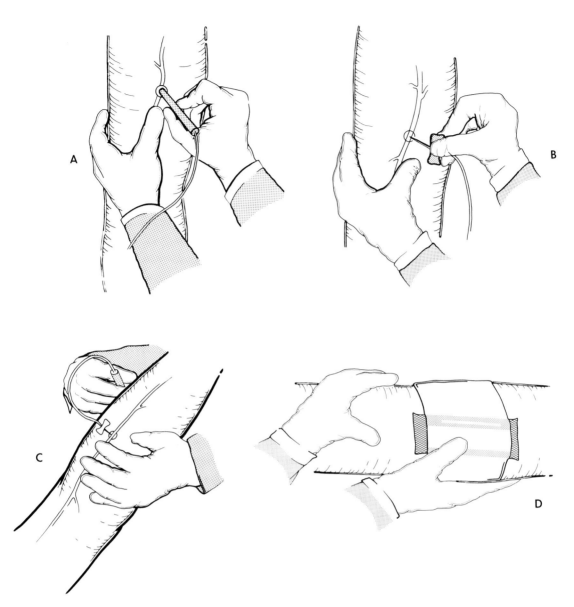

**Fig. 9-4** **A,** Localization of an incompetent perforating vein through the use of a hand-held Doppler. **B,** Cannulation of the incompetent communicating vein with a 26-gauge butterfly needle. **C,** The leg is then elevated 45 degrees and 0.5 to 1.0 ml of sclerosing solution is placed into the now empty communicating vein under minimal pressure. Note placement of a finger distal to the injection site to feel for extravasation of solution (which would indicate improper placement of the needle and necessitate immediate discontinuance of treatment and infiltration of the injection site with lidocaine 1%). **D,** Immediate compression of the treated vessel with an STD foam pad and tape dressing.

blood, the sclerosing solution is injected and the vein compressed, as described above, with stocking and/or bandage. Since Sigg uses mainly iodinated iodine solutions, he developed this technique to ensure continual intravascular placement of the sclerosing solution (see Chapters 7 and 8).

For both the Fegan and Sigg methods described, the needles are either all positioned and inserted while the varicose veins are distended or each needle is inserted separately, one at a time before each injection. When the latter is performed, distal compression prevents dilation of the preceding vein segment when the leg is lowered for each subsequent needle insertion.

**Reclining.** Another method for injection advocated since the 1920s is that of having the patient remain horizontal throughout the procedure.[42] If the varicose veins easily collapse in this position, they can be marked with indelible ink while the patient is standing before the procedure. Radiologic study has shown that a 0.5 ml bolus of contrast medium injected into a varicose tributary of the LSV travels proximally for 8 cm and remains within the vessel for about 2 minutes before being drawn into the deep venous system.[37] The relaxation of the calf muscles permits the injected fluid to stay within the vein since blood flow in this position is slow. Therefore, this position produces the longest lasting and most uniform contact between the injected solution and the vein wall.

To produce a relatively bloodless vein during injection in the horizontal position, some authors[42] advocate rubbing along the vein in both a proximal and distal direction away from the injection site. Manual compression is then maintained at the proximal and distal sites along the vein to prevent the vein segment from filling up with blood. After the injection a compression pad and bandage is immediately applied to the treated vein segment.

## Variations on Injection Technique

**Air-bolus.** The air-bolus technique was first advocated by Orbach[42] to ensure that sclerotherapy treatment of varicose veins occurred with minimal thrombosis. The rationale for instilling air before injecting the sclerosing solution is that clearing the vessel of blood will allow undiluted contact to occur between the solution and the vessel wall. This procedure was thought to minimize the concentration and quantity of solution required to produce endothelial injury. A comparative evaluation of this technique demonstrated enhanced efficacy of treatment regardless of the type of sclerosing agent used.[43] The potential complications of air embolism are addressed in Chapter 8. Unfortunately, there are many theoretical disadvantages of this technique. First, air proximal to the sclerosing solution in the syringe will cause compression of the solution producing leakage of solution from the needle after depression of the plunger has stopped. This may result in extravasation of solution upon needle withdrawal.

Air-bolus injections into large varicose veins in the area of the LSV have been shown in radiologic studies to be ineffective in clearing the vessel of blood even when 0.5 ml of air is injected immediately before the injection of contrast medium.[37] In addition, the air inhibits complete and even filling of the varix both proximal and distal to the injection site. In smaller varicosities, injected air forms several bubbles and does not act as a bolus. It also moves independently of the position of the patient and is not totally under the influence of gravity. Therefore, the air-bolus technique may not be an advantageous technique for use in varicose veins.

**Foam sclerotherapy.** It has been shown that shaking a solution of STS in the syringe to produce a foam increases the thrombogenic activity of the sclerosing solution fourfold.[44] STS foam is made by shaking a vial of STS for 30 seconds. The foam is then aspirated into a syringe. The amount of solution needed to make 1 ml of foam is approximately 0.05 ml.[45] The advantage of the foam is thought to be the result of the STS concentration in the walls of the bubbles, which continually bombard the intima and exert a continuous corroding effect on the vein wall. Therefore, unlike injection of a solution that is rapidly carried away and diluted in the blood stream, the foam acts longer at the point of injection.[45] A comparison of this technique versus the air-block technique has not been performed.

**Use of a tourniquet.** The use of a tourniquet is not recommended as an aid to injection. Although it may distend the vein for easier cannulation, the increased pressure in the varicose vein may force sclerosing solution into normal veins. In addition, the tourniquet will also impede flow in the normal vein, thus limiting the normal dilution of sclerosing solution. However, the tourniquet may be used just to facilitate placement of the needle into the vein. It is then removed, ensuring that the intended vein has been cannulated, and the solution is then injected.

## RECOMMENDED SCLEROSING SOLUTION AMOUNTS AND CONCENTRATIONS

Although the exact concentration of sclerosing solution depends on the caliber and location of the varicose vein, the following suggestions can serve as an initial guide to therapy. When diluting nonosmotic sclerosing solutions, dilution with sterile water will cause the sclerosing agent to sting at injection. Therefore, dilutions should be performed with bacteriostatic normal saline, which will not impart an additional "sting."

The *first principle* of determining solution amounts and concentrations is concentrations used should be stronger at the highest point of reflux. Therefore, with saphenofemoral reflux, the concentration should be strongest at the upper thigh and weakest at the ankle. Likewise, with ankle or calf perforating veins, the concentration should be highest at the perforator. For example, Vin[46] recommends that 1 ml of STS 1.0% be used at the proximal thigh, 0.5 ml of STS 1.0% be used at the medial thigh, and 0.3 ml of STS 0.5% be used at the medial knee location to treat a moderately sized varicose vein.

The *second principle,* as described by Tournay in 1949,[47] is, "It is not the concentration of the sclerosing agent in the syringe that matters, but the concentration within the vein." Sackmann[48] expanded on this principle by demonstrating in polyvinyl tubes that the local conditions of "time and space" regarding contact of the sclerosing solution with the vessel wall were also important. He demonstrated that the zone of contact diminishes as the caliber of the vessel increases. In tubes with a diameter less than or equal to 4 mm, the liquid flowed in a laminar fashion. In tubes with a diameter greater than or equal to 8 mm, turbulent flow was produced. At tubes of 6 mm in diameter a mixed flow occurred with a transition between a laminar and turbulent appearance. In contrast, the caliber and position of the needle, the speed of injection, and the viscosity of the solution did not seem to influence the time of contact of the sclerosing solution with the tube.

A study by Cornu-Thenard[49] suggests the following sclerosing concentrations for varicosities of various diameters:
    4 mm = STS 0.25%
    5 mm = STS 0.5%
    6 mm = STS 1.0%
He recommends injections of 0.5 ml placed every 6 to 10 cm along the varicose vein. Additional recommended concentrations for injection of Polidocanol and Variglobin into various types and diameters of veins are found in Chapter 7.

The *third principle* is the amount of sclerosing solution injected into a single site should not be more than 1.5 ml (usually 0.5 ml). Venography studies of direct injections into varicosities of the leg have demonstrated that if more than 1.5 ml of solution is injected at a single site, it is likely to spill over into the deep veins.[50] In addition, the patient should not move the leg for a few minutes so that the sclerosing solution can remain in contact with the varicose vein. This is important since any movement of the leg will rapidly move the sclerosing solution into the deep venous system.

## POSTSCLEROTHERAPY COMPRESSION

After injections of varicose or telangiectatic veins, the treated veins are immediately compressed to minimize significant thrombosis. The patient is instructed to walk immediately after the injection session to help prevent DVT and reduce venous reflux into the treated veins. Calf muscle movement produces a rapid blood flow in the deep venous system, which dilutes out any sclerosing solution that may have migrated into the area.

Postsclerosis compression is perhaps the most important advance in sclerotherapy treatment of varicose veins since the introduction of relatively safe synthetic sclerosing agents in the 1940s. Primarily, compression eliminates a thrombophlebitic reaction and substitutes a "sclerophlebitis" with the production of a firm fibrous cord.[10] The advantages of postsclerotherapy compression are discussed in detail in Chapter 6.

In addition to providing external compression to the treated vessel, one should also try to minimize forces that act to distend the vessel. Obviously, taking hot baths or saunas will dilate the cutaneous venous network and should be avoided for 2 to 6 weeks after sclerotherapy or until such time as the treated vessel is fully sclerosed. Also, any activity that increases abdominal pressure may act to force blood in a retrograde manner through the saphenofemoral junction or incompetent perforating veins producing venous dilation. Heavy weight lifting is therefore to be discouraged, as are any exercises that use the abdominal musculature. One such activity that increases abdominal pressure by about 22 mm Hg is running, pressure apparently produced to splint the trunk and pelvis.[51] Therefore, aerobic exercises, jogging, and running should be limited for 1 to 2 weeks.

Patients should be examined 2 weeks after injection so that any area of thrombosis can be evacuated early.[52] Each individual area should not be treated again sooner than 6 to 8 weeks after initial injection to allow adequate healing between treatments.

## CONTRAINDICATIONS TO TREATMENT
### Pregnancy

Besides the risk of absorption of the sclerosing solution by the fetus, pregnancy is associated with dilation of the entire venous system through multiple mechanisms (see Chapter 3).[53] Therefore, although sclerotherapy can and has been successfully performed by many authors on pregnant women,[54-58] the increase in venous distensibility counteracts the desired contraction of the treated varicose vein (see Chapters 3, 4, and 8). Finally, varicose veins may decrease in size and may disappear after delivery (see Chapters 3 and 4).[59] Thus waiting may eliminate the need for the procedure.

### Inability to Ambulate

Walking after treatment is very important because it ensures a rapid dilution of the sclerosing solution, which may enter normal deep veins. Walking also lessens the possibility of excessive thrombosis by liberating thrombolytic factors during muscle contraction and thereby avoids stagnation of blood flow. Walking also decreases physical distension of the vein caused by reflux.

## History of Thrombophlebitis and Deep Vein Thrombosis

Patients with a history of certain venous diseases may be predisposed to the development of excessive thrombosis with injection of a sclerosing agent, that is, development of an excessive phlebitic reaction (see Chapter 8). Also, in rare patients the dilated superficial system may serve as a conduit for carrying blood to the heart. Interruption of the superficial system then may increase venous insufficiency. Therefore, photoplethysmography, both with and without application of a superficial tourniquet or even with a trial of 30-to-40 mm Hg graduated compression stockings, will help determine which patients will benefit and which may be harmed by sclerotherapy treatment.

## Allergic Reaction

Rarely, patients may be allergic to a sclerosing solution, but one usually can substitute it for a different solution. If the allergic reaction consists of some generalized urticaria, with or without an erythematous papulosquamous appearance, French authors advocate continuing treatment with the offending sclerosing solution with the addition of antihistamines before and after treatment[60] (see Chapter 8).

Infrequently, patients may develop periorbital edema and a maculopapular cutaneous eruption even with the use of unadulterated hypertonic saline solutions. In this case, the "allergic reaction" may be the result of histamine release by intravascular basophils or perivascular mast cells that are directly damaged by the sclerosing solution (see Chapter 7).[61] Under this circumstance, before and after treatment with antihistamines appears safe while continuing therapy.

## Patients on Antabuse

Patients taking Antabuse should not be treated with Polidocanol or Sclerodex since these sclerosing solutions contain ethyl alcohol.

## CASE HISTORIES

The following case histories demonstrate my technique of sclerotherapy for different varicose veins (see box below).

---

**SCLEROTHERAPY OF VARICOSE VEINS**

**Sequence of Events**

1. Physical examination
2. Noninvasive diagnostic examination
3. If findings are abnormal, consider duplex scanning, varicography, or photoplethysmography
4. Eliminate the high pressure inflow points
   a. Saphenofemoral/saphenopopliteal junction
   b. Incompetent perforators
5. Sclerotherapy of the largest-diameter varicose veins
6. Sclerotherapy of communicating or reticular veins that feed "spider" telangiectasia
7. Sclerotherapy of "spider" telangiectasia
8. Candela pulsed dye laser treatment of remaining fine telangiectasia and arteriolar telangiectasia

**CASE 1: INCOMPETENT PERFORATOR VEINS TREATED WITH FEGAN'S TECHNIQUE**

*This 35-year-old woman developed varicose veins during the second trimester of her second pregnancy and wore an over-the-counter light compression stocking during the remainder of her pregnancy. At delivery she developed thrombophlebitis that was treated with hot packs only. She came for evaluation and treatment 6 months after delivery. Physical examination showed a 4-to-6 mm varicose tributary of the LSV originating at the medial midthigh and extending to the medial calf with continuation across the anterior tibia (Fig. 9-5, A and B). Venous Doppler examination revealed a continuous venous sound with distal augmentation at the level of the posterior tibial vein at the left ankle. There was no evidence of saphenofemoral reflux or other abnormalities. Photoplethysmography revealed a normal venous refilling time in the right leg. The venous refilling time was abnormal in the left leg (<20 seconds). The venous refilling time normalized with placement of a tourniquet at the level of the left upper calf and left lower thigh. Therefore, the physical and noninvasive examinations were consistent, showing incompetence of the Hunterian and superior calf perforating veins.*

*Because of the localized abnormality (incompetent perforator veins) producing the varicose vein, Fegan's technique of perforator interruption was used. Sclerotherapy was performed with the injection of 0.5 to 1.0 ml of STS 1.0% at the midthigh, medial superior calf, and anterior distal tibia point of fascial depression. The needles were inserted with the patient standing, and the patient then assumed the supine position with the leg elevated to 45 degrees. After aspiration to confirm proper needle placement, the sclerosing solution was injected while proximal pressure was maintained. STD E-foam pads were placed over the entire course of the varicose vein and secured with 3-M Microfoam tape. A 30-to-40 mm Hg graduated compression stocking was applied and worn continuously for 7 days, after which it was only worn while ambulatory for an additional week.*

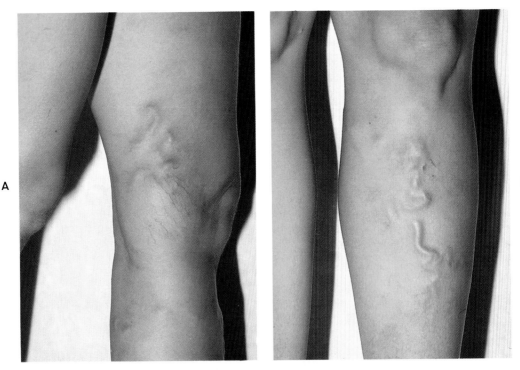

**Fig. 9-5**   Varicose tributary of LSV originating at medial midthigh, **A**, and extending to medial calf and continuing across anterior tibia, **B**.

*The patient was next seen 2 weeks later, at which time physical examination revealed total resolution of the varicosity at the midthigh (Fig. 9-5, C) and persistence of a thrombosed varicosity at the anterior tibial level (Fig. 9-5, D). This was drained and the pressure stocking was prescribed for use while the patient was ambulatory for another week. On follow-up examination 6 weeks later the vessel had resolved (Fig. 9-5, E). One-year follow-up demonstrates total obliteration of the varicosity and posttreatment hyperpigmentation (Fig. 9-5, F and G). This case illustrates Fegan's principle that interuption of the incompetent perforating veins alone will result in normalization of the entire varicose vein.*

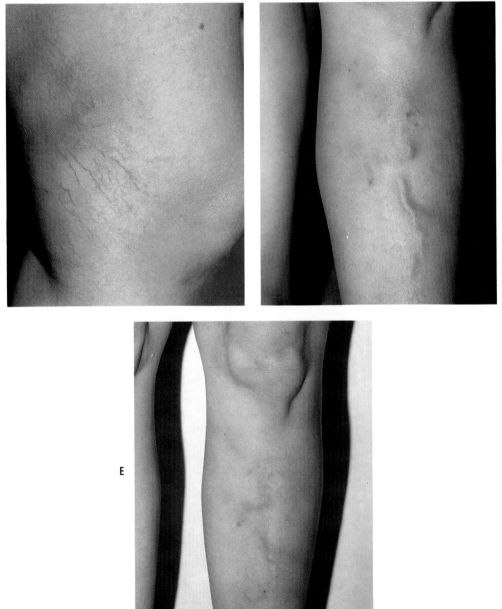

**Fig. 9-5, cont'd.**    C, Two weeks after sclerotherapy total resolution of varicosity is shown at midthigh but, **D,** persistence of thrombosed varicosity is visible at anterior tibial level. **E,** Complete resolution 6 weeks after sclerotherapy.                    *Continued.*

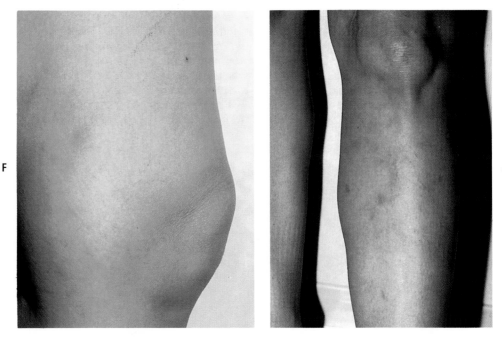

**Fig. 9-5, cont'd.** F, Lateral and G, anterior views of vein normalization 1 year after treatment.

### CASE 2: INCOMPETENT PERFORATING VEIN AT THE MIDCALF TREATED WITH MODIFIED FEGAN TECHNIQUE

*This 40-year-old woman noticed the gradual development of a varicose vein over the last 4 years without any predisposing factors. Physical examination showed a varicose tributary of the LSV 3 to 5 mm in diameter extending from the midanterior tibial surface to the medial calf and thigh ending in the lower anterior thigh (Fig. 9-6, A and B). Venous Doppler examination was remarkable only for an incompetent perforating vein at the right midmedial calf.*

*Since fascial depressions could not be felt, the classic Fegan technique could not be performed. Therefore, 25-gauge butterfly catheters were randomly placed into the varicosity at the level of the anterior midtibia, medial superior tibia, and the lateral knee with the patient standing. After the patient assumed the supine position, STS 0.5% was injected into these sites after proper needle placement was confirmed with blood aspiration. A total of 0.5 ml was injected at the anterior midtibia, 1 ml at the medial superior tibia and 2 ml at the lateral knee while pressure was maintained on the vein proximally. STD E-foam pads were placed over the entire vessel and secured with Coban tape applied with moderate pressure. A 30-to-40 mm Hg graduated compression stocking was applied with two stockings being worn on top of each other while the patient was ambulatory and one stocking being worn at night for 1 week. During the second week the dressing was removed and the graduated support stocking was then worn only while the patient was ambulatory for another week. The varicosity was completely resolved on follow-up examination at 2 weeks, and a few thrombi were drained. Fig. 9-6, C and D, were taken 11 months after treatment.*

*This latter technique used the principles of Fegan except that the entire area of presummed perforator incompetence was sclerosed. If one were to use Sigg's technique, the sclerosing solution would have been more randomly injected throughout the entire coarse of the varicose veins. The classic Fegan technique could have been performed if the sites of incompetent perforator veins were localized with Duplex imaging. Duplex-controlled injections may have limited the quantity of sclerosing solution injected to very specific sites but probably would not have affected the clinical outcome.*

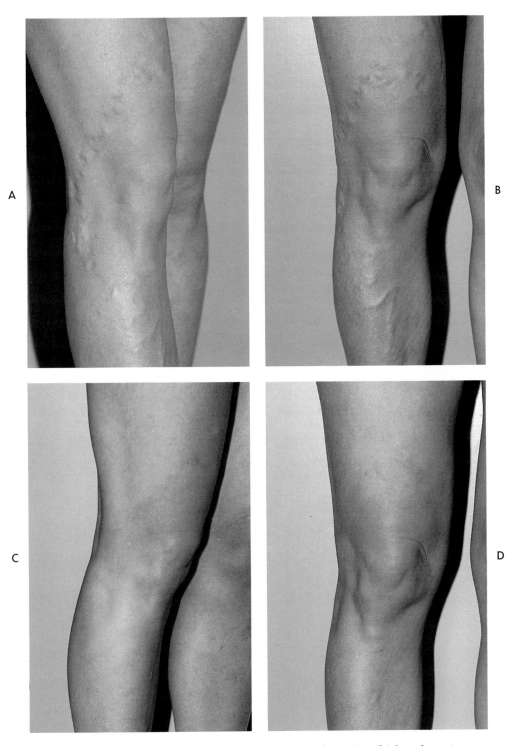

**Fig. 9-6**   Varicose tributary of LSV extending from midanterior tibial surface, **A,** to medial calf and thigh ending in lower anterior thigh, **B. C,** Midanterior tibial surface and medial calf and thigh and, **D,** lower anterior thigh views of vein normalization 11 months after treatment.

**CASE 3: RETICULAR VARICOSITIES WITHOUT PERFORATING VEIN REFLUX TREATED WITH TOTAL-VEIN SCLEROTHERAPY (SIGG'S TECHNIQUE)**

*This 34-year-old woman first noticed the appearance of varicose veins with her second pregnancy 3 years before treatment. The veins were symptomatic after prolonged standing and were thought to be enlarging over the past year. Physical examination showed a set of 3-to-4 mm varicose reticular veins coursing from the posterior midthigh to the posterior midcalf bilaterally (Fig. 9-7, A and B). There was no evidence of incompetence in either perforating veins or the saphenofemoral junctions on venous Doppler examination.*

*While the patient was lying horizontal on her abdomen, multiple injections of STS 0.5% were made into the varicose veins. Approximately 0.5 ml was injected into each site every 4 to 6 cm for a total of 8 ml of solution per leg. Continuous compression was maintained for 7 days only with a 30-to-40 mm Hg graduated compression stocking overlying STD E-foam pads over the varicose veins. Follow-up examination did not disclose excessive bruising or pigmentation. No thrombosis occurred. Fig. 9-7, C and D, show the appearance of the treated vessels at 1-year follow-up.*

*Since points of venous relux could not be found either at the saphenofemoral junction or in perforating veins, it was assumed that the varicose vein was essential in nature. Therefore, since it was serving no useful function it was obliterated in its entirety. This forms the rationale for Sigg's technique.*

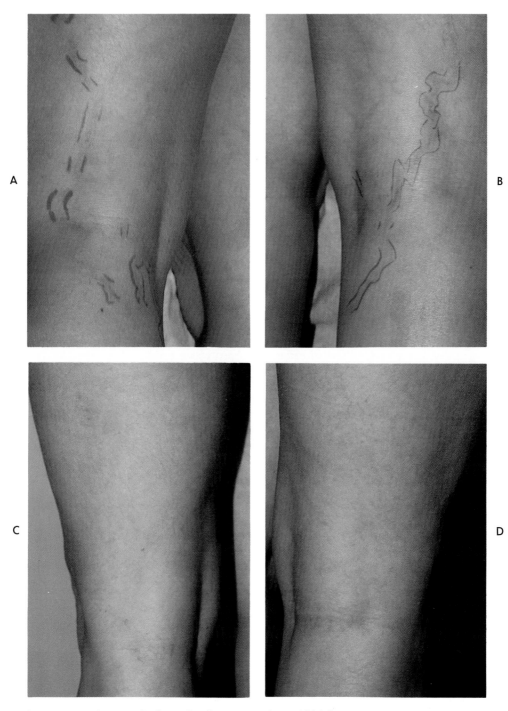

**Fig. 9-7**   Varicose reticular veins from posterior midthigh, **A**, to posterior midcalf, **B. C,** Posterior midthigh to **D**, posterior midcalf normalization of veins 1 year after treatment.

**CASE 4: POSTERIOR THIGH VARICOSE LSV TRIBUTARY ASSOCIATED WITH AN INCOMPETENT SAPHENOFEMORAL JUNCTION TREATED WITH SCLEROTHERAPY ALONE USING THE AIR-BOLUS TECHNIQUE.**

*This 36-year-old woman developed a varicose vein during her second pregnancy 3 years before our evaluation and treatment. The vein was symptomatic during prolonged standing, and she reported associated ankle edema. Physical examination showed a 5-to-8 mm diameter varicose vein coursing from the midposterior thigh to the midcalf (Fig. 9-8, A). Venous Doppler examination demonstrated gross incompetence of the right saphenofemoral junction and a positive Trendelenburg test in the lower thigh. The remainder of the examination was otherwise normal.*

*Surgical ligation and limited stripping were recommended but refused by the patient. Therefore, sclerotherapy of the involved varicose vein was performed using an air-block technique. The air-block was used in an attempt to concentrate the sclerosing solution in the injection site without dilution or inactivation of blood. Butterfly needles, 25-gauge, were placed in the vein at areas of fascial depression — two sites on the thigh and one site on the calf — while the patient was standing. These areas were not found by venous Doppler to represent incompetent perforator veins. With the patient lying horizontal and the leg elevated to 45 degrees, 1 ml of STS 1.0% was injected into each site after injection of 0.5 ml of air. STD E-pads were immediately placed and secured with 3-M Microfoam tape and a single 30-to-40 mm Hg graduated compression stocking was worn continuously for 2 weeks. Follow-up examinations at 2 and 6 weeks showed persistent resolution of the vein with a slightly palpable cord. A small amount of coagula was drained at 6 weeks. The vein has continued to remain fibrosed 2 years after treatment (Fig. 9-8, B).*

*Treatment in this patient consisted of a modified Fegan and Sigg technique. The entire varicosity was obliterated using fascial depression areas as injection sites. Alternatively, one could have used the French technique with injection of sclerosing solution into the saphenofemoral junction. However, this was not performed because of the unavailability of Variglobin. Alternatively, STS 3% could have been injected under Duplex control at the saphenofemoral junction. Refer to the excellent articles by Raymond-Martimbeau[27] and Schultz-Ehrenburg et al.[28] for a description of these latter techniques.*

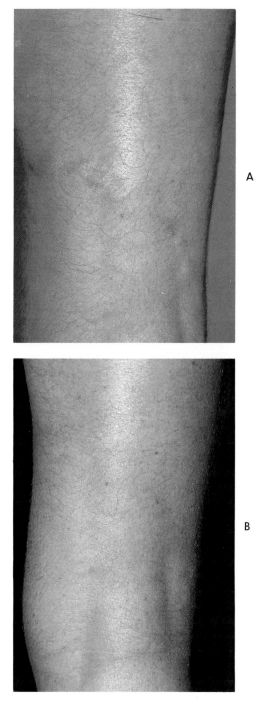

**Fig. 9-8**    A, Varicose vein from midposterior thigh to midcalf. B, Vein remains sclerosed 2 years after treatment.

**CASE 5: INCOMPETENT SSV VARICOSE TRIBUTARIES TREATED WITH TOTAL-VEIN SCLEROTHERAPY ALONE**

*This 31-year-old woman noted the onset of varicose veins over the right lower leg at 10 years of age. With each of her succeeding three pregnancies, the veins enlarged and became more painful while standing. Physical examination showed a clustered varicose vein 5 to 10 mm in diameter over the right anterior and medial calf (Fig. 9-9, A). Venous Doppler examination demonstrated marked reflux of the right SSV throughout the varicosity.*

*The patient refused surgical ligation and limited stripping. Therefore, sclerotherapy with STS 1.0% was performed while the patient was horizontal. One ml of solution was slowly injected at each of nine separate locations followed by application of STD foam pads and a double layer of 30-to-40 mm Hg graduated compression stockings worn continuously while ambulatory for 2 weeks. One stocking was removed while sleeping. A mild phlebitic reaction was clinically apparent 2 weeks after injection (Fig. 9-9, B) and compression was maintained another 2 weeks. Four weeks after the first injection, multiple thrombi were drained from the medial calf and two more injections of STS 1%, 1 ml each, were made into persistent varicose dilations on the medial and anterior superior calf (Fig. 9-9, C). At 1-year follow-up, the leg continued to be pain free and showed persistent resolution of the treated veins (Fig. 9-9, D). Venous Doppler examination disclosed an incompetent 4-mm diameter varicose vein just below the right anterior tibia and another incompetent varicosis over the inferior midposterior calf. These veins were successfully sclerosed with STS 1%. At 2 years follow-up the multiple new varicosities became apparent after resolution of sclerotherapy-induced hyperpigmentation. Interestingly, the patient has remained pain free and is very happy with the results of treatment. Her wish is to continue sclerotherapy treatment even with the understanding that new or recurrent varicose veins may later occur.*

*This patient represents two common findings in my practice. First, many patients would rather undergo multiple (perpetual?) sclerotherapy treatments rather than limited surgical ligations or strippings. And, second, the resolution of symptoms, if very important to patients, may occur despite a reappearance of the varicose vein. It appears that in many patients, incomplete treatment is enough to alleviate symptoms.*

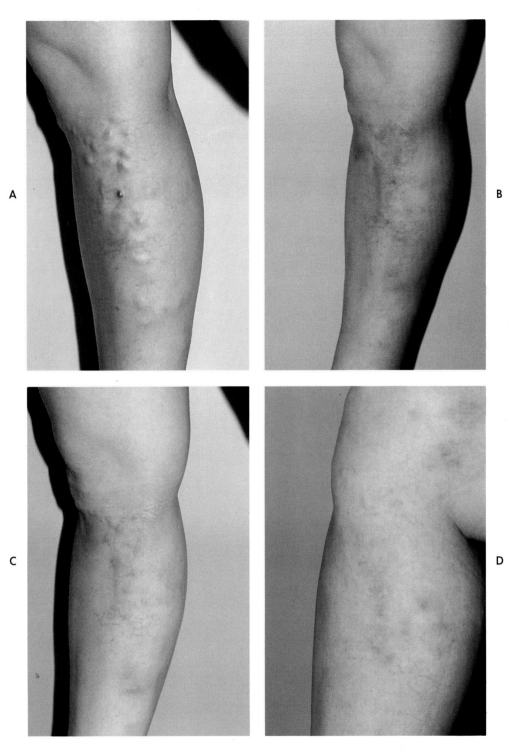

**Fig. 9-9**   **A,** Clustered varicose vein over right anterior and medial calf. **B,** Mild phlebitic reaction 2 weeks after treatment. **C,** Further treatment 4 weeks after first injection. **D,** Resolution of vein continues at 1 year after treatment.

**CASE 6: INCOMPETENT PERFORATOR VEIN UNDERLYING ANKLE ULCERATION.**

*A 27-year-old woman sought treatment for a 3-year history of a cutaneous ulceration over the right medial mallear region (Fig. 9-10, A). The patient was previously seen by the infectious disease service and was prescribed multiple courses of systemic antibiotic treatments which did not produce significant change in the appearance of the ulceration. She was also evaluated by the plastic surgery department and treated with the placement of full-thickness pinch grafts, which did not heal. Physical examination was remarkable for pedal edema extending to the midcalf and associated truncal varicosities. Venous Doppler examination demonstrated a normal deep venous system, saphenofemoral and popliteal junctions and an incompetent perforating vein at the base of the ulcer (marked X in Fig. 9-10, A). The perforating vein was injected through the ulcer. A 23-gauge butterfly needle was inserted into the perforating vein while the patient was standing, and the leg was elevated while the patient reclined. STS 1.0%, 1 ml, was slowly injected while the leg was blocked proximally and distally with hand pressure 3 cm in either direction. Immediately afterwards compression was applied with an STD foam pad under microfoam tape and two 30-to-40 mm Hg graduated compression stockings. The stockings were worn for 2 weeks. Double stockings were worn during the day, and the outer stocking was removed when the patient was supine.*

*Follow-up examination at 3 months showed complete healing of the ulceration and resolution of associated venous stasis changes (Fig. 9-10, B). The patient remains free of ulceration at 2 years after treatment.*

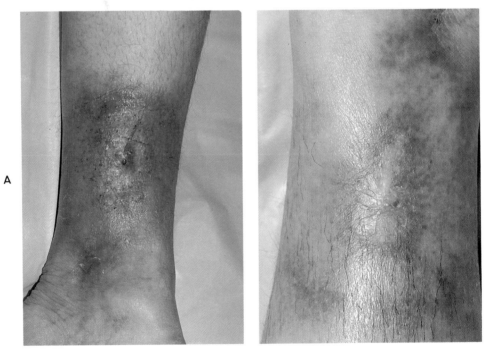

**Fig. 9-10**   A, Cutaneous ulceration over right medial mallear region. B, Complete healing of ulceration and resolution of venous stasis changes 3 months after treatment.

## REFERENCES

1. Goldman MP and Fronek A: Anatomy and pathophysiology of varicose veins, J Dermatol Surg Oncol 15:138, 1989.
2. Goldman MP and Bennett RG: Treatment of telangiectasia: a review, J Am Acad Dermatol 17:167, 1987.
3. de Groot WP: Treatment of varicose veins: modern concepts and methods, J Dermatol Surg Oncol 15:191, 1989.
4. Tournay R et al: La sclerose des varices, ed 4, Paris, 1985, Expansion Scientifique Francaise.
5. Heyerdale WW and Stalker LK: Management of varicose veins of the lower extremities, Ann Surg 114:1042, 1941.
6. Moszkowicz L: Behandlung der Krampfadern mit Zuckerinjektionen kombinurt mit Venenligatur, Zentralbl f Chir 54:1732, 1927.
7. de Takats G and Quint H: The injection treatment of varicose veins, Surg Gynecol Obstet 50:545, 1930.
8. Sigg K: Neure Gesichtspunkte zur Technik der Varizenbehandlung, Therap Unschau, vol 6, 1949.
9. Dodd H and Cockett FB: The pathology and surgery of the veins of the lower limbs, London, 1956, ES Livingstone Ltd.
10. Reid RG and Rothnie NG: Treatment of varicose veins by compression sclerotherapy, Br J Surg 55:889, 1968.
11. Fegan WC, Fitzgerald DE, and Milliken JC: The results of simultaneous pressure recordings from the superficial and deep veins of the leg, Ir J Med Sci 6:363, 1964.
12. Quill RD and Fegan WG: Reversibility of femorosaphenous reflux, Br J Surg 55:389, 1971.
13. Schalin L: Arteriovenous communication localized by thermography and identified by operative microscopy, Acta Chir Scand 147:109, 1981.
14. Kakkar VV, Howe CT, and Flanc C: Compression sclerotherapy for varicose veins — a phlebographic study, Br J Surg 56:620, 1969.
15. Tolins SH: Treatment of varicose veins: an update, Am J Surg 145:248, 1983.
16. Doran FSA and White M: A clinical trial designed to discover if the primary treatment of varicose veins should be by Fegan's method or by operation, Br J Surg 62:72, 1975.
17. Hobbs JT: Surgery and sclerotherapy in the treatment of varicose veins: a random trial, Arch Surg 109:793, 1974.
18. Tretbar LL and Pattisson PH: Injection-compression treatment of varicose veins, Am J Surg 120:539, 1970.
19. Sladen JG: Compression sclerotherapy: preparation, technique, complications, and results, Am J Surg 146:228, 1983.
20. Hobbs JT: A random trial of the treatment of varicose veins by surgery and sclerotherapy. In Hobbs JT, editor: The treatment of venous thrombosis, Philadelphia, 1977, JB Lippincott Co.
21. Kerner J and Schultz-Ehrenburg U: Funktionele Auswirkungen unterschiedlicher Angriffspunkte bei der Sklerosierungstherapie, Phlebol Proktol 17:101, 1988.
22. Kerner J and Schultz-Ehrenburg U: Functional meaning of different injection levels in the course of sclerotherapy, Phlebology 4:123, 1989.
23. Goldman MP: Rational treatment of varicose and spider leg veins. In Robbins P, editor: Surgical gems in dermatology, vol 2, New York, 1991, Journal Publishing Group (in press).
24. Cooper WM: The treatment of varicose veins, Ann Surg 99:799, 1934.
25. Butie A: Experience with injections at the saphenofemoral junction in the United States. In Davy A and Stemmer R, editors: Phlebologie '89 Montrouge, France, 1989, John Libbey Eurotext Ltd.
26. Boyd AM and Robertson DJ: Treatment of varicose veins: possible danger of injection of sclerosing fluids, Br Med J 2:452, 1947.
27. Raymond-Martimbeau P: Two different techniques for sclerosing the incompetent saphenofemoral junction: a comparative study, J Dermatol Surg Oncol 16:626, 1990.
28. Schultz-Ehrenburg U, Weindorf N, and Tourbier H: Moderne, hamodynamisch orientierte Richtlinien fur die Sklerosierung der Stamm- und Seitenastvaricosis der V saphena magna und parva, Phlebol Proktol 17:83, 1988.
29. Bjordal RI: Circulation patterns in incompetent perforating veins in the calf and in the saphenous system in primary varicose veins, Acta Chir Scand 138:251, 1972.
30. McCaffrey J: An approach to the treatment of varicose veins, Med J Aust 1:1379, 1969.
31. Sigg K: The treatment of varicosities and accompanying complications, Angiology 3:355, 1952.
32. Foote RR: Varicose veins, St Louis, 1949, The CV Mosby Co.
33. Lufkin H and McPheeters HQ: Pathological studies on injected varicose veins, Surg Gynecol Obstet 54:511, 1932.
34. Orbach EJ: A new approach to the sclerotherapy of varicose veins, Angiology 1:302, 1950.

35. Meisen V: A lecture on injection-treatment of varicose veins and their sequelae (eczema and ulcus cruris), clinically and experimentally, Acta Chir Scand 60:435, 1926.
36. Kinmonth JB and Boyd A: Discussion on primary treatment of varicose veins, Proc R Soc London 41:631, 1948.
37. Steinacher J and Kammerhuber F: Weg und Verweildauer eines Kontrastmittels im oberflachlichen Venesystem unter Bedingungen der Varicenverodung: Eine Studie zur Technik der Varicenverodung, Zschr Haut-Geschl-Krkh 43:369, 1968.
38. Heyn G, Waigand J, and Tamaschke C: Flow behaviour of sclerosants in the treatment of primary varicose veins. In Davy A and Stemmer R, editors: Phlebologie '89, Montrouge, France, 1989, John Libbey Eurotext Ltd.
39. Fegan WG: Continuous compression technique of injecting varicose veins, Lancet 2:109, 1963.
40. Perchuk E: Injection therapy of varicose veins: a method of oblitering huge varicosities with small doses of sclerosing agent, Angiology 25:393, 1974.
41. Fegan WG: Personal communication, 1990.
42. Orbach EJ: Sclerotherapy of varicose veins: utilization of intravenous air block, Am J Surg 66:362, 1944.
43. Orbach EJ: Clinical evaluation of a new technique in the sclerotherapy of varicose veins, J Int Coll Surgeons, 11:396, 1948.
44. Orbach EJ and Petretti AK: Thrombogenic property of foam synthetic anionic detergent (sodium tetradecyl sulfate, NNR), Angiology 1:237, 1950.
45. Orbach EJ: Has injection treatment of varicose veins become obsolete? JAMA 166:1964, 1958.
46. Vin F: Principles, technique, and results of treatment of the greater saphenous vein by sclerotherapy. Paper presented at the second annual International Congress of the North American Society of Phlebology, New Orleans, Feb 25, 1989.
47. Merlen JF et al: Histologic study of a sclerosed vein, Phlebologie 31:17, 1978.
48. Sackmann LA: Etude physique de l'injection sclerosante, Soc Fran Phlebol 22:149, 1969.
49. Cornu-Thenard A: Sclerotherapy of varicose veins: value of measurement of vessel diameter before the first injection. Paper presented at the second annual International Congress of the North American Society of Phlebology, New Orleans, Feb 25, 1989.
50. Kinmonth JB and Robertson DJ: Injection treatment of varicose veins: radiological amd histological investigations of methods, Br J Surg 36:294, 1949.
51. Stegall HF: Muscle pumping in the dependent leg, Circ Res 19:180, 1966.
52. Orbach EJ: The importance of removal of postinjection coagula during the course of sclerotherapy of varicose veins, Vasa 3:475, 1974.
53. Barwin BN and Roddie IC: Venous distensibility during pregnancy determined by graded venous congestion, Am J Obstet Gynecol 125:921, 1976.
54. McPheeters HO: Prophylactic injection treatment of varicose veins during pregnancy, Lancet 51:589, 1931.
55. Kilbourne NJ: Varicose veins of pregnancy, Am J Obstet Gynecol 25:104, 1933.
56. Mullane DJ: Varicose veins of pregnancy, Am J Obstet Gynecol 63:620, 1952.
57. McCausland AM: Varicose veins in pregnancy, West J Surg 47:81, 1939.
58. Fegan G: Varicose veins: compression therapy, London, 1967, Heinemann Medical.
59. Mantse L: The treatment of varicose veins with compression sclerotherapy: technique, contraindications, complications, Am J Cosmetic Surg 3:47, 1986.
60. Passas H: One case of tetradecyl-sodium sulfate allergy with general symptoms, Soc Fran Phlebol 25:19, 1972.
61. Stroncek DF et al: Sodium morrhuate stimulates granulocytes and damages erythrocytes and endothelial cells: probable mechanism of an adverse reaction during sclerotherapy, J Lab Clin Med 106:498, 1985.

# 10 The Role of Surgery in Treatment of Varicose Veins and Venous Telangiectasias

*John J. Bergan*

Jean Van der Stricht has called attention to the fact that some observations made in the late 19th century are applicable to treatment of varicose veins in the late 20th century. Specifically, he has cited Quenu who said in 1890, ". . . the continuation of the disorder is inevitable. . . . The only real cure is the treatment which would restore the normal structure to the vascular walls." Before 1900, at the time of Quenu, the various therapeutic possibilities included elastic compression, sclerotherapy, and surgery. These remain mainstays of treatment today. Another observation from the 1890s discussed sclerotherapy particularly and said that "any method whose main characteristic is that it provokes phlebitis is bad." Surgical therapy then was treated no more kindly by opinions, which said that "most varicose vein patients do not need surgery." Finally, the overall conclusion of workers in the field that treated venous stasis 100 years ago was that "the surgical solution is perhaps only palliative."

With the above observations in mind, it is possible in this chapter to touch on the current contribution of surgery to the care of patients with varicose veins and cutaneous telangiectasias.

## HISTORICAL LESSONS

For many years after 1950, the bible and textbook for varicose vein surgery was the monumental contribution by Harold Dodd and Frank Cockett: *Pathology and Surgery of the Veins of the Lower Limbs.* The foreword was written by R.R. Linton, and thus the three most famous names in vein surgery were linked inseparably.[1] That text was greatly concerned with the techniques of operative surgery. Detailed results of operations developed in the first half of this century are found there and are still relevant to present-day surgery.

### Types of Operations Performed

The operations detailed in Dodd and Cockett's text include proximal ligation and division of the saphenous vein at the groin, ligation of the saphenous vein in the groin combined with retrograde injection of sclerosing solution, ligation of the saphenous vein above the knee either with or without distal sclerosing injections, and operative sclerosing solutions injected into various segments of the LSV alone. Interestingly, among the sclerosing solutions used was hypertonic saline (30%), recently rediscovered in its 23.4% incarnation. Finally, it can be emphasized that after 1950, stripping of the LSV was by far ". . . the most satisfactory after three to eight years' follow-up." The operation, as depicted in photographs and drawings, was the standard surgical procedure from that time until approximately 1980.

### Long and Short Saphenous Vein Stripping

Lessons learned from the standard long and short saphenous stripping operation are as follows: First, the long incisions at groin, ankle, and over large varicosities in the thighs and legs were anticosmetic. Even as late as 1983, at least one author advocated a "6-to-8 cm incision placed 3 to 4 cm below and lateral to the pubic tubercle." This was too much incision placed too low. Its saving grace was that its length allowed wide exploration, but the resulting scar was simply too obvious. Next, passing the stripper internally was frequently quite easy, and consequently, the surgeon was able to remove long lengths of vein from the body. Unfortunately, these veins were often found to have competent valves, absence of dilation, and absence of elongation and tortuosity — in short, these were normal saphenous veins.

## Recurrent Varicosities

It became apparent to many physicians that a large body of literature on the subject of recurrent varicose veins was accumulating. The only logical conclusion to be drawn from such an expanse of literature was that the vein stripping operation, which often removed a normal vein, failed to cure the patient of the condition for which it was designed. It is that operation, now greatly modified and to some extent abandoned, that is the subject of criticism by nonsurgeons today.

## MODERN SURGERY
## Stripping and Stab Avulsion Varicectomy

As a reaction to the above-mentioned lessons learned, many surgeons modified the technique of varicose vein removal in an attempt to remove the end organ, varicose veins, while at the same time preserving normal axial veins. Some pressures came from cardiac and arterial surgeons who decried standard stripping because it removed a vein that might later be used as an arterial substitute.

The crux of the modern operation is a careful assessment, made by the noninvasive techniques described in Chapter 5, of the function of the superficial veins. Thus saphenofemoral and saphenopopliteal competence can be assessed and a more cosmetic and conservative operation can be performed that is specifically designed to remove the offending varicosities and preserve the saphenous vein if possible.

Ultimately, the modern operation is resolved into three stages: (1) preoperative evaluation including a thorough history and physical examination supplemented by meticulous noninvasive testing, thereby comprehensively studying the superficial and deep veins; (2) accurate marking of the offending varicosities to allow careful planning with the objective of removing virtually all of the subcutaneous varicosities (A direct correlation has been established between good results and thorough varicosity removal[2]); and (3) the operation itself. It is frequently performed with the patient's legs elevated to decrease blood loss, sometimes under tourniquet control.[3] Incisions are limited in length and are made with a fine-bladed, narrow (No. 11) scalpel. Varicosities are avulsed, and skin closure is accomplished with tape strips.[4-6]

## High Tie and Distal Sclerotherapy

There has been some tendency in recent years to avoid stripping the LSV. Some surgeons now advocate proximal division without stripping. Instead, they perform sclerotherapy with compression. Compression is added for a number of reasons, including that after saphenous vein division at the groin with retrograde injection of sclerosing agents, if no compression bandage is applied, the results are unsatisfactory. This operation of groin tie and compression sclerotherapy leads to two thirds of patients receiving a satisfactory result when assessed at 3 years. These good results deteriorate to only 40% satisfactory results at 5 years.[7] A mid-1980s review of this subject has been performed, and this is important to note because of current advocacy of high tie and distal sclerotherapy for saphenous vein insufficiency. This, in some ways, is retrogressive. When this combined technique was performed and objectively evaluated at the University of Lund, Neglen, Einarsson, and Eklof[8] reported that "when mainstem insufficiency is present, high tie combined with compression sclerotherapy is a poor treatment in the long-term and is no replacement for surgery." Surgery in this instance refers to local saphenous removal from groin to distal thigh or upper leg. Therefore, when saphenofemoral incompetence is present, resection of the LSV down to the distal thigh or upper leg should be done. Many physicians have come to this conclusion and condemn operations limited to the saphenofemoral junction. Among these physicians is Van der Stricht[9] who says that ". . . any correct saphenectomy will include the resection of the saphenofemoral junction. This is practiced where there is an open (incompetent) saphenofemoral junction and in clear cases of incompetence in the saphenous axis." Van der Stricht continues, saying that indications for simple resection of the saphenofemoral junction are rare except in second operations after incomplete previous surgery. He does open the door to a simplified operation in cases of aesthetic saphenous removal. This operation is chosen for selected patients today because simple resection of the saphenous vein at its termination avoids distal disfiguring scars in the thigh and leg.[9] It also allows brief outpatient surgery performed with the patient under local anesthesia at a minimal cost, an important fact when third party payors deny benefits.

## Telangiectasias and Their Treatment

Intradermal, dilated venules and arterioles (termed *telangiectasias*), alone and in combination, are of great concern to many patients. Being common, they are known by many names including "spider veins," "spider web veins," "rocket bursts," "starbursts," "venous stars," and "arborizing telangiectases." They are described elsewhere in this volume. Many are asymptomatic but at least an equal number produce local aching, heaviness, and fatigue. These symptoms are more likely caused by deeper veins that, being unsupported, have dilated under the pressures of hormonal cycling, pregnancy, aging, and upright posture. They, in turn, transmit their hypertension to their feeding dermal venules. These dilate to the point of disrupting the capillary barrier that allows arteriolar pressure to be exerted on primary dermal venules. When symptomatic, this vascular arborization can be treated by sclerotherapy, and such therapy may be effective for the dermal tip of the "iceberg" and the iceberg itself, the subcutaneous, blue, incompetent communicating vein. The "glacier," to continue the metaphor, is incurable. Surgery cannot treat the intradermal dilated vessels but may, in some instances, remove the subcutaneous 2-to-4 mm veins that are in direct continuity with the dermal reticular blemishes.

## PREOPERATIVE PREPARATION

Preoperative evaluations are as important as surgical technique; they consist of photoplethysmography, varicography, Doppler examination, and skin marking.

## Photoplethysmography and Light Reflection Rheography

Photoplethysmography (PPG) and light reflection rheography (LRG) make use of the fact that the subdermal tangle of blood vessels is largely a venous pool. Infrared light beamed through the epidermis into this pool can be reflected back and give a semiquantitative evaluation of the emptying of that pool and its refilling. Refill time, as assessed by PPG and LRG, correlates well with venous pressure refill time. When performing the examination with the patient in a comfortable sitting position (legs dependent), in a warm room, and with tourniquets placed at below-knee and above-knee positions, accurate differentiation between deep venous reflux and superficial venous reflux can be ascertained. This is the entire purpose of this examination. If only superficial incompetence is present, the patient can be cured. The effect of tourniquets on reflux gives an estimate of beneficial effects of superficial venous stripping.

## Varicography

Varicography is planned and used only when the surgical situation is complex. Several indications for this procedure are (1) after previous major vein stripping, (2) in the presence of massive, recurrent varicose veins, (3) in identifying tributaries to the lesser saphenous system, and (4) in identifying popliteal fossa and gastrocnemius veins described below. Furthermore, identification of the termination of the SSV at the popliteal vein is well accomplished with on-table varicography if preoperative Duplex imaging has failed to reveal this junction.

## Doppler Examination

Surgery is also preceded by Doppler examination. The patient is examined standing, supported by an adjacent chair or table. The Doppler probe is placed on the LSV in the thigh, at the femoral vein, the SSV, and the popliteal vein sequentially. The patient is asked to breathe deeply, cough, and Valsalva as each site is examined. Reflux during inspiration, coughing, or Valsalva is a reliable index of reflux. If LSV reflux is present, this vein must be removed if surgical benefit is to be long-lasting.

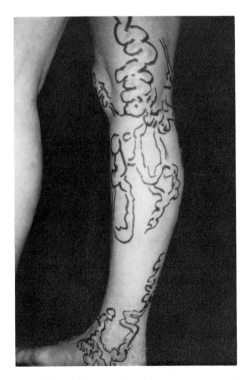

**Fig. 10-1** Preoperative marking of the varicosities as completely as possible will ensure that operative incisions are placed exactly where desired and all offending varicosities are removed. In this instance, a limited LSV stripping to the below-knee position was planned with stab avulsion of varicose clusters. The SSV was found to be competent and was left intact.

## Marking Varicosities

Preoperative marking is done with a felt-tipped, indelible marking pen; the relative size of the varix is indicated by the breadth of the line, and individual palpable fascial defects are marked by circles (Fig. 10-1). Accurate marking is an absolute requisite to successful varicosity removal. Subsequently, during the surgical procedure such markings may dictate the placement of surgical incisions.

## SURGICAL TECHNIQUE
### Long Saphenous Vein Stripping

At surgery, the LSV and SSV are ignored if Doppler studies show their terminations to be competent. This point deserves emphasis because surgical literature contains many descriptions of removal of the saphenous veins and very few details of preservation of these structures.

Surgeons have no difficulty identifying the LSV termination when viewed through a short, oblique groin incision made at the groin crease in patients who do need removal of this vein. The incision is begun at the medial edge of the femoral pulse and is carried medially as far as is necessary (2 to 3 cm). Distal stripping extends only to the distal thigh or upper anteromedial calf as indicated previously (Fig. 10-2). Removal of the saphenous vein below the upper calf level is

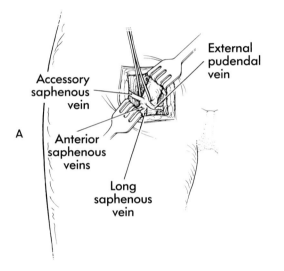

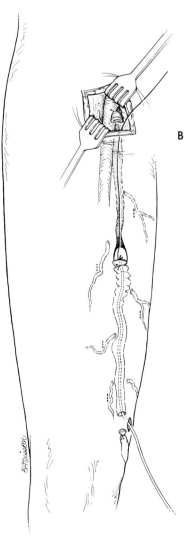

Fig. 10-2 Surgical removal of the LSV through a groin and distal incision are illustrated in these diagrams. A shows an enlarged view of the groin incision placed high in the groin crease. Note that this exposes the common femoral vein and its tributaries. In **B** the stripper within the proximally and distally divided saphenous vein is pulled distally to, but not through, the distal incision. It is then retrieved proximally by means of a heavy ligature or 3-mm polyester umbilical tape.

usually unnecessary and is occasionally associated with damage to the saphenous nerve. Removal of the LSV for gross incompetence automatically removes the midthigh communicating veins (Hunterian perforators), which are a source for recurrent venous insufficiency. A short vertical incision in the distal thigh or upper anteromedial calf allows the stripping instrument to be removed from the lumen of the vein at this point. The stripping head is brought down to that point, the vein is fixed to the stripper by ligature, and the stripper, stripper head, and vein are retrieved proximally at groin level. This allows the distal incision to be very small and quite cosmetic. The device for retrieving the stripper and vein is a simple, heavy ligature or 3-mm umbilical tape.

## Short Saphenous Vein Stripping

Stripping of the SSV is required in a minority of cases and should always be preceded by identification of the termination of the SSV by Duplex or color-flow imaging or intraoperative varicography. The SSV origin is approached at the lateral aspect of the ankle (Fig. 10-3). This is done with great care because the sural nerve is intimately associated with the SSV at this point and may lie within the layers of fascia rather than deep to the fascia (see Chapter 1). At the termination

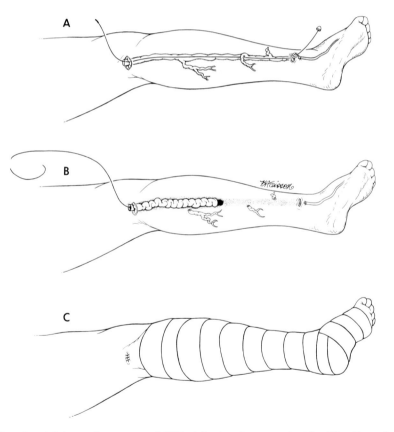

**Fig. 10-3**    Crucial to performance of SSV stripping is accurate identification of true saphenopopliteal reflux (by continuous wave Doppler) and accurate determination of saphenous venous termination (by Duplex). Otherwise, the operation is straightforward with intraluminal cannulation, **A**; proximal removal of stripper and vein, **B**; and avulsion of varices as in Fig. 10-4, *A* and *B*. Postoperative pressure bandaging after cosmetic skin closure completes the operation, **C**.

of the SSV in the popliteal fossa, the vein should never be ligated until the surgeon has seen the popliteal junction clearly. This dissection may be difficult and complicated by large tributaries. Some of these join the SSV from above and some may come from varicosities within the nerve. It is essential that the popliteal vein and peroneal nerve be carefully preserved during this part of the dissection.

## Stab Avulsion

When long and short saphenous stripping was abandoned as the cornerstone of the operation for varicosities, it was replaced by the stab avulsion technique of varicosity removal. Because of the meticulous marking that precedes the surgical procedure today, each of the varicose veins, singly or in clusters, can be removed through minimal incisions. Associated incompetent perforating veins are treated simultaneously. The incisions are made with a sharp-pointed blade (No. 11) directly over the vein, and the varicosity is lifted through the wound with fine-pointed forceps (Fig. 10-4, *A*). After surrounding fat is cleared away, the loop of vein that appears through the wound is doubly clamped and divided (Fig. 10-4, *B*). Each end is teased out through the incision as the areolar tissue on the surface is dissected off (Fig. 10-4, *C*). The forceps are always placed close to the skin to prevent the vein from breaking. Traction on the skin itself allows tributaries to be broken and greater lengths of the varicosity to be removed. Observation has shown that varicosities are divided clinically into two types — those that are white on their surface avulse well, those that are blue often tear easily. Distal or proximal incisions are made within the markings to ensure that total removal of offending varicosities is accomplished. Varicosities removed by this technique are inevitably tributaries to axial veins and do not require ligation except if they terminate into the axial vein itself and that vein is to be left in place. Perforator

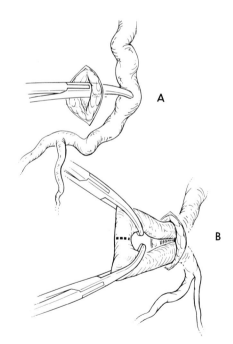

**Fig. 10-4**    A, The grasping of previously marked varicosities. The incision is a 2-to-3 mm stab made with a No. 11 blade. After the varicosity is exteriorized, **B**, it is divided and each end is carefully avulsed to remove as much varix as possible.                    *Continued.*

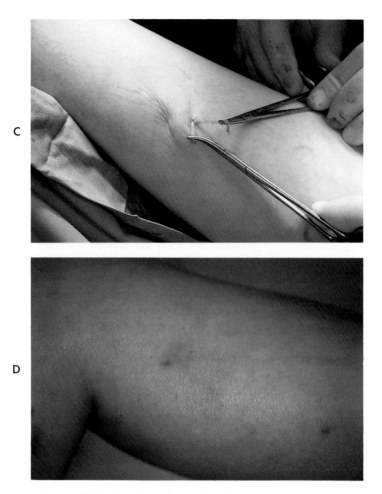

**Fig. 10-4, cont'd.**   C, With the limb elevated 30 degrees, 2-mm cutaneous incisions can be made, the varicosity brought to the surface by the hook technique, and after division of the vein, each end can be avulsed selectively. Placement of subsequent incisions will depend on the length of varicosity excised. **D,** This photograph, taken 10 days after surgery, shows the location of a distal medial calf incision through which the LSV has been stripped from the groin to this level.

veins associated with clusters of varices are ligated, of course. Incisions made for local varicosity removal are made small enough that sutures are unnecessary and tape closure can be used. If an individual incision is made longer than the average, it can be closed by an inverted, absorbable suture and covered over with the usual tape closure. Fig. 10-4, *D*, shows the appearance 10 days after surgery.

## Recurrent Varicosities

Surgery has a definite place in the treatment regimen for removal of recurrent varicose veins. These veins may be residual varicosities left as a result of incomplete sclerotherapy, new veins not treated at sclerotherapy or a previous operation, or residual veins overlooked at prior surgery. It would be most correct to refer to varicose veins present after therapy as being either residual veins missed at the time of original therapy, or recurrent veins that were formerly normal and then became varicose because of an underlying genetic or physiologic abnormality that was not corrected.

Varicography or Duplex scanning may be very important for accurate removal of residual or recurrent varicosities. Complications introduced by prior surgery can be diagnosed by using such direct imaging of offending incompetent veins. At the groin level, a number of causes of recurrence have been identified. These include failure to complete flush ligation of the saphenous vein, failure to remove terminal tributaries to the saphenous vein, failure to identify duplicated saphenous veins or their tributaries, and failure to remove the termination of the saphenous vein, thus allowing midthigh communicating veins to develop recurrent saphenous incompetence. At the popliteal level, recurrent varicosities frequently develop in scar tissue through transgastrocnemius communicating veins not ligated at the initial operation and also through secondary muscular communicating veins. Isolated, recurrent, superficial varicosities are also a major reason for failures of primary therapy. These are best managed by careful marking and simple avulsion through multiple incisions, as indicated above, or through sclerotherapy, as described elsewhere in this volume.

It should be emphasized that not all recurrent veins are caused by inadequate primary operations or sclerotherapy. Clearly, abnormal veins can develop after primary therapy; they can even develop in the absence of deep venous abnormalities. The stab avulsion surgical technique lends itself well to treatment of such veins.[10]

## Perforating Veins

Surgery on the perforating veins is not simple surgery. Apart from division of perforating veins incidental to varicose vein removal, planning surgery on major perforating veins in cases of severe chronic venous insufficiency is a formidable decision to make. Underlying difficulties in judgment is the startling fact that from 15% to 50% of such operations are failures. Even when failure is judged by the harshest criteria, recurrence of venous ulcer, this fact is true.

Principles that act as a guide in deciding whether to perform perforator interruption include the following: (1) Classical anatomic studies by surgeons in the first half of the twentieth century are informative but inaccurate.[11] The perforating veins tributary to the posterior arch vein, so carefully mapped out in such studies, are found to lie on a lane rather than a line and are extremely variable in importance and location; (2) surgery performed to interrupt such perforating veins and remove associated varicosities is plagued by wound healing failure and secondary infection; (3) classic subfascial perforator interruptions produce a formidable operative procedure frequently followed by immediate wound complications and later ulcer recurrence; and (4) the subcutaneous or Cockett approach causes skin slough if undermining is performed. Therefore, careful identification of perforating veins associated with venous ulceration is requisite. This is done with the hand-held Doppler even before ulcer healing is complete, knowing that sclerotherapy to obliterate such perforating veins may accelerate ulcer healing. Objectives of sclerotherapy intended to interrupt perforator veins include improving skin nutrition in the hope that ulcer recurrence may be delayed. This, in combination with careful patient adherence to instructions, minimizes treatment failures. The subject of perforator interruption by surgery is so vast that this mention of it serves only as parenthetical information for this chapter, which deals more with primary varicosities than with the severe chronic venous insufficiency that is often secondary.

## ALTERNATIVE OPERATIONS
### Babcock Internal Stripping

When Babcock of Philadelphia described his new operation for removal of varicose veins in 1907, he said, "the cause of varicose veins is pressure acting upon imperfect or damaged venous walls." How prescient that statement was has been demonstrated over the years. New information has only confirmed Babcock's observations.[12]

Babcock described the previous methods of varicose vein extraction including that of Schede in which an incision was made circumcising the leg down to the muscular aponeurosis at the junction of the middle and upper thirds of the thigh. Predictably, the superficial venous circulation was reestablished after that operation by collateral venous anastomoses, and the scar produced disconcerting areas of anesthesia, paresthesia, and sometimes even ischemia of the foot. Subsequently, the same operation was accomplished instead by making interrupted incisions, leaving bridges of undivided skin, and eventually by extracting long axial venous trunks by raising large flaps of skin.

### Mayo External Stripping

Later, Charles Mayo described the external vein stripper; the instrument, shaped like a dull ring, was pushed down over the vein tearing it free from adjacent tissues and venous branches.

Although Mayo's external stripper is still in use, Babcock described its shortcomings by saying, "in our own experience, the method is valuable. But fragile, very tortuous or adherent vessels often embarrass the operator."

### Keller Inversion Stripping

Babcock went on to describe Keller's method. Stripping the saphenous vein was described before 1910 by Keller[12] and then cited by Rivlin[13] in 1975 and by Van der Stricht[14] in 1982. Nevertheless, the procedure is still unfamiliar to most surgeons in North America. Keller's method consisted of passing a stout thread through the vein by means of a probe or twisted wire, tying it firmly to one of the divided ends, and then pulling the other end of the thread, causing the vein to be turned inside out and then removed through the upper or lower incision (Fig. 10-5). Saphenous stripping by invagination is ingenious and has great theoretic appeal. However, Babcock said this method was disadvantaged because, "unfortunately, the vein often tears in two before the inversion has proceeded very far" (Fig. 10-6). The article concluded with a long description of the intraluminal vein stripper similar to that in use today.

The article, in the style of the early 1900s, described 11 cases in which this method had been used, gave the author's address, and no supporting references. Despite this, it was a truly landmark article and set the stage for surgical treatment of varicose veins for the next 50 years.

### Myers' Internal Stripper

By 1954, varicose vein surgery had been consolidated into intraluminal stripping supplemented by extraluminal stripping and injection of residual venous radicals.[15] At that time, T.T. Myers, writing from the "Section of Peripheral Vein Surgery" of the Mayo Clinic, described his experience with an instrument modestly named the Myers' vein stripper. His device took advantage of technology developed during World War II: flexible steel aircraft cables were developed that were extremely strong and of small external diameter. The procedure performed was essentially that of Babcock, described 40 years earlier. As was typical of descrip-

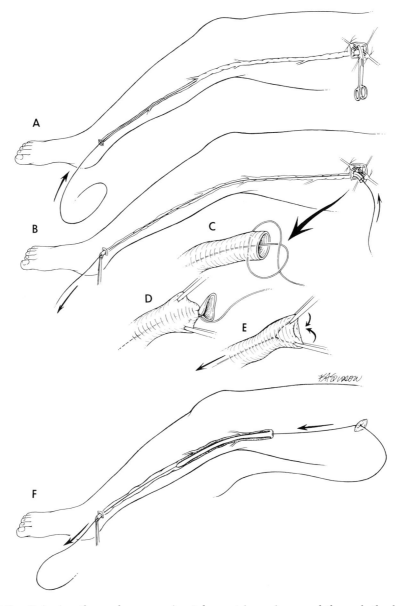

**Fig. 10-5** Stripping the saphenous vein. A long stripper is passed through the lumen of the saphenous vein from ankle to groin. **A,** The stripper can be passed from below upward, and **B,** a long suture can be attached to the stripper to fully traverse the saphenous vein from groin to ankle. The suture is knotted about the vein as in **C,** and the vein is invaginated with the aid of hemostats, **D,** so that it can be removed from above downward as in **E** and **F.**

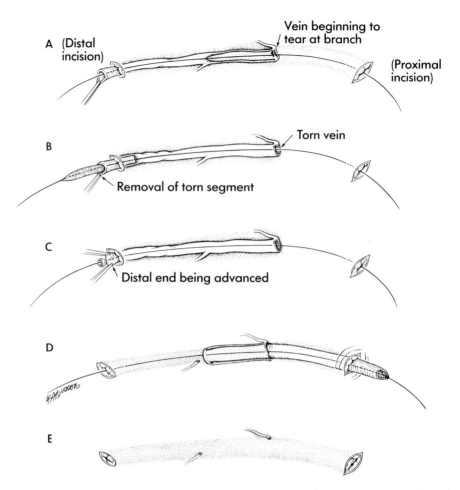

**Fig. 10-6**  One solution to the problem of vein tearing. As the vein tears, **A**, it is avulsed distally, **B**, the long suture is knotted about the distal end of the vein, **C**, the vein is invaginated and removed proximally, **D**, leaving very small proximal and distal incisions for closure, **E**.

tions of procedures in the 1950s, no objective data regarding results was provided, and of course, application of statistical methods was unheard of.

## Proximal Ligation and Distal Injection

Even as late as 1970, the surgical fashion was to describe operations without giving accurate, observational, objective data and without applying critical statistical methods, and it is for these reasons that varicose vein surgery remained crude and anticosmetic. For example, in Nabatoff's presentation,[16] operations on 3000 patients were described in which "all incompetent saphenous veins had been stripped out and all other incompetent perforating veins ligated flush with the deep veins." Clearly, these are objectives impossible to accomplish. Although the thesis of his presentation was that this could be done on a semiambulatory basis, our present-day focus is not on advantages of 1-day hospitalization, but instead on minimizing postoperative morbidity and providing the patient with a cosmetic surgical result.

Attempts to apply the principles espoused by Babcock, Myers, Nabatoff, and others, and also to perform the operation in a cosmetic fashion were being undertaken simultaneously. Stanley Rivlin's presentation[13] in 1975 describes in detail just how this could be accomplished. To achieve better cosmetic results, emphasis was placed on the belief that ". . . a prime requisite of successful varicose vein surgery is a detailed clinical examination." From such examinations would come the knowledge that lesser saphenous system varicosities caused by lesser saphenous valvular incompetence were present in as many as 14% of patients operated on.

Furthermore, by the time of Rivlin's 1975 report, it was recognized that the standard operations then in vogue, which consisted of LSV vein stripping from groin to ankle, produced dramatic short-term effects but contributed very little to long-term success. Rivlin pointed out correctly that removal of the LSV was only necessary from groin to within 1 cm of the tibial tuberosity at the knee where the upper calf perforating vein contributed to anteromedial leg varicosities. Rivlin's observations have been corroborated in subsequent experiences.

Discussion of varicose vein operations performed before 1980 would be incomplete without a mention of Geza de Takats.[17] His contributions were intellectual and philosophical, couched in excellent English even though it was his third or fourth language. It may be said that de Takats introduced intelligence into the surgery of varicose veins.

Disappointment with results of saphenous vein stripping as referred to by Rivlin led to the combination of proximal ligation and retrograde injection of varicosities and ligation and stripping combined with injection of residual varicosities as referred to earlier in this chapter.[18,19]

## OBJECTIVE EVALUATION OF RESULTS

Thus, during the military lull between World War II and the Korean War, operations for removal of varicose veins included LSV stripping from groin to ankle; SSV stripping from knee to ankle, alone or in combination with ligation and division of perforating veins; and excision of varicosities with or without intraoperative, retrograde sclerosing injections, supplemented by postoperative transcutaneous sclerosing injections with or without permanent wearing of elastic support stockings. A complex series of choices, indeed. Clearly, there was a need for evaluation of techniques and standardization of operations.

Lofgren, Ribisi, and Myers[20] provided an evaluation in the late 1950s, but their analytic methods were flawed by lack of objective data collection. As scientific evaluation of surgical results became more sophisticated through the 1970s and as techniques of measurement of venous dynamics became available, objective data was obtained.[21] Data collection and evaluation by statistical methods was then applied to the two radically opposing forms of treatment so that conclusions could be drawn. John Hobbs[22] of London early on contributed his trial of surgery versus sclerotherapy in treatment of varicose veins, and his observations were later confirmed by Jakobsen[23] of Copenhagen.

A précis of Jakobsen's observations suffices to summarize the experience of the two studies. In his study, 516 patients were divided into three treatment groups. Those in the first underwent a radical operation under full anesthesia, those in the second were treated with saphenous vein ligation and division followed by injection compression, and those in the third group were treated by injection compression alone. The radical operation required over 1 hour of anesthesia for bilateral procedures, and an average of eight incisions. The minor procedures varied from patient to patient, but consisted of proximal ligation, usually with distal perforator interruption but without full-length stripping. Injection compression was applied according to the Swiss method of Sigg.[24]

Objective evaluation of the results was done at 3 months and 3 years. It was found that the best results occurred after combined treatment; the worst results occurred with injection compression therapy alone.

When saphenofemoral valvular incompetence was present, all authors agreed that the LSV should be ligated and divided at the groin. However, disagreement occurred with regard to the necessity for distal stripping. Dormandy, operating at St. George's Hospital, performed a prospective, randomized study to determine whether stripping the LSV was essential. His 200 patients were randomly allocated to have either high saphenous ligation with stripping of the LSV and avulsion of calf varices or high saphenous ligation and thigh perforator ligation only. Residual varicosities were treated by injection sclerotherapy. The conclusion of the study was that, "there was no subjective or objective advantage to stripping the LSV in management of primary varicose veins."[25]

Dormandy's presentation was vigorously criticized at the time, but the criticism had to do mostly with technique rather than follow-up. In fact, no answers were provided regarding the fundamental question: Is there need of or any value in performing high ligation combined with limited stripping to the knee region.

This question was addressed in the early 1980s when a double-blind control trial of surgery for varicose veins was completed.[26] By using accurate data collection and objective evaluation and applying statistical methods to a study of randomly allocated patients, acceptable conclusions could be drawn. Unfortunately, full stripping to the ankle was employed, not the limited stripping advocated by Hobbs and by Rivlin.

In summary, this study showed that, ". . . stripping conferred a significant advantage, but the incidence of paresthesia and pain biased patient opinions against stripping." Pain and paresthesias occurred in the region of the saphenous nerve distal to the tibial tuberosity, thus confirming Rivlin's observation made 10 years earlier. In fact, stripping needs to be carried out only to knee level before the nerve becomes intimately associated with the saphenous vein at the upper calf.[27]

More recent evaluations of high ligation versus limited stripping have also supported the limited stripping operation strongly advocated first by Rivlin. The surgical group at Lund, Sweden, for example, compared compression sclerotherapy with high ligation with division and limited stripping of the incompetent LSV.[28,29] These studies can all be summarized in a quotation from the latter article: "The results emphasize the importance in following patients for at least five years and compression sclerotherapy combined with high tie cannot replace surgery (saphenous vein removal) in patients with mainstem insufficiency."

Although there is now agreement that limited saphenous vein stripping is a contribution to treatment in patients with saphenofemoral incompetence and SSV division is a contribution to patients with saphenopopliteal incompetence, there is no agreement on the actual methods of removal of the saphenous vein. In practice, both the intraluminal and extraluminal stripping techniques can be used.

The intraluminal invagination technique has some potential. It has been modified and used extensively by Paul Ouvry of Dieppe. In his modification, a gauze strip, 5 to 10 cm in width, is inserted with the invagination so that the risk of breaking and tearing the vein is decreased. Ouvry describes directing the stripper in the LSV from groin to the upper leg. This stripper is then attached to a gauze strip with fishline. A 10-cm wide strip is used for large saphenous veins and a 5-cm strip for moderate or small saphenous veins. As the vein is stripped, the gauze strip remains in the venous pathway until the very end of the operation. In this way, it aids in hemostasis, decreasing hematoma formation. Residual

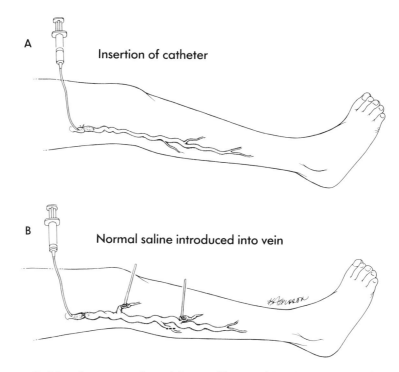

**Fig. 10-7** Simkin advocates stab avulsion as illustrated in Fig. 10-4, *A* and *B*. However, he eases the technique by the performance of intraluminal cannulation and distention of the veins using normal saline as shown in this figure. **A,** Insertion of the catheter. **B,** Distention of the vein for removal by crochet-hook technique or by stab avulsion with hemostats.

varicose veins untreated by the stab avulsion or stripping technique are then treated by sclerotherapy beginning 3 weeks after the operation.

Other techniques of varix removal are less well known. Fig. 10-7 shows the method advocated by Simkin.[30] In his method the varicosities are enlarged by injection before avulsion by the stab avulsion techniques.

Modern alternatives to vein stripping include plication of the vein wall at the proximal incompetent valve to restore valve competency.[31,32] Although there is no doubt that valve competency can be restored, it is doubtful that this technique will allow long-term successful eradication of distal varicosities either by compression sclerotherapy or satisfactory stab avulsion.

**REFERENCES**

1. Dodd H and Cockett FB, editors: Pathology and surgery of the veins of the lower limbs, Edinburgh, 1956, E&S Livingstone Ltd.
2. Large J: Surgical treatment of saphenous varices with preservation of the main saphenous trunk, J Vasc Surg 2:886, 1985.
3. Corbett R and Njayakumar K: Cleanup varicose vein surgery — use a tourniquet, Ann R Coll Surg Engl 71:57, 1989.
4. Samuels PB: Technique of varicose vein surgery, Am J Surg 142:239, 1981.
5. Royle JP: Recurrent varicose veins, World J Surg 10:944, 1986.
6. Haeger K: The anatomy of the veins of the leg. In Hobb JT, editor: The treatment of venous disorders, Lancaster, England, 1977, MTP Press Limited.
7. Jakobsen BH: The value of different forms of treatment for varicose veins, Br J Surg 66:182, 1979.

8. Neglen P, Einarsson E, and Eklof B: High tie with sclerotherapy for saphenous vein insufficiency, Phlebology 1:105, 1986.

9. Van der Stricht J: La Crossectomie, Quant Et Pourquoi? Extrait de Phlebologie n 39(1):47, 1986.

10. Browse NL, Burnand KG, and Thomas ML: Disease of the veins: pathology, diagnosis, and treatment, London, 1988, Edward Arnold.

11. Sherman RS: Varicose veins: further findings based on anatomic and surgical dissections, Ann Surg 130:219, 1949.

12. Babcock WW: A new operation for extirpation of varicose veins, NY Med J 86:1553, 1907.

13. Rivlin S: Surgical care of primary varicose veins, Br J Surg 62:913, 1975.

14. Van der Stricht J: Saphenectomie, Presse Med 71:1081, 1963.

15. Myers TT and Cooley JC: Varicose vein surgery in management of the postphlebitic limb, Surg Gynecol Obstet 99:733, 1954.

16. Nabatoff RA: 3000 operations for varicose veins, Surg Gynecol Obstet 130:497, 1970.

17. de Takats G: Ambulatory ligation of the saphenous vein, JAMA 94:1194, 1930.

18. McPheeters HO and Anderson JK: Injection treatment of varicose veins, Surg Gynecol Obstet 81:355, 1945.

19. Waugh JM: Ligation and injection of great saphenous veins, Proc Staff Meet Mayo Clin 16:832, 1941.

20. Lofgren KA, Ribisi AP, and Myers TT: An evaluation of stripping versus ligation for varicose veins, Arch Surg 76:310, 1958.

21. Norgren L: Foot volumetry before and after surgical treatment of patients with varicose veins, Acta Chir Scand 141:129, 1975.

22. Hobbs JT: Surgery and sclerotherapy in treatment of varicose veins, Arch Surg 109:793, 1974.

23. Jakobsen BH: The value of different forms of treatment for varicose veins, Br J Surg 66:182, 1979.

24. Sigg K: Treatment of varicose veins by injection sclerotherapy. In Hobbs JT, editor: Treatment of venous disorders, Lancaster, England, 1977, MTP Press.

25. Woodyer AB et al: Should we strip the long saphenous vein? In Negus D and Jantet G, editors: Phlebology '85, London, 1986, John Libbey & Co Ltd.

26. Munn SR et al: To strip or not to strip the long saphenous vein? A varicose vein trial, Br J Surg 68:426, 1981.

27. Holme JB, Holme K, and Schmidt-Sorenson L: Anatomic relationship between the long saphenous vein and saphenous nerve, Acta Chir Scan 154:631, 1988.

28. Einarsson E, Eklof B, and Norgren L: Compression sclerotherapy or operation for primary varicose veins? Proceedings of seventh International Congress of Phlebology, vol I, Copenhagen, 1980.

29. Neglen P, Einarsson E, and Eklof B: High tie with sclerotherapy for saphenous vein insufficiency, Phlebology 1:105, 1986.

30. Simkin R: Enfermeda des enfermedades venosas, Buenos Aires, 1979, Lopez Liberos.

31. Jones JW, Elliot F, and Kerstein MD: Triangular venous valvuloplasty, Arch Surg 117:1250, 1982.

32. Belcaro G: Plication of the saphenofemoral junction: an alternative to ligation and stripping? Vasa 18:296, 1989.

# Clinical Methods for Sclerotherapy of Telangiectasias

## HISTORICAL REVIEW OF TECHNIQUES

Sclerosing treatment for telangiectasias was ignored until the 1930s when Biegeleisen[1] injected sclerosing agents intradermally or subcutaneously into the general area of capillary enlargement. However, this resulted in severe necrosis and lack of effect on the telangiectasias. Biegeleisen then developed and popularized a method of "micro-injection" of telangiectasias with sclerosing agents through the use of an "extremely fine metal needle" (later described as a hand-made 32- or 33-gauge needle).[2] Unfortunately, he used sodium morrhuate (SM) in the treatment of these fragile small vessels, which produced multiple complications including pigmentation, cutaneous necrosis, and allergic reactions. Thereafter, sclerotherapy treatment of leg telangiectasias was thought of disparagingly by most practitioners until the 1970s when Alderman,[4] Foley,[5] Tretbar,[6] and Shields and Jansen[7] published reports of procedures that had achieved excellent results with few adverse sequelae. In these procedures solutions that were less caustic to the telangiectasia were used, and techniques that ensured accurate placement of the solution into the blood vessels were employed.

## INDICATION

Microsclerotherapy is indicated for, theoretically, any small telangiectatic vessel or venule on the cutaneous surface. Best results are obtained on superficial linear or radiating vessels on the lower extremities. Telangiectasias on the face are less reliably responsive to microsclerotherapy because they probably have more of an arteriolar component and are the result of active vasodilation (see Chapter 4). In addition, bright-red telangiectasias on the leg that have a rapid refilling time after diascopy (applying pressure with a glass slide) (Fig. 11-1) are probably also supplied through arteriolar flow.[8] These vessels are relatively recalcitrant to usual therapy and tend to recur after treatment. More importantly, these arteriolar leg veins are more likely to develop overlying cutaneous necrosis if sclerosing solutions reach the arteriolar feeding loop (see Chapter 8). They may be more effectively treated with the pulsed dye laser (see Chapter 12).

The description in Chapter 9 of the injection of varicose veins by first closing off the high pressure reflux points with a small volume of sclerosing solution and then by sclerotherapy of remaining abnormal vessels forms the basis for rational compression sclerotherapy of varicose veins. The treatment of "spider" leg veins can be just as rational.

In the vast majority of cases, spider veins are in direct connection to underlying varicose veins either directly or through tributaries.[9] Tretbar[10] found on Doppler examination that all visible, blue reticular veins were connected to telangiectasia when they were large enough for flow to be perceived in them. Therefore, as with varicose veins, treatment should first be directed at "plugging" the leaking high pressure outflow at its point of origin. An appropriate analogy is to think of spider veins as the "fingers" and of the feeding varicose vein as the "arm." Treatment should first be directed to the feeding arm and then, only if necessary, directed to the spider fingers. There are a number of advantages to

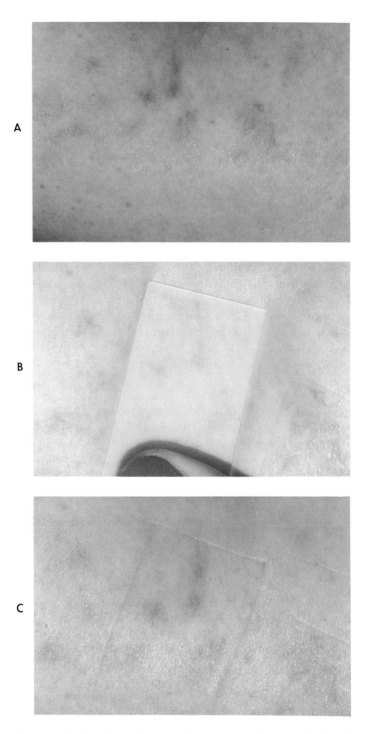

**Fig. 11-1** Bright-red telangiectasias may have an arteriolar origin. In this series the telangiectasia was located on the medial thigh. **A,** Appearance while the leg is raised 45 degrees. **B,** Blanching with pressure under a glass slide. **C,** Immediate reappearance on removal of the glass slide while the leg is still elevated.

this systematic approach to sclerotherapy. When sclerotherapy is performed in this manner, the spider veins often disappear without being directly treated, thus limiting the number of injections into the patient. The larger feeding vein is both easier to cannulate and less likely to rupture when injected with the sclerosing solution, thus minimizing the extent of extravasated red blood cells and solution. Theoretically, this method should minimize the development after sclerotherapy of hyperpigmentation, cutaneous necrosis, and telangiectatic matting (see Chapter 8).

# INJECTION TECHNIQUE
## Preinjection Procedure

After a physical examination including the use of noninvasive diagnostic techniques (see Chapter 5), the patient is scheduled for a sclerotherapy session and given a questionnaire (Appendix C), consent form (Appendix D), and instructional material (Appendix G) to be read and completed at home. Questions regarding the procedure are answered and all possible complications and adverse sequelae addressed. An estimate of the approximate number of treatment sessions and cost of treatment is given in writing to prevent any future misunderstandings. Insurance reimbursement policies are discussed. Documentation of the relief of symptoms with compression stockings is helpful in gaining preauthorization of treatment from insurance companies. Since graduated compression stockings should be worn in most cases after treatment, they are fitted at this time and given to the patient to be worn before treatment. If the stockings produce a resolution of symptoms, one can be assured that successful sclerotherapy will give the same result.

On the day of treatment, legs should not be shaved because burning may result when alcohol is applied to the areas to be treated. Moisturizers should also not be applied the day of treatment since they cause unnecessary slipperiness of the skin. Patients are instructed to eat a light meal or drink juice an hour or so before the procedure in an effort to prevent a vasovagal reaction. Shorts, a bathing suit, or a leotard should be worn during the procedure since some vessels may be near the groin.

With the patient standing on a low stool, a complete set of photographs of the legs are taken from four different views, and the individual areas to be treated are photographed close up. Photographic documentation is important because patients often will not remember exactly how their legs appeared before treatment. Any pretreatment pigmentation irregularities and scars may later be blamed on the sclerotherapy treatment, since patients usually look more closely at their legs once treatment has begun.

At the end of the treatment session, the treated areas are recorded on a diagrammatic chart to help check progress at follow-up examinations (see Appendix E).

## Preparation and Visualization of the Vessels

Microsclerotherapy of spider veins is performed with the patient in the supine position. Gravitational dilation of telangiectasias is usually unnecessary. The skin is wiped with alcohol, making the telangiectasias more visible because of a change in the index of refraction of the skin. The glistening effect of alcohol renders the skin more transparent and also helps clean the injection site. In addition, alcohol may cause some vasodilation of the telangiectasias. Alternatively, Sadick[11] recommends that the skin be wiped with a solution of 70% isopropyl alcohol with ½% acetic acid. He finds this solution to improve the angle of refraction better than alcohol alone. Scarborough and Bisaccia[12] recommend rubbing a few drops of the sclerosing solution on the skin overlying the venules with a gloved finger. They use polidocanol, which also contains alcohol in water as the dilutant. I agree that visualization is enhanced with this technique once the initial effects of the isopropyl alcohol has worn off through evaporation. Whether this holds for other solutions is unknown. To further enhance visualization of the vessels, I recommend the use of magnifiers from, $\times 2\frac{1}{4}$ to $\times 5$ (see Chapter 13).

If the vessels are too small to be injected, having the patient stand for approximately 5 minutes and then placing him or her in a reverse Trendelenburg position may result in some vessel dilation. Alternatively, inflating a blood pressure cuff to about 40 mm Hg proximal to the injection site may also result in some distention of the vessels.

## Equipment

**Needle and syringe.** Although visualization of the vessel is important in ensuring proper needle placement, one actually enters the vessel "by feel." This is particularly true when injecting reticular varices. In this situation it is best to rapidly pierce the skin and advance the needle superficially over the vessel at a slight angle. Penetration of the vessel is "felt" even when one uses a 30-gauge needle. Some authors state that the "feel" is enhanced with the use of a 26- or 27-gauge needle.[13] In this regard the use of a glass syringe would best reflect an impedance to flow if a vessel was not properly cannulated. However, glass syringes are more cumbersome to use. With the availability of high quality plastic syringes, a good "feel" can be obtained, and the risk of transmitting blood-borne diseases obviated (see Chapter 13).

Ideally, the goal of microsclerotherapy is to cannulate the vessel, injecting sclerosing solution within and not outside of the vessel wall. Usually, a 30-gauge needle will suffice for most vessels, although some physicians[14-17] recommend the use of a 32-to-33 gauge needle to decrease the likelihood of inadvertent perivenular injection in the treatment of the smallest diameter vessels. The disadvantages of using a 32-gauge needle are that it is not disposable, dulls rather quickly, and easily bends (see Chapter 13).

I find the use of a 3-ml syringe filled with 2 ml of sclerosing solution to be ideal. It fits well in the palm of the hand and can be easily manipulated. In addition, the quantity of solution is usually satisfactory for injecting either larger venules with 0.5 ml each or multiple smaller vessels. Alternatively, for those with small hands, a 1-ml syringe filled with 0.5 ml may be easier to handle, although a large number of syringes will be needed per treatment session. One theoretical disadvantage to multiple injections with the same needle is that it will become dull.[15] However, this was found not to occur on microscopic examination of the needle tips after eight injections into the skin (see Chapter 13).

**Table and lighting.** Direct lighting should be avoided during treatment since this may produce a glare from the alcohol-soaked skin. Indirect lighting allows for the best visualization.

The ideal treatment table is one that can be easily raised or lowered to provide a comfortable position for the physician to ensure injection accuracy. Also, it is helpful if the physician can easily maneuver around the table on a stool so the best approach to a given vessel is attainable. Finally, tables that can be positioned in Trendelenburg or reverse Trendelenburg positions can help in the treatment of an early vasovagal reaction and in effecting vessel dilation.

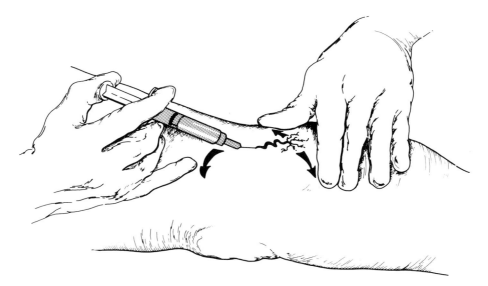

**Fig. 11-2**  Illustration of proper hand placement to exert three-point traction to aid in needle insertion. Injection is made into the feeding "arm" of the "fingers" of the spider vein.

## Skin Tension

To facilitate cannulation of the vessel it is important to have the skin taut. This can be accomplished with the help of an assistant who stretches the patient's skin in at least two directions. Alternatively, with proper hand placement, three-point tension can be produced by the physician alone. Fig. 11-2 illustrates my recommended technique for injection. The nondominant hand is used to stretch the skin adjacent to the treated vessel in two directions. Then the fifth finger of the dominant hand exerts countertraction in a third direction. With a little practice, even the most lax skin, such as that on the thighs, can be brought under tension with this technique. Obviously, skin laxity varies with patient age, adiposity, and location on the leg.

## Depth of Injection

It is important to remember that the location of most leg telangiectasias is in the upper dermis (see Chapter 1). The most common error in technique is to place the needle tip deep to the vessel. To allow one to enter the vessel at a less acute angle, almost parallel to the skin surface, the needle should be bent to 145 degrees with the bevel up (Fig. 11-3).[18] If the needle is not within the vessel, the solution will either leak out onto the skin or produce an immediate superficial wheal. At times gentle upward traction can be applied as the needle is being advanced to ensure superficial placement.

Injecting with the bevel of the needle up has the advantage of minimizing the chance of transecting the vessel. Inserting the needle bevel down may be easier. This is thought to be the result of the vacuum produced by the bevel on the skin surface.

When using a sclerosing solution that does not cause cutaneous necrosis on extravasation (such as STS 0.1% to 0.25%, POL 0.25% to 1.0%, and Scleremo), one can even inject as the needle is being inserted into the vessel. As soon as the bevel is within the vessel, the telangiectasia blanches. This technique allows one

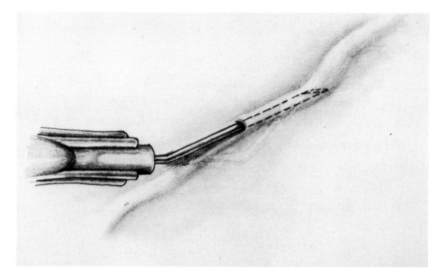

**Fig. 11-3**  The needle is bent to 145 degrees with the bevel up to facilitate accurate insertion into the superficial telangiectasia. (From Goldman MP and Bennett RG: J Am Acad Dermatol 17:167, 1987.)

to inject vessels with diameters less than the diameter of the needle because the tip of the bevel is thinner than the needle shaft and with injection the telangiectasia dilates, allowing complete insertion to occur.

### Air-Bolus (Block)/Foam Technique

Bodian,[16] Alderman,[4] and Foley[5] recommend the air-bolus technique: injecting a small amount of air to clear the vessel before instilling the sclerosing solution. This is thought to minimize the risk of inadvertent intradermal injection. This, however, may not occur, since once the vessel is cleared of blood, it is more difficult to see the progress of the sclerosing solution within its lumen. Therefore, I and many other physicians[15,17] have abandoned this technique. Another theoretical advantage of the air-bolus technique is the decreased risk of intravascular thrombosis. It is thought that if the vessel is cleared of blood by first injecting air, the risk of extravasation of red blood cells may also be minimized. However, antegrade and retrograde filling of the treated vessel occurs after the injection. Thus the air-bolus technique may not prevent or lessen the incidence of postsclerosis pigmentation.

Another variant of the air-bolus technique that helps visualize clearing of the vessels is that of creating a foamy solution before injection. This can be performed with the use of any "detergent" class of sclerosing solution such as sodium tetradecyl sulfate (STS) or polidocanol (POL) (see Chapter 7). Another method described by Green and Morgan[19] is to add Haemacel to STS to accentuate bubble formation.

### Quantity of Sclerosing Solution per Injection Site

The maximum quantity of sclerosing solution that can be safely injected into a single site when treating varicose veins is detailed in Chapter 9. In short, one should not inject a volume that would easily travel undiluted into the deep venous system. The maximum amount of sclerosing solution that can be injected into leg telangiectasias is unclear. Although Duffy[15] places little emphasis on limiting the amount of solution injected at a single site and Lary[20] recommends the injection of up to 3 ml at a single site when injecting a reticular 3-mm diameter vein, excessive inflammation and inadvertent flow of the solution into a feeding varicose vein or arteriole can produce complications (Chapter 8). Ouvry and Davy[21] recommend that the amount injected should be sufficient to produce a blanching of vessels 1 to 2 cm around the point of injection. No more than 0.5 ml should be used to avoid the risk of initiating the formation of new telangiectasias around the edge of the treated area because of excessive inflammation. In this regard, the same area should not be retreated sooner than every 4 to 6 weeks. In my practice it appears that telangiectatic matting occurs more frequently if reinjections are given to a previously treated area that is still undergoing resolution. This unresolved state can be appreciated clinically by slight inflammation and evidence of microthrombosis of vessels.

In addition to limiting the inflammatory reaction of sclerotherapy treatment, limiting the amount of solution may also prevent pain and cramping when hypertonic solutions are used. Sadick[11] has found that volumes greater than 0.3 ml of HS 23.4% caused the most pain and cramping.

Finally, some areas, especially the ankles, should not be injected with more than 1 ml of any sclerosing solution. In this area the skin is thinnest, the distance between the deep and superficial venous system is the least and swelling after treatment is common (see Chapter 8).

## Concentration and Strength of Sclerosing Solutions

This subject is discussed in detail in Chapter 7, but a few points should be mentioned here. The most important concept in sclerotherapy is that of optimal destruction of the blood vessel wall; too much will lead to excessive complications and adverse sequelae (see Chapter 8). Inadequate destruction leads to rapid recanalization of the treated vessel. One should always estimate conservatively when choosing the concentration and type of sclerosing solution.

There are only three randomized double-blind, double-paired comparative human studies that compare the results of different sclerosing solutions and concentrations in the treatment of leg telangiectasia. Carlin and Ratz[22] tested POL 0.25%, STS 0.5%, and HS 20% with Heparin 100 U/ml (Heparsal) in the treatment of leg telangiectasia and found that whereas HS and STS gave a quicker clearing of telangiectasia with fewer injections, the overall level of improvement was identical for all agents. Interestingly, POL was the best-tolerated sclerosing solution with the fewest number of adverse sequelae. In a follow-up study comparing POL in four concentrations — 0.25%, 0.5%, 0.75%, and 1.0% — Norris, Carlin, and Ratz[23] found that all concentrations were equally effective in treating leg telangiectasia. POL 0.5% was shown to be ideal, with the least number of adverse effects and the most rapid clearing in their patients with leg telangiectasia 0.2 to 1.0 mm in diameter. Sadick[24] compared HS in three concentrations — 23.4%, 11.7% and 5.8% — and found that HS 11.7% appears to be the minimal concentration of saline that will produce the most effective vein sclerosis of vessels 1.0 mm in diameter, while producing the least discomfort and morbidity.

I recommend that leg telangiectasia less than 1.0 mm diameter be treated with either POL 0.5%, STS 0.2%, chromated glycerin, or HS 11.7%. Vessels between 1.0 mm and 3.0 mm should be treated with POL 0.75%, STS 0.4%, or HS 23.4%. The treatment of larger vessels is discussed in Chapter 9.

## Pressure of Injection

Another variable of technique is the pressure and rapidity of injection. If leg telangiectasias are injected under excessive force, they may rupture and result in extravasation of solution (see Chapter 8). Therefore, injections should be made with minimal pressure. This may be difficult when injecting sclerosing solutions of high viscosity such as chromated glycerin and Sclerodex, since more pressure is required to push these through a 30-gauge needle. Duffy[15] likens the proper injection pressure to that which is needed to fix a postage stamp to an envelope. In addition, the slower one injects, the longer the solution will be in contact with the vessel wall. When treating varicose veins, patient position and movement determines the length of time that the solution will be in contact with the endothelium (see Chapter 9). But, with the injection of telangiectasias, the blood flow is not determined by muscle movement or body position, but by many other factors including environmental temperature, nervous stress, and their association with arterioles and underlying veins. Therefore, injections should be made slow enough that it takes about 5 to 10 seconds to fill the vessel. Many times the vessel will remain filled with sclerosing solution if the plunger of the syringe is held with almost zero force while the needle remains motionless.

## POSTTREATMENT TECHNIQUES

Immediately after injection of the sclerosing solution, the perivascular tissues may swell producing a clinically visable occlusion of the vessel, or the vessels may go into spasm. This usually occurs if the injection is given slowly and if the sclerosing solution is of adequate strength. Indeed, I and others recommend that a given vessel be treated until such an effect occurs.[13] This may require a second injection of a more concentrated solution (+25%) into the same vessel during the same sclerotherapy session.

After injecting hypertonic solutions, the injected area should be massaged to minimize the stinging and help alleviate the associated muscle cramping by rapidly diluting the hyperosmotic solution outside of the treated vessel.[15-17,25] The slower the injection, the less cramping occurs. Also, when withdrawing the needle, a small amount of sclerosing solution may be deposited under the skin causing a burning sensation. This usually occurs only with hypertonic solutions and chromated glycerin. Massaging for 30 to 60 seconds alleviates the pain and prevents necrosis from the hypertonic saline.[16]

All sclerosing solutions will produce some degree of erythema and/or urtication with injection (see Chapter 8). Pruritus may be associated with this effect, especially when associated with urticarial lesions. This probably occurs as a result of histamine release caused by perivascular release of mast cell mediators because of perivascular irritation or as a result of intravascular degranulation of basophils and other white blood cells destroyed by the direct toxic effects of the sclerosing solution. This reaction and its associated pruritus can be minimized by the application of a potent topical corticosteroid cream, thereby providing a welcome relief to the patient, especially if injected areas are to be occluded with compression pads and/or stockings.

For telangiectasias that do not respond to standard compression sclerotherapy, added vasoconstriction induced by cold temperature may be helpful. Orbach[26] finds that vessels respond better to the injection of refrigerated sclerosing solution. Marteau and Marteau,[27] using similar logic, advise applying cold compression pads after injection. Although these two techniques seem logical, I have not found them to be helpful.

## POSTTREATMENT COMPRESSION

Compression of the sclerosed vessel with 30 to 40 mm Hg should be maintained for a minimum of 24 to 72 hours after treatment of leg telangiectasias. Postsclerosis compression serves a number of purposes. First, the pressure helps seal the irritated vascular lumen. Second, the pressure helps decrease the likelihood of recanalization of the sclerosed vessel, especially if compression is maintained for 1 to 2 weeks. Third, the possibility of clinical and symptomatic thrombosis will be minimized, thus minimizing hyperpigmentation and telangiectatic matting after sclerosis. Although some physicians[7,11,15,16,27,28] do not advocate postsclerosis compression, the procedure is so simple and the benefits theoretically so great that its routine use is recommended. In addition, most patients actually like the feel of the compression stocking while they are ambulatory. (A complete discussion on the use of compression in the treatment of varicose and telangiectatic leg veins is presented in Chapter 6.)

## REPEAT TREATMENT SESSIONS

All patients are informed that successful treatment of a given telangiectasia may require more than one treatment. As previously mentioned, the same vessel or immediate area is not retreated for 4 to 6 weeks to allow resolution of the endosclerosis or controlled phlebitis to occur. Waiting also allows one to appreciate the effectiveness of treatment with a given solution and concentration. If little change is apparent 6 weeks after injection, the second treatment can be performed with a stronger sclerosing agent or more concentrated solution. Obviously, different areas can be treated as often as every day. The only real limiting factor is the patient and physician motivation for treatment and adherence to the maximal daily recommended amounts of sclerosing solution that can be injected (see Chapter 7). In addition, if compression is used, it may be best to wait until the pressure stocking has been removed for a few days before continuing treatment on the same leg.

Although we as physicians think of medicine as a science, it is also an art. Therefore, the sclerotherapy technique just mentioned should not be perceived as dogma. Rather, it should serve as a logical outline for the physician in planning individualized treatment.

## CASE HISTORIES

The treatment of telangiectatic matting is discussed in Chapter 12.

### CASE 1: Traumatic telangiectatic patch

*This 46-year-old woman was accidentally hit by a tennis ball while she was playing the net. The telangiectatic patch on the posterior medial thigh developed after resolution of the bruise 4 to 6 weeks after the initial injury and did not change in size or color over the following 4 years (Fig. 11-4, A). The patch was treated one time only with injections of POL 0.5% in three locations to completely blanch the lesion. A total of 1 ml was used. A localized pressure dressing with an STD foam pad was placed and secured with Medi-Rip tape for 3 days. Fig. 11-4, B, shows the same area 10 months after initial treatment.*

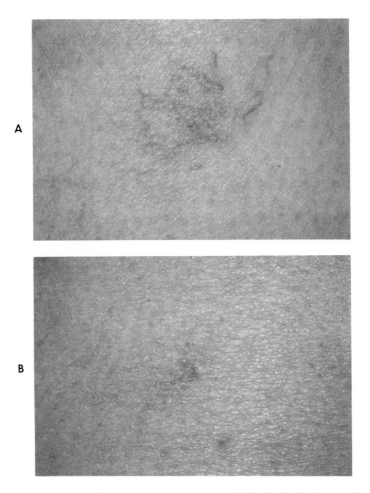

**Fig. 11-4**    A, Telangiectatic patch on posterior medial thigh; **B,** 10 months after treatment.

**CASE 2: Unassociated telangiectasia**

*Fig. 11-5, A, shows the appearance of linear telangiectasia on the medial thigh of a 46-year-old woman that were noted during her second pregnancy 22 years previously. The area was asymptomatic and treatment was requested for cosmetic improvement. The appearance 6 months after a single treatment using approximately 3 ml of POL 0.5% is shown in Fig. 11-5, B. A 30-to-40 mm Hg graduated compression stocking was worn for 3 days after the injection. Note some mild hyperpigmentation in one of the treated vessels.*

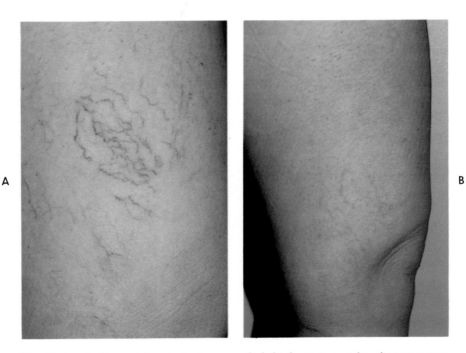

**Fig. 11-5**    **A,** Linear telangiectasia on medial thigh; **B,** 6 months after treatment.

CASE 3: **Reticular vein unassociated with the saphenous system**

*Appearance of a reticular vein 2 to 3 mm in diameter on the popliteal fossa in a 32-year-old woman is shown in Fig. 11-6, A. The same area 18 months after one treatment with 1 ml of POL 0.75% is shown in Fig. 11-6, B. The area was compressed for 72 hours after treatment with an STD foam pad under a 30-to-40 mg Hg graduated compression stocking, after which the compression stocking alone was worn for one more week while the patient was ambulatory. In the intervening 18 months the patient wore a 20-mm Hg graduated compression stocking while ambulatory on a fairly consistent basis.*

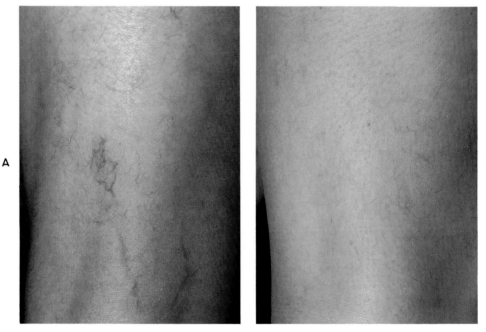

**Fig. 11-6**  A, Reticular vein on popliteal fossa; B, 18 months after treatment.

CASE 4: **Mixed reticular and telangiectatic veins**

*Reticular veins, approximately 2 mm in diameter, associated with multiple telangiectasias on the lateral distal thigh in a 32-year-old woman appeared during her second pregnancy 10 years previously (Fig. 11-7, A). The patient requested treatment because of a dull aching that occurred in the area during menses and after prolonged standing. The treated veins are shown immediately after injection with 0.5 ml total of POL 0.75% in Fig. 11-7, B. Fig. 11-7, C, shows the treated area 1 day after injection after removal of the STD pad and 30- to-40 mm Hg graduated compression stocking. Note the ecchymosis induced by the pressure dressing. Fig. 11-7, D, shows the area 1 week after injection. Intravascular thrombi were noted and drained at that time. Eight weeks after injection the vessels were almost totally resolved. Some mild pigmentation was present in the distal aspect where thrombosis was most extensive (Fig. 11-7, E). Fig. 11-7, F, shows the area 22 months after initial treatment, demonstrating sustained resolution of the telangiectasia, reticular veins, and pigmentation.*

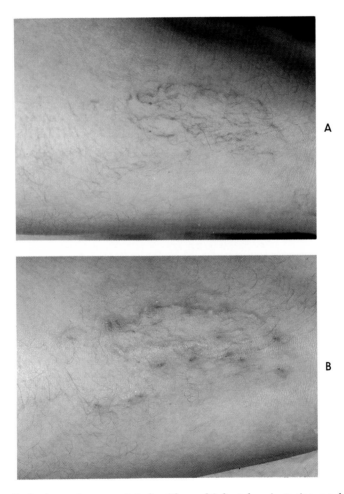

**Fig. 11-7** **A,** Reticular veins associated with multiple telangiectasias on lateral distal thigh. **B,** Immediately after injection. *Continued.*

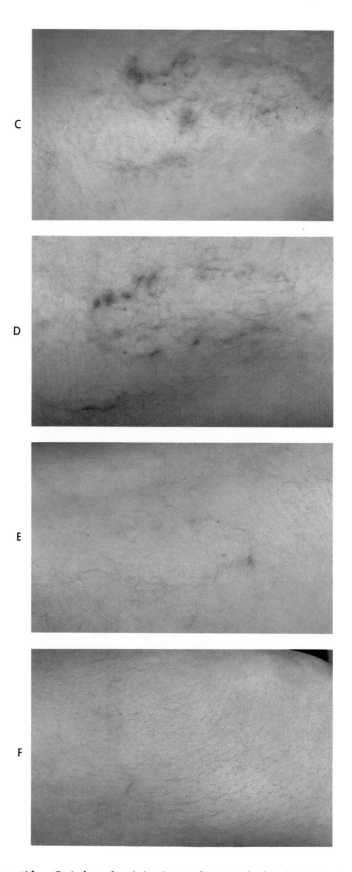

**Fig. 11-7, cont'd.** C, 1 day after injection and removal of pad and graduated pressure stocking; **D**, 1 week after injection; **E**, 8 weeks after injection; **F**, 22 months after treatment with complete resolution.

## CASE 5: Extensive reticular and telangiectatic veins

*This 53-year-old woman had a 30-year history of asymptomatic leg veins that had been stable in appearance since her last of two pregnancies 20 years previously. She sought treatment for cosmetic reasons (Fig. 11-8, A). A total of 10 ml of POL 0.75% was injected into all feeding reticular veins on the proximal and distal lateral thigh. POL 0.5%, 2 ml, was injected into the portion of the telangiectatic mats on the lateral calf and knee, which did not blanch with the previous injection. STD foam pads were placed under a 30-to-40 mm Hg graduated support stocking that was continually worn for 7 days after the procedure. When the stocking was removed, multiple small thrombi were drained. Fig. 11-8, B, shows the appearance of the treated area 25 months after the single treatment session.*

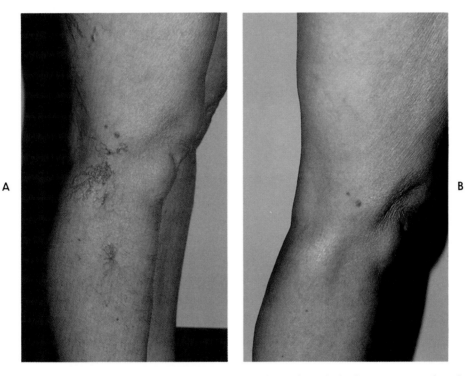

**Fig. 11-8** A, Reticular veins on proximal and distal lateral thigh; **B,** 25 months after treatment.

**CASE 6: Treatment of cherry hemangioma**

*This 48-year-old woman had multiple cherry hemangioma on the abdomen and thighs and a 4-mm diameter hemangioma located on the anterior thigh (Fig. 11-9, A). Fig. 11-9, B shows the appearance 5 months after injection with 0.1 ml of POL 0.75%. Note the slight indented and hypopigmented scar, which was acceptable to the patient.*

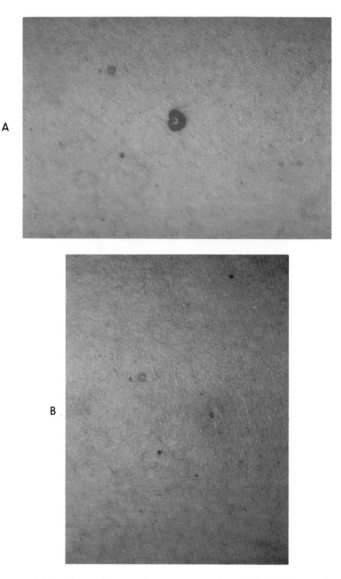

**Fig. 11-9** A, Multiple cherry hemangioma on anterior thigh; **B**, 5 months after injection.

## REFERENCES

1. Biegeleisen HI: Telangiectasia associated with varicose veins: treatment by a micro-injection technique, JAMA 102:2092, 1934.
2. Biegeleisen HI: Varicose veins, related diseases, and sclerotherapy: a guide for practitioners, Canada, 1984, Eden Press.
3. Higgins TT and Kittel PB: Injection treatment with sodium morrhuate, Lancet 1:68, 1930.
4. Alderman DB: Therapy for essential cutaneous telangiectasias, Postgrad Med 61:91, 1977.
5. Foley WT: The eradication of venous blemishes, Cutis 15:665, 1975.
6. Tretbar LL: Spider angiomata: treatment with sclerosant injections, J Kansas Med Soc 79:198, 1978.
7. Shields JL and Jansen GT: Therapy for superficial telangiectasias of the lower extremities, J Dermatol Surg Oncol 8:857, 1982.
8. Merlen JF: Red telangiectasias, blue telangiectasia, Soc Fran Phlebol 22:167, 1970.
9. de Faria JL and Moraes IN: Histopathology of the telangiectasias associated with varicose veins, Dermatologia 127:321, 1963.
10. Tretbar LL: The origin of reflux in incompetent blue reticular/telangiectasia veins. In Davy A and Stemmer R, editors: Phlebologie '89, Montrouge, France, 1989, John Libby Eurotext Ltd.
11. Sadick N: Treatment of varicose and telangiectatic leg veins with hypertonic saline: a comparative study of heparin and saline, J Dermatol Surg Oncol 16:24, 1990.
12. Scarborough DA and Bisaccia E: Sclerotherapy — translucidation of the skin prior to injection, J Dermatol Surg Oncol 15:498, 1989.
13. Marley W: Low dose sotradecol for small vessel sclerotherapy. Newsletter North Am Soc Phlebol 3:3, 1989.
14. Eichenberger H: Results of phlebosclerosation with hydroxy-polyethoxydodecane, Zentralbl Phlebol 8:181, 1969.
15. Duffy DM: Small vessel sclerotherapy: an overview. In Callen et al, editors: Advances in dermatology, vol 3, Chicago, 1988, Year Book Medical Publishers Inc.
16. Bodian E: Sclerotherapy, Dialogues in Dermatology 13(3), 1983.
17. Green D: Compression sclerotherapy techniques, Dermatol Clin 7:137, 1989.
18. Goldman MP and Bennett RG: Treatment of telangiectasia: a review, J Am Acad Dermatol 17:167, 1987.
19. Green AR and Morgan BDG: Sclerotherapy for venous flare, Br J Plast Surg 38:241, 1985.
20. Lary BG: Varicose veins and intracutaneous telangiectasia: combined treatment in 1500 cases, S Med J 80:1105, 1987.
21. Ouvry P and Davy A: Le traitement sclerosant des telangiectasies des membres inferieurs, Phlebologie 35:349, 1982.
22. Carlin MC and Ratz JL: Treatment of telangiectasia: comparison of sclerosing agents, J Dermatol Surg Oncol 13:1181, 1987.
23. Norris MJ, Carlin MC, and Ratz JL: Treatment of essential telangiectasia: effects of increasing concentrations of polidocanol, J Am Acad Dermatol 20:643, 1989.
24. Sadick N: Sclerotherapy of varicose and telangiectatic leg veins: minimal sclerosant concentration of hypertonic saline and HS relationship to vessel diameter, J Dermatol Surg Oncol 17:65, 1991.
25. Weiss R and Weiss M: Resolution of pain associated with varicose and telangiectatic leg veins after compression sclerotherapy, J Dermatol Surg Oncol 16:333, 1990.
26. Orbach J: A new look at sclerotherapy, Folia Angiologica 25:181, 1977.
27. Marteau J and Marteau J: Contribution de la cryotherapie en phlebologie, Phlebologie 31:191, 1978.
28. Chrisman BB: Treatment of venous ectasias with hypertonic saline, Hawaii Med J 41:406, 1982.

# 12 Laser Treatment of Leg Telangiectasias with and without Sclerotherapy

The laser was first conceived in the imagination of H.G. Wells who described the use of a light gun in 1896 as an outer-space weapon. Albert Einstein then transformed imagination into a theoretical possibility in the early 1900s. He described the process of stimulated emission as an offshoot in his quest to show the inherent singular nature of the four basic forces of the universe. However, it was not until 1960 that the first laser was actually constructed (ruby laser).

The acronym *LASER* stands for Light Amplification by the Stimulated Emission of Radiation. In short, a laser emits a beam of monochromic, coherent, collimated photons of a specific wavelength. The emitted wavelength is produced by exciting an atom or molecule to release particles, or photons, at a wavelength specific for that type of molecule. This ability to produce a laser light at a specific wavelength is one key factor in producing selective damage. By tuning the laser to the absorption wavelength of a particular substance, such as oxygenated hemoglobin, only that substance will be affected, theoretically, by the laser energy.

With proper usage, lasers are very safe and have not been associated with long-term side effects. Laser radiation used in medicine is in or near the range of visible light in the electromagnetic spectrum. Therefore, its radiant energy level is at a much longer wavelength than the high-energy ionizing type of radiation associated with x-rays or radiation therapy (Fig. 12-1) and is not associated with the commonly perceived radiation hazards.[1] (A complete practical discussion of laser physics can be found in other sources.[1]) Four types of lasers have been

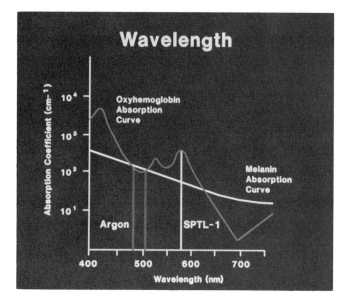

**Fig. 12-1** Absorption spectrum for hemoglobin and melanin. Note the specific targeted wavelengths for the argon and yellow, 577 to 585 nm, pulsed dye laser (SPTL-1) types of lasers. (Courtesy Candela Laser Corporation.)

324

used to treat telangiectasias: carbon dioxide, neodymium-YAG, argon, and yellow, 577-to-585 nm pulsed dye and continuous wave. They each act in a different manner to effect vessel destruction.

## LASER MODALITIES
### Carbon Dioxide

The carbon dioxide ($CO_2$) laser, developed in 1964, has been used for the obliteration of venules and telangiectatic vessels.[2-5] The $CO_2$ laser emits light energy at 10,600 nm in the infrared portion of the electromagnetic spectrum. At this wavelength, vaporization occurs through a conversion of intracellular and intravascular water to steam. Thus the $CO_2$ laser produces total vaporization of all targeted tissue.

The rationale for using the $CO_2$ laser in the treatment of telangiectasias is that it can produce a precise vaporization of a blood vessel without causing significant damage to tissue structures adjacent to the penetrating laser beam. However, since tissue destruction is nonselective when produced by vaporization of water within cells, the skin surface, as well as the dermis overlying the blood vessel, is also destroyed. $CO_2$ laser penetration of vessels was also reported to cause occasional brisk bleeding from the vessel, which required pressure bandages for 48 hours.[4] Pain during treatment is moderate to severe, but of short duration. It is not surprising therefore that all reported studies demonstrate unsatisfactory cosmetic results. Treated areas show multiple hypopigmented punctate scars with either minimal resolution of the treated vessel or neovascularization adjacent to the treatment site (Fig. 12-2). Because of this nonselective action, the $CO_2$ laser has no advantage over the electrodesiccation needle and has not been successfully used in treating telangiectasias on the leg. When given a choice, patients prefer sclerotherapy to $CO_2$ laser therapy.[5] The box on p. 326 summarizes the disadvantages of the $CO_2$ laser.

### Neodymium-YAG

The neodymium-YAG laser has been studied recently as a treatment for leg telangiectasias.[4] This laser light has a wavelength of 1060 nm. Therefore, the wavelength used by the YAG laser is not absorbed well by melanin, hemoglobin,

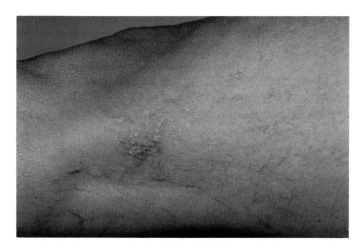

**Fig. 12-2** Hypopigmented scars with skin textural changes 5 years after treatment of leg telangiectasia with the $CO_2$ laser.

---

**DISADVANTAGES OF CARBON DIOXIDE LASER TREATMENT**

Nonselective tissue damage
Hypopigmented punctate scars
Brisk bleeding may occur
Procedure is painful

---

**DISADVANTAGES OF NEODYMIUM-YAG LASER TREATMENT**

Relatively nonselective tissue damage
Significant risk of scar formation
Hypopigmented linear scars
Procedure is painful

---

or any cutaneous chromophores but is absorbed much better by water. So, just as with the $CO_2$ laser, tissue damage is relatively nonspecific. The average depth of penetration of this laser in human skin is 0.75 mm; a reduction of the incident power to 10% occurs at a depth of 3.7 mm.[6] Thus this laser is well suited to treat blood vessels (and all cutaneous structures) to the depth of the middermis.

When used to treat facial vascular lesions, the tissue destruction that occurs requires up to 4 weeks to heal. In addition, scar formation is more likely to occur with this laser than when similar lesions are treated with the argon laser.[7]

Recently, Apfelberg et al.[4] treated leg telangiectasias with a neodymium-YAG laser equipped with a 1.5-mm sapphire contact probe. Problems encountered included linear hypopigmentation and depressions overlying the skin of the treated vessel and the need to retreat the vessels at 6-week intervals. Also, the cost of the procedure is high because the disposable sapphire tips are very expensive. In summary, as reported with the $CO_2$ laser, this modality produces unsatisfactory cosmetic results and has yet to be found useful in treating leg telangiectasias. The disadvantages of the neodymium-YAG laser are summarized in the box above.

### Argon

The argon laser is theoretically better suited for treating telangiectasias than are the modalities previously mentioned. The blue-green light of this laser emits 80% of its energy at 488 and 514 nm. The red-purple oxygenated hemoglobin located in the superficial dermal ectatic blood vessels has absorption peaks at 418, 542, and 577 nm and therefore, for the most part, is selectively absorbed by the argon laser spectrum. However, the argon laser light is not entirely hemoglobin specific. The epidermis absorbs the 488- and 514-nm wavelengths about half as strongly as blood does and is therefore nontransparent.[8] Epidermal melanin also absorbs a variable portion of argon laser light. This may result in hypopigmentation of the treated areas. Thus the specificity of argon laser−induced damage appears to be much less than originally hypothesized.

Argon laser light passes through the skin surface into the upper reticular dermis for a distance of about 1 mm in white skin.[9] The depth of laser absorption can be increased by cooling the tissue. When experimentally excised tissue is cooled, the depth of effective vascular coagulation increases from 1.7 to 3.5 mm.[10] Unfortunately, tissue cooling may also affect thermal energy absorption so high laser energies are necessary to effect tissue destruction. Thus the increased laser energy required to offset the decrease in efficiency of thermal damage to the targeted tissues may result in nonselective tissue damage.

In addition to the relative specificity of the argon laser wavelength for oxygenated hemoglobin, presently available argon lasers deliver energy exposures with pulse durations as short as only 20 to 50 ms. This minimal exposure still allows time for extensive radial diffusion and dissipation of heat generated in the treated blood vessels, thereby resulting in a relatively nonselective thermal destruction.[11] In practice, for the argon laser to produce clinically effective results, pulses are delivered until tissue whitening occurs.[12] This whitening represents nonspecific thermal damage to the epidermis and dermis and not simply blanching of the vascular bed. In fact, Arndt[12] has demonstrated that there is no clinical difference between continuous-wave therapy and 50-ms pulse therapy. Thus there is a risk of hypertrophic or atrophic scarring caused by nonspecific epidermal and upper dermal necrosis and subsequent fibrosis. This is noted clinically by epidermal sloughing postoperatively followed by crusting and gradual reepithelialization over 1 to 2 weeks.[13] This may be minimized through the use of lower laser energies.

Although satisfactory treatment results have been reported with the use of the argon laser for facial telangiectasias, a number of adverse effects also occur. Typically, pitted, hypertrophic, and depressed scars have been observed.[14-22] "Unexpected pigmentary changes" have been noted by 43% of physicians using the argon laser.[23] Hypopigmentation has been reported to occur in up to 32% of women having port-wine stain treatment.[14] Hyperpigmentation, occurring in up to 20% of patients, has been demonstrated to be the result of an increased production of melanin by a normal population of melanocytes.[24] The authors speculate that this pigmentation is induced by thermal stimulation of melanocytes as the argon laser produces a superficial burn. Again, these adverse sequelae are decreased somewhat with the use of lower laser energies.

A number of techniques have been developed in an attempt to limit thermal-induced complications. Before and after treatment cooling of the skin offers no improvement in the rate of frank hypertrophic scarring.[25-27] A grid or checkerboard pattern of treatment has been shown to offer no advantage by some,[28] but may be of some benefit when produced through a robotized scanning laser handpiece.[29] Apfelberg et al.[14] have also reported on the use of a stripping technique that produces unacceptable sequelae. Finally, Apfelberg et al.[30] have described a dot or pointillistic method that may offer some improvement over standard treatment techniques, but it still produced scarring in 3 of 8 patients treated on the upper or lower extremity and 2 of 25 evaluable patients with treatments on the upper lip or nasolabial folds. Thus variations in treatment technique have failed to significantly minimize the complications of argon laser treatment.

Telangiectasias or superficial varicosities of the lower extremities are much less responsive than are facial lesions to argon laser treatment. Apfelberg and McBurney[31] and Craig et al.[32] caution that the treated areas in this location usually appear purple or depressed, often leaving a worse cosmetic appearance than the untreated condition. In a report of 38 patients treated by Apfelberg et al.,[33] 49% had either poor or no results from treatment; only 16% had excellent or good results. In addition, almost half of the patients had hemosiderin bruising.[33] In another series, Dixon et al.[34] noted significant improvement in only 49% of patients. They speculated that after initial improvement, incomplete thrombosis, recanalization, or new vein formation produced reappearance of the vessels after 6 to 12 months.[35] Thus the argon laser has been demonstrated to result in a relatively high percentage of unsatisfactory treatment outcomes when used to treat leg telangiectasias (Table 12-1; Fig. 12-3).

Recently, Keller[36] has reported on the use of a microcontact argon laser probe to treat "spray telangiectasias" of the leg. Fifteen patients were treated with this devise using an argon laser energy of 1 to 2 W with a pulse duration of 0.1 seconds. This treatment was performed as "spot welding" along the coarse of the blood vessel; 100% effectiveness and no notable complications were reported. We have not achieved the same success rate as Keller[37] and await further reports of this novel form of therapy. Thus, at the present time, argon laser therapy appears to be a satisfactory method for treating selected facial telangiectasias but is much less effective in treating leg telangiectasias. A summary of the disadvantages of the argon laser appears in the box below.

---

### DISADVANTAGES OF ARGON LASER TREATMENT

Partially selective vascular damage  
Hypopigmentation and hyperpigmentation after treatment  

Atrophic and hypertrophic scarring  
Procedure is painful

---

**Table 12-1** Results of treatment of leg telangiectasias with argon laser

| Study | No. of sites treated | <90% faded | 100% faded | Adverse sequelae |
|---|---|---|---|---|
| Arndt (1982)[19] | 8 | 37% | 27% | 37% |
| Dixon (1984)[20] | 24* | 48% | none | 4+% |
| Apfelberg (1984)[3] | 38 | 89% | 11% | 6+% |
| Craig (1985)[32] | 4 | 100%† | none | none |

*51% of patients would not undergo additional treatment.
†"Poor response."

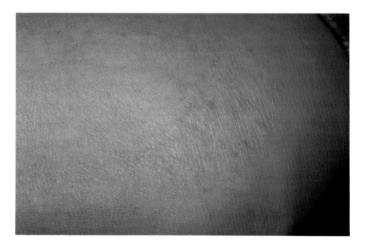

**Fig. 12-3** Hypopigmented scars with skin textural changes 4 years after treatment of leg telangiectasia with the argon laser. Specific laser parameters unknown.

## 577-585 nm Dye Laser and Pulsed Dye Laser

In an effort to produce highly selective laser destruction with less interference from overlying melanin, lasers using various dyes at wavelengths at the longer oxygenated hemoglobin absorption peaks were developed. The main chromophore in the blood vessel is oxyhemoglobin.[38] The oxyhemoglobin absorption spectrum has three major bands, the largest at 418 nm and two smaller peaks at 542 and 577 nm. Although there are stronger oxyhemoglobin bands at shorter wavelengths, competing absorption by epidermal melanin overlying the dermal vessels tends to dominate.[39] However, when tuned to 577 nm, corresponding to the alpha band of oxyhemoglobin, the laser energy penetrates to the depth of dermal blood vessels (1 mm)[38,40] with little interfering absorption by melanin in light skin types.[41,42]

A restriction of the application of the 577-nm wavelength in the treatment of vascular lesions has been its penetration to only approximately 0.5 mm in depth from the dermal-epidermal junction.[43] Recently, Tan et al.[44] found that the depth of vascular damage increases from 0.5 to 1.2 mm by changing the wavelength from 577 to 585 nm while maintaining the same degree of vascular selectivity as that previously described for 577-nm irradiation. This study confirmed calculated predictions that 585-nm light would penetrate approximately 0.75 mm into the dermis.[45] A change in wavelength from 577 to 585 nm has been reported to result in a more complete clearance of vascular cutaneous lesions in patients.[46]

In addition to thermal damage produced by the absorption of the 577-nm wavelength, "shock-wave" damage resulting from rapid absorption of energy by the oxyhemoglobin molecules has also been demonstrated.[42,43,47] Recently, in vitro studies by Glassberg et al.[48,49] have demonstrated that the 577-nm pulsed dye laser produces a direct destructive effect on endothelial cell cultures. Therefore, in addition to thermal absorption of laser energy by erythrocytes, resulting in "shock-wave" and thermal-induced destruction of the blood vessel, direct laser effects on endothelial cells may also contribute to the highly specific vessel damage.

Besides matching the wavelength of the laser to the target tissue, it would be ideal to limit the laser energy absorption and contain it within the targeted structure. This is accomplished by pulsing the laser. Limiting the duration of laser exposure ensures that highly specific laser energy is delivered in a period of time less than that required for the cooling of the target vessel, that is, less than the thermal relaxation time.

For superficial cutaneous blood vessels, thermal relaxation times range from 0.1 to 10 ms, depending on the size and type of the vessel,[38,50] and average 1.2 ms.[38] Therefore, a pulsed dye laser has been developed in an attempt to perfect selective vascular injury. Nakagawa, Tan, and Parrish[43] and Garden et al.,[51] have found that a 1.5-μs pulse is absorbed almost entirely by the erythrocyte resulting in microvaporization with endothelial and pericyte damage, vessel rupture, and hemorrhage. In contrast to the destruction in these specific cellular structures, mast cells, fibroblasts, and even collagen fibers in the perivascular tissues remain unaltered.[43]

Because the 1-μs pulse width (approximately a thousandfold faster than the thermal relaxation time for microvessels) produces evidence of microvascular hemorrhage, longer pulse widths within the thermal relaxation times were studied. Garden et al.[51] found a relative lack of microvessel rupture and hemorrhage at pulse widths of 20 μs or greater. Tan et al.[52] using 300-μs pulses, demonstrated specific intravascular damage with destruction of endothelial cells. Garden et al.[51] subsequently confirmed that a 360-μs pulse duration was more efficacious than a 20-$\mu$s laser impulse. Most recently, the SPTL-1 model of the Candela pulsed dye laser* (PDL), which delivers the laser energy in 450 $\mu$s, has been found to be as efficacious as the 300-$\mu$s unit.[49] The advantage of using longer pulse durations that are still within the thermal relaxation times for the targeted blood vessels is that larger diameter blood vessels may be treated. Studies are presently being conducted to test even longer pulse durations with the hope of extending the treatment parameters of the pulsed dye laser.

Studies using a 577-nm dye laser with a 300-$\mu$s pulse demonstrate minimal perivascular or epidermal damage.[52-54] In fact, Garden, Polla, and Tan[55] noted no evidence of scarring after treating 52 patients with port-wine stains, including a number of retreatments. Glassberg et al.[49] reported that 27 of 28 patients with port-wine stains experienced definite clinical fading, and only 5 patients developed hyperpigmentation, which resolved within 6 to 8 weeks. However, although very effective for facial port-wine hemangiomas, telangiectasias, spider ectasia, and capillary hemangiomas,[54-57] telangiectasias over the lower extremities have not responded as well; they show less lightening and more hyperpigmentation after therapy.[58] Polla et al.[59] treated 35 superficial leg telangiectasias with the Candela PDL. The exact laser parameters were not given except for information that vessels were treated an average of 2.1 times with a maximum of four separate treatments. These vessels were described as being either red-purple and raised or blue and flat. No mention was made regarding the association of reticular or varicose veins. No mention was made of the vessel diameter. Of vessels treated, 15% had greater than 75% clearing, and 73% of treated areas showed little response to treatment. The only lesions that responded at all were the red or pink tiny telangiectasias. Almost 50% of the treated patients developed a persistent hypopigmentation or hyperpigmentation of treated sites (Fig. 12-4). Table 12-2 lists the advantages and disadvantages of the PDL.

Recently, Smith et al.[60] reported on the use of a 532-nm green laser beam treatment on "nonpalpable," smooth, fine-linear, purple-to-red leg telangiectasias. The 100-$\mu$m spot-size beam was directed along the vessel in a continuous mode until tissue whitening appeared. Moderate to severe pain during the procedure and a 1 to 2 week wound healing time were observed, and only 50% of patients received a satisfactory result. The incidence of postlaser scarring and pigmentation was not described; the diameter of the treated vessels was also omitted. Compression was not used after treatment.

Unfortunately, it is difficult to compare the clinical and experimental studies of laser treatment of leg telangiectasias with that of port-wine stains. Laser studies on the treatment of leg telangiectasias typically do not report the diameter, location, or type of vessel treated. In addition, no mention is made of "feeding" varicosities or of postlaser compression. Therefore, we systematically examined the clinical effects of various powers of the PDL in specific leg telangiectasias. We chose type 1 red telangiectasia less than 0.2 mm in diameter and vessels arising as a function of telangiectatic matting for examination since these vessels are the most difficult to treat with standard sclerotherapy techniques.

In addition, we hypothesized that the use of subtherapeutic concentrations of sclerosing solutions in combination with highly specific laser-induced endothelial damage may result in an enhanced efficacy with laser treatment of larger blood vessels. The combination of PDL and sclerotherapy technique (PDL/SCL) was hypothesized to result in a decreased incidence of extravasation of erythrocytes and a decrease in perivascular inflammation. Thus PDL/SCL may result in a

---

*Candela Laser Corporation, Wayland, Mass.

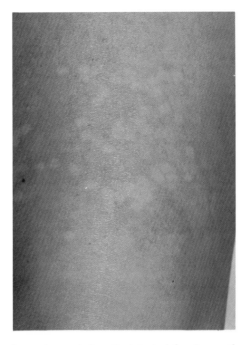

**Fig. 12-4**  Temporary hypopigmentation that lasted for 6 months developed in this 32-year-old woman with type III tan skin treated on the anterior thigh with the SPTL-1 at 7.5 J/cm².

**Table**   Pulsed dye laser treatment of leg telangiectasia

| Advantages | Disadvantages |
|---|---|
| Extremely selective vascular destruction | Variable success rate (high energies necessary) |
| Rare temporary pigmentary changes | Only effective on small-diameter blood vessels |
| No telangiectatic matting | Expensive |
| No scarring | Mildly painful |

decreased incidence of adverse sequelae (postsclerotherapy hyperpigmentation and telangiectatic matting).

Before using PDL/SCL treatment on patients, it was first necessary to demonstrate that this novel form of treatment was efficacious. Therefore, before performing clinical studies, an experimental analysis of the clinical and histologic effects of both PDL alone and PDL/SCL in the rabbit ear vein was performed. Using this animal model has been demonstrated previously to be an accurate method of comparing different sclerosing solutions and concentrations and was used also as a guide in choosing the most clinically appropriate laser parameters.[61] The results of these experimental and clinical studies were recently reported.[62,63]

All vessels in the rabbit ear vein model treated with the PDL alone demonstrated an immediate clinical thrombosis. After 10 days, vessels treated with 8 to 9.5 J/cm² returned to a clinically normal appearance. Only the vessels treated with 10 J/cm² remained clinically sclerosed at 45 days.

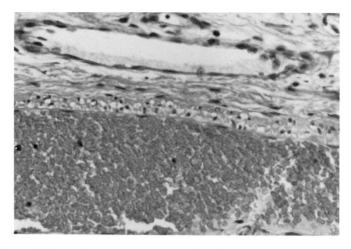

**Fig. 12-5** Vessel 1 hour after treatment with PDL alone at 8 J/cm². Endothelium is vacuolated. (Hematoxylin-eosin, original magnification ×200.) (Goldman MP et al: J Am Acad Dermatol 23:23, 1990.)

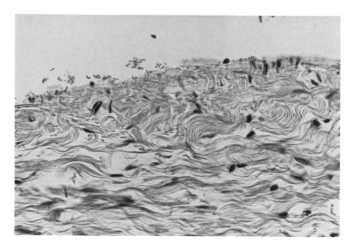

**Fig. 12-6** Vessel 1 hour after treatment with PDL alone at 9.5 J/cm². There is focal endothelial necrosis with adherence of platelets to damaged endothelium. (Hematoxylin-eosin, original magnification ×400.) (Goldman MP et al: J Am Acad Dermatol 23:23, 1990.)

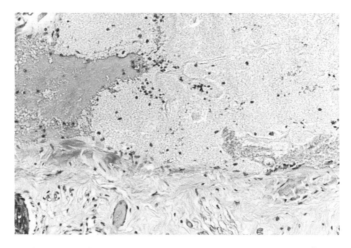

**Fig. 12-7** Vessel 1 hour after treatment with PDL alone at 10 J/cm². Perivascular heat denaturization of collagen is apparent. Also, there is extensive homogenization of red blood cells with intravascular fibrin deposition. (Hematoxylin-eosin, original magnification ×200.) (Goldman MP et al: J Am Acad Dermatol 23:23, 1990.)

Histologically, no evidence of laser-induced vascular damage was apparent at 1 hour or at 2 days in vessels treated with PDL at 8 and 8.5 J/cm$^2$ except for some mild endothelial vacuolization (Fig. 12-5). At 9.0 and 9.5 J/cm$^2$, focal endothelial necrosis was apparent with intravascular fibrin deposition, thrombosis, and adherence of platelets to the damaged endothelium (Fig. 12-6). At 10 J/cm$^2$, perivascular heat denaturization of collagen was demonstrated (Fig. 12-7; Table 12-3).

At the study's conclusion on day 45, vessels treated with 8 and 9 J/cm$^2$ were histologically normal. The previously noted vessel treated with 8.5 J/cm$^2$ showed endosclerosis with microangiopathic recanalization. Endosclerosis and full recanalization were present in the vessel treated with 9.5 J/cm$^2$ (Fig. 12-8), and complete endosclerosis was present in the vessel treated with 10 J/cm$^2$ (Fig. 12-9; Table 12-4).

The PDL produces vascular injury in a histologic pattern that is different than that produced by sclerotherapy (see box below). An examination of the PDL specific histologic effects may explain its theoretically enhanced clinical efficacy. We hypothesized two advantages to be gained from this form of treatment: a decreased incidence and/or extent of postsclerosis pigmentation and a decreased incidence and/or extent of telangiectatic matting.

Table  Pulsed dye laser treatment of 0.4-mm diameter rabbit ear vein: immediate effects

| Laser energy | Immediate histologic effects |
|---|---|
| 8-8.5 J/cm$^2$ | Endothelial vacuolization |
| 9-9.5 J/cm$^2$ | Focal endothelial destruction |
| 10 J/cm$^2$ | Perivascular thermal effects |

Table [ 12-4 ] Pulsed dye laser treatment of 0.4-mm diameter rabbit ear vein: effects after 48 hours

| Laser energy | Histologic effects after 48 hours |
|---|---|
| 8-10 J/cm$^2$ | Intravascular fibrin strands |
| 8-10 J/cm$^2$ | Minimal perivascular inflammation |
| 9-10 J/cm$^2$ | Thrombosis |
| 10 J/cm$^2$ | Endosclerosis |

## SPECIFIC HISTOLOGIC EFFECTS OF PULSED DYE LASER TREATMENT IN THE RABBIT EAR VEIN

Platelet adherence to endothelium
Perivascular heat denaturization of collagen
Intravascular fibrin strands

Relative decrease in perivascular inflammation
Relative decrease in extravasated red blood cells

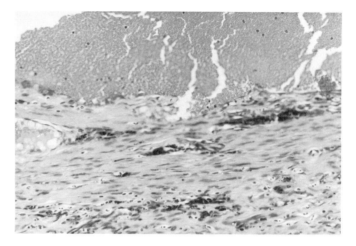

**Fig. 12-8** Vessel 2 days after treatment with PDL alone at 9.5 J/cm². Focal endothelial necrosis and thrombus formation is present along with margination of white blood cells. (Hematoxylin-eosin, original magnification ×200.) (Goldman MP et al: J Am Acad Dermatol 23:23, 1990.)

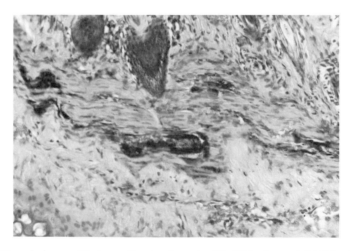

**Fig. 12-9** Vessel shown 10 days after treatment with PDL alone at 10 J/cm². Advanced endosclerosis is present within organizing thrombosis. (Hematoxylin-eosin, original magnification ×200.) (Goldman MP et al: J Am Acad Dermatol 23:23, 1990.)

## PDL TREATMENT OF LEG TELANGIECTASIA: CLINICAL STUDIES

Patients with red leg telangiectasias less than 0.2 mm in diameter were treated with a Candela SPTL-1 pulsed dye laser (PDL) tuned to 585 nm with a pulse duration of 450 $\mu$s at energies ranging from 6.0 to 8.5 J/cm$^2$ delivered through a 5-mm spot size to the entire length of the telangiectasia. PDL spots were overlapped slightly with every effort made to treat the entire vessel.

Patients were initially evaluated approximately 2 to 4 weeks after treatment and had a follow-up visit at between 4 and 16 months. Garden, Polla, and Tan[55] have previously discussed the difficulty of objectively evaluating lesional lightening either by the investigator or patient and with or without the use of photographic documentation. Since we have found it to be difficult to accurately reproduce identical quality photographs of lesions to be compared by independent investigators, we have elected to use a rigid criteria in judging successful outcome of treatment (Fig. 12-10). Therefore, patients and investigators graded the response to therapy as 90% to 100% faded, <90% faded, or no change. Pigmentation was also noted. This basic yes-or-no question appears to be a more accurate way for both investigator and patient to evaluate treatment outcome. In truth, patients usually are not satisfied with only partial resolution of their leg veins. Therefore, this all or none criteria appears to be practical for the practicing clinician.

### Complications

The most significant outcome of PDL treatment of leg telangiectasias was the relative lack of adverse sequelae and complications. With PDL treatment alone, there were no episodes of telangiectatic matting in the 101 treated sites. All patients with hyperpigmentation induced by PDL experienced complete resolution within 4 months. There were no episodes of cutaneous ulceration, thrombophlebitis, or other complications (Fig. 12-11).

### Effective Energy Levels

Unlike the effective PDL energy requirement for the successful treatment of rabbit ear veins, PDL treatment of human telangiectasia demonstrates that the most effective laser energy is that between 7.0 and 8.0 J/cm$^2$ (Table 12-5). At these laser parameters, 48% to 67% of telangiectatic patches totally fade within 4 months.

**Table 12-5**  Results of pulsed dye laser treatment of leg telangiectasia

| Laser energy (J/cm$^2$) | No. of sites treated | No change | <90% faded | Total fade |
|---|---|---|---|---|
| 6.0 | 1 | 100% | | |
| 6.5 | 4 | 25% | 50% | 25% |
| 6.75 | 7 | 42% | 16% | 42% |
| 7.0 | 25 | 24% | 28% | 48% |
| 7.25 | 30 | 10% | 23% | 67% |
| 7.5 | 23 | 13% | 39% | 48% |
| 7.75 | 6 | 17% | 33% | 50% |
| 8.0 | 3 | 23% | | 67% |
| 8.5 | 2 | 100% | | |

Modified from Goldman MP and Fitzpatrick RE: Pulsed dye laser treatment of telangiectasia: with and without simultaneous sclerotherapy, J Dermatol Surg Oncol 16:338, 1990.

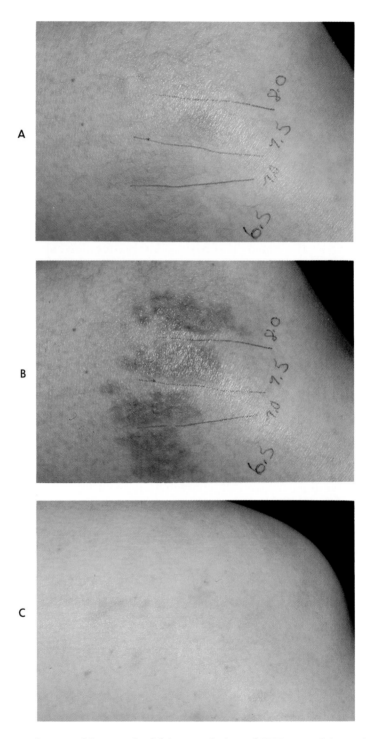

**Fig. 12-10** Photographic record of false resolution of PDL-treated leg veins. **A,** Treatment site at medial distal thigh with parameters of experimental treatment marked. **B,** Immediately after PDL treatment; note extent of purpura. **C,** Same treatment site immediately before marking the skin with laser parameters. (Taken at different F-stop exposure.) Note "false" clearing of vessels.

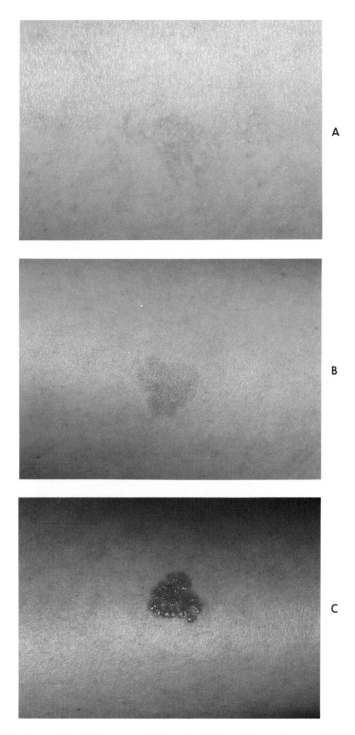

**Fig. 12-11**   Photographic follow-up of telangiectatic patch on the medial thigh treated with the PDL at 7.5 J/cm², 15 pulses. **A,** Immediately before treatment. **B,** Immediately after treatment; **C,** 2 days after treatment. Note some nonspecific vesiculation of the skin.

*Continued.*

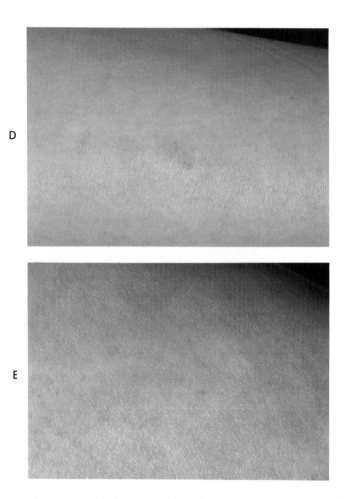

**Fig. 12-11, cont'd.** D, Vessel shown 11 days after treatment. Note some hypopigmentation and fading of the telangiectasia; purpura no longer present. E, Eleven months after treatment showing complete vessel elimination without pigmentary or textural skin changes.

The percent of telangiectasia that totally fade increases when only vessels without reticular feeding veins are considered (Table 12-6; Figs. 12-12 and 12-13). There appears to be no difference in the response to PDL in telangiectatic matting vessels (Fig. 12-14).

## Vessel Location

Many physicians have found that vessel location may affect treatment outcome, vessels on the medial thigh being the most difficult to completely resolve.[66-68] However, with the PDL, vessel location appears to be unrelated to treatment outcome if telangiectatic patches with untreated feeding reticular veins are excluded (Table 12-7; Fig. 12-15).

*Text continued on p. 345.*

**Table 12-6** Pulsed dye laser treatment of leg telangiectasia: results of vessels without reticular veins

| Laser energy (J/cm²) | No. of sites treated | No change | <90% faded | Total fade |
|---|---|---|---|---|
| 7.0 | 22 | 23% | 23% | 54% |
| 7.25 | 27 | 11% | 15% | 74% |
| 7.5 | 20 | 10% | 35% | 55% |
| 7.75 | 3 | 0% | 0% | 100% |
| 8.0 | 2 | | | 100% |
| TOTAL | 74 | 13% | 19% | 68% |

Modified from Goldman MP and Fitzpatrick RE: Pulsed dye laser treatment of telangietasia: with and without simultaneous sclerotherapy, J Dermatol Surg Oncol 16:338, 1990.

**Table 12-7** Results of pulsed dye laser treatment by vessel location of leg telangiectasia (laser energy: 7-7.75 J/cm²)

| Vessel location | No. of sites treated | No change | <90% faded | Total fade |
|---|---|---|---|---|
| Thigh | 35 | 26% | 40% | 34% |
| Thigh* | 22 | 15% | 20% | 65% |
| Knee | 9 | 11% | 11% | 78% |
| Calf | 28 | 14% | 18% | 68% |
| Ankle | 6 | 0% | 50% | 50% |
| Foot | 13 | 23% | 8% | 69% |
| TOTAL | 91 | 19% | 25% | 56% |

Modified from Goldman MP and Fitzpatrick RE: Pulsed dye laser treatment of telangiectasia: with and without simultaneous sclerotherapy, J Dermatol Surg Oncol 16:338, 1990.
*Less patients with untreated feeding reticular veins.

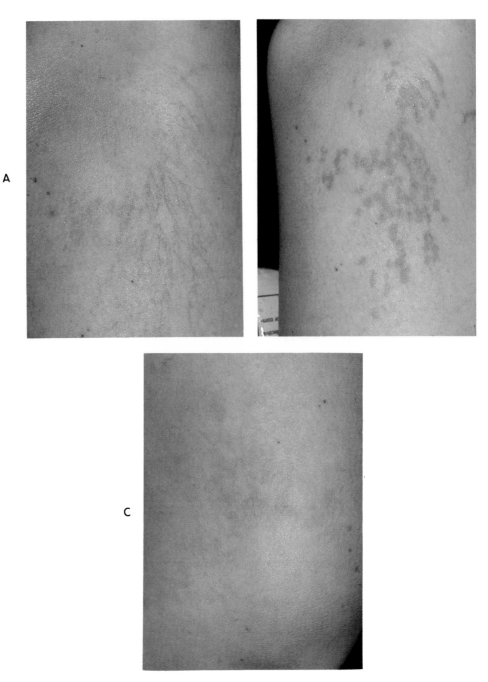

**Fig. 12-12**   Photographic follow-up of telangiectatic flair on the lateral thigh treated with the PDL at 7 J/cm$^2$, 125 pulses. **A,** Immediately before treatment. **B,** Immediately after treatment. **C,** Six weeks after treatment; note slight hyperpigmentation and total resolution of telangiectasia. Pigmentation completely faded after 2 to 4 more weeks.

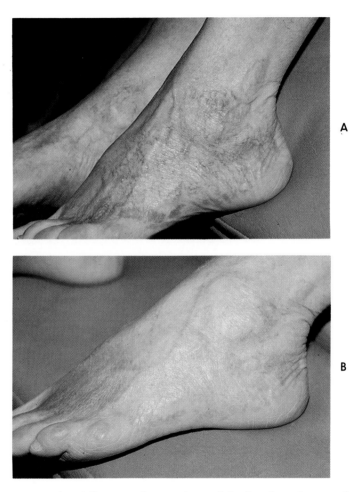

**Fig. 12-13**    Photographic follow-up of extensive pedal telangiectasia treated on 2 occasions with the PDL at 7.25 J/cm$^2$, 84 pulses and 115 pulses. **A,** Before treatment. **B,** Six months after initial treatment; 3 months after second treatment. (Courtesy Richard Fitzpatrick, M.D.)

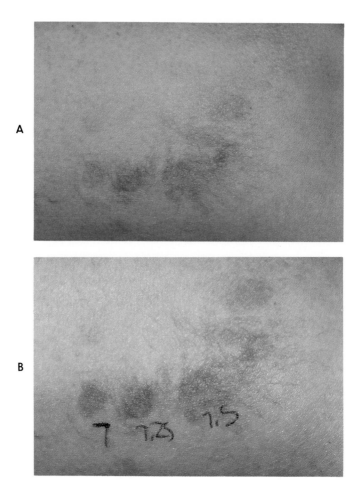

**Fig. 12-14**   Telangiectatic matting 9 months after sclerotherapy treatment of leg telangiectasia on the medial thigh. **A,** Immediately before treatment. **B,** Immediately after patch tests were performed with the PDL, 9 pulses to each site.

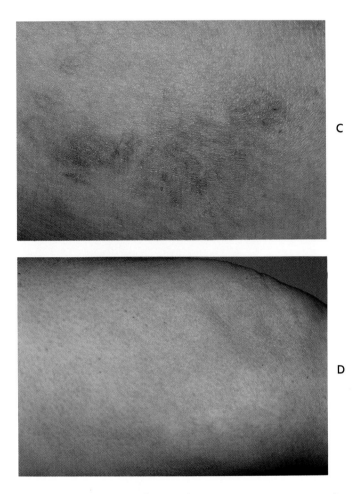

**Fig. 12-14, cont'd.** C, Two months after patch test treatment; note complete vessel resolution in areas treated at laser parameters of 7.25 and 7.5 J/cm$^2$. Only partial resolution occurred at 7.0 J/cm$^2$. Some hyperpigmentation is noted. **D,** One year after treatment of the entire area with PDL at 7.25 J/cm$^2$, 46 pulses; note complete resolution of the telangiectatic mat without pigmentary or textural skin changes.

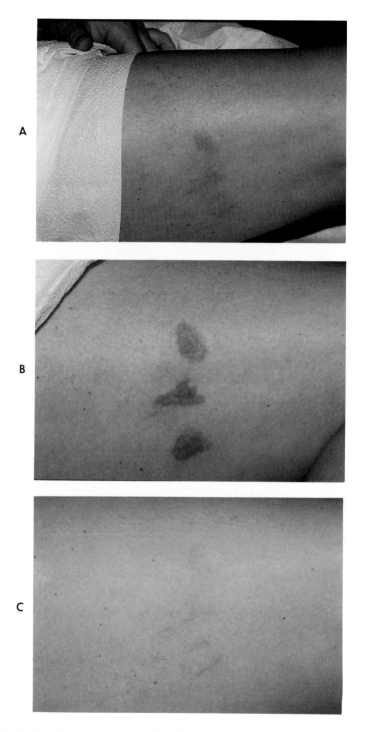

**Fig. 12-15** Telangiectatic patches with a feeding reticular vein 2 mm in diameter on the lateral thigh. **A,** Immediately before treatment. **B,** Immediately after treatment with the PDL, 20 pulses to each patch; 7.25 J/cm², superior patch; 7.5 J/cm², medial patch; 7.75 J/cm², inferior patch. **C,** Nine months after treatment. Note only partial resolution of the treated areas with persistence of the untreated reticular vein. (Courtesy Richard Fitzpatrick, M.D.)

**Table** [ 12-8 ] Effect of compression combined with pulsed dye laser treatment (laser energy: 7.0-8.0 J/cm$^2$)

| | No. of sites treated | No change | <90% faded | Total fade |
|---|---|---|---|---|
| Compression | 39 | 26% | 20% | 54% |
| No compression | 44 | 4% | 23% | 73% |

Modified from Goldman MP and Fitzpatrick RE: Pulsed dye laser treatment of telangietasia: with and without simultaneous sclerotherapy, J Dermatol Surg Oncol 16:338, 1990.

## Compression

Goldman[69] hypothesized and Goldman et al.[70] found that compression of telangiectatic leg veins improves sclerotherapy treatment outcome and promotes a decreased incidence of adverse sequelae. With pulsed dye laser, there appeared to be no obvious difference in treatment efficacy between telangiectatic patches that were treated with compression and those that were not (Table 12-8).

## Conclusions

In conclusion, the Candela SPTL-1 pulsed dye laser at 585 nm is an effective modality for treatment of red leg telangiectasia less than or equal to 0.2 mm in diameter. PDL treatment is efficacious for both essential telangiectasia and vessels that arise through the phenomenon of telangiectatic matting. This form of treatment used alone has a remarkably low incidence of adverse sequelae.

The optimal clinically useful laser energy with the Candela SPTL-1 laser in the treatment of red, 0.2-mm diameter telangiectatic mats is between 7.0 and 8.0 J/cm$^2$. Treatment is most efficacious if all vessels larger than 0.2 mm in diameter, especially varicose and reticular feeding veins, are treated first. Treatment results are not effected by vessel location. And, compression of the vessels after treatment appears to be unnecessary.

## COMBINED LASER AND SCLEROTHERAPY TREATMENT
### Experimental Evaluation of the Clinical and Histologic Effects of Combined PDL and Sclerotherapy (PDL/SCL) in the Rabbit Ear Vein Model

Combined PDL/SCL therapy has two theoretical advantages: an increase in efficacy of treatment allowing for successful sclerosis of blood vessels with a diameter >0.2 mm and a decrease in the most common adverse sequelae of sclerotherapy alone (pigmentation and telangiectatic matting). In addition, the combination of PDL and SCL treatments, by its synergistic endosclerotic action, may effectively treat previously untreatable cutaneous telangiectasias (those associated with arteriolar feeding vessel communication).

To summarize, PDL/SCL produces cumulative damage that leads to an enhanced efficacy of the sclerosing agent. However, a comparison of the degree and type of endothelial damage histologically does not demonstrate a significant difference between treatment with PDL and PDL/SCL (Table 12-9).[62] Pilot studies using a combination of sclerotherapy with POL 0.25% and PDL with laser energies of 6 and 7 J/cm$^2$ demonstrated no endothelial damage in vessels treated with PDL alone at 8 days. The combination of PDL at 6 and 7 J/cm$^2$ with SCL did demonstrate endothelial vacuolization. Thus it is possible that PDL energies less than 8 J/cm$^2$ may be successfully combined with sclerotherapy in human leg veins to provide effective therapy.

**Table** | **12-9** | Comparison of endothelial damage resulting from PDL and PDL/SCL

| | Laser energy used | |
| Type of damage | PDL alone | PDL + SCL with POL 0.25% |
| --- | --- | --- |
| Vacuolization | 8-8.5 J/cm$^2$ | 8 J/cm$^2$ |
| Necrosis | 9-9.5 J/cm$^2$ | 8.5-9.5 J/cm$^2$ |
| Perivascular collagen denaturization | 10 J/cm$^2$ | 10 J/cm$^2$ |

## PDL Treatment Combined with Sclerotherapy of Leg Telangiectasia

A study was conducted with 27 patients who had either bilaterally symmetrical telangiectatic patches or a large "starburst" telangiectatic flair that could be divided into two separate treatment sites (Fig. 12-16).[63] These patients were treated at one site only with a Candela SPTL-1 pulsed dye laser tuned to 585 nm with a pulse duration of 450 µs at energies ranging from 6.0 to 8.5 J/cm$^2$ delivered through a 5-mm spot size to the entire length of the telangiectasia. The other site was treated with laser energies of between 5.5 and 8.0 J/cm$^2$ immediately before injection of the telangiectasia with POL 0.25%, 0.5%, or 0.75%, a volume of 0.1 to 0.25 ml per injection site.

Of areas treated, 44% completely resolved (Table 12-10; Fig. 12-17). There appeared to be little difference in efficacy and adverse sequelae produced with concentrations of POL 0.25% and POL 0.5% (Table 12-11). When two areas were treated with POL 0.75%, ulceration occurred at 7.0 J/cm$^2$, and <90% fade was noted at 7.5 J/cm$^2$. There did appear to be an increased efficacy of treatment with

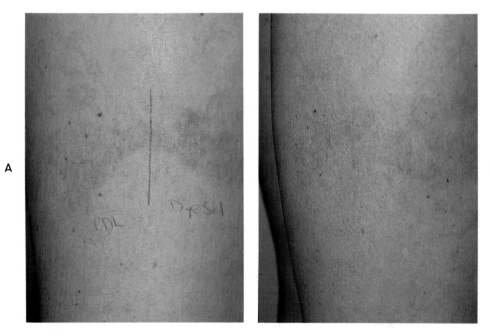

**Fig. 12-16**   Telangiectatic flair on lateral thigh divided into two treatment sites. Anterior aspect treated with PDL 6 J/cm$^2$, 50 pulses, immediately before sclerotherapy with POL 0.25%, 2 ml. Posterior aspect treated with PDL 7 J/cm$^2$, 34 pulses. **A,** Immediately before treatment. **B,** Three months after treatment.

**Table** 12-10   Results of PDL/SCL treatment of leg telangiectasia (all POL concentrations)

| Laser energy (J/cm²) | No. of sites treated | No change | <90% faded | Total fade | Ulceration/matting |
|---|---|---|---|---|---|
| 5.5 | 3 | | 100% | | |
| 6.0 | 10 | 20% | 30% | 40% | 10% |
| 7.0 | 4 | | 25% | 25% | 50% |
| 7.25 | 2 | | 50% | 50% | |
| 7.5 | 7 | 14% | 14% | 72% | |
| 7.75 | 1 | | | 100% | |
| TOTAL | 27 | 11% | 33% | 44% | 11% |

Modified from Goldman MP and Fitzpatrick RE: Pulsed dye laser treatment of telangiectasia: with and without simultaneous sclerotherapy, J Dermatol Surg Oncol 16:338, 1990.

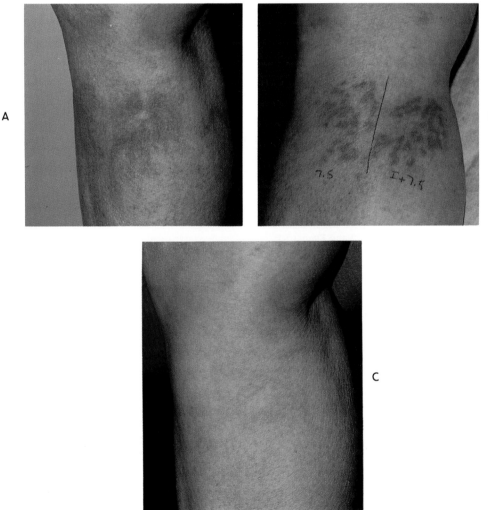

**Fig. 12-17**   Telangiectatic matting on medial knee/calf 6 months after sclerotherapy. **A,** Immediately before treatment. **B,** Immediately after treatment with PDL to anterior aspect at 7.5 J/cm², 51 pulses; posterior aspect treated with PDL 7.5 J/cm², 41 pulses, followed by sclerotherapy with POL 0.5%, 1 ml. **C,** Eleven months after treatment.

**Table** ⟦ **12-11** ⟧  Results of PDL/SCL treatment with POL 0.25% and POL 0.5%

| Laser energy (J/cm²) | No. of treatment sites | No change | <90% | Total fade | Ulceration/matting |
|---|---|---|---|---|---|
| **POL 0.25%** | | | | | |
| 5.5 | 1 | | 100% | | |
| 6.0 | 6 | 17% | 33% | 33% | 17% |
| 7.0 | 1 | | | 100% | |
| | | | | | |
| **POL 0.5%** | | | | | |
| 5.5 | 2 | | 100% | | |
| 6.0 | 2 | 50% | | 50% | |
| 7.0 | 2 | | 50% | | 50% |
| 7.25 | 2 | | 50% | 50% | |
| 7.5 | 6 | 17% | | 83% | |
| 7.75 | 1 | | | 100% | |

Modified from Goldman MP and Fitzpatrick RE: Pulsed dye laser treatment of telangiectasia: with and without simultaneous sclerotherapy, J Dermatol Surg Oncol 16:338, 1990.

**Table** ⟦ **12-12** ⟧  Results of PDL/SCL treatment (all POL concentrations) by vessel location

| Vessel location | No. of sites treated | No change | <90% faded | Total fade | Ulceration/matting |
|---|---|---|---|---|---|
| Thigh | 8 | 12% | 25% | 63% | |
| Knee | 7 | 28% | 28% | 14% | 28% |
| Calf | 7 | | 28% | 72% | |
| Ankle | 3 | | 33% | 33% | 33% |
| Foot | 1 | 100% | | | |

Modified from Goldman MP and Fitzpatrick RE: Pulsed dye laser treatment of telangiectasia: with and without simultaneous sclerotherapy, J Dermatol Surg Oncol 16:338, 1990.

laser energies of 7.5 to 7.75 J/cm². As with PDL alone, treatment site location did not appear to significantly affect treatment outcome except for an increased incidence of complications in the ankle and knee area (Table 12-12; Fig. 12-18).

## Complications

The most significant difference between PDL alone and PDL/SCL was the incidence of complications. With PDL/SCL treatment, posttreatment ulceration and telangiectatic matting occurred in 11% of patient treatment areas. Six of 23 nonulcerated treatment sites developed persistent pigmentation that remained unresolved beyond 1 year. Two of 27 sites developed telangiectatic matting that lasted over 1 year. Four of 27 treatment sites developed superficial ulceration. In these patients with ulceration, laser energies were equal to or greater than 6.5 J/cm² and Polidocanol concentration was equal to or greater than 0.5% (Fig. 12-19).

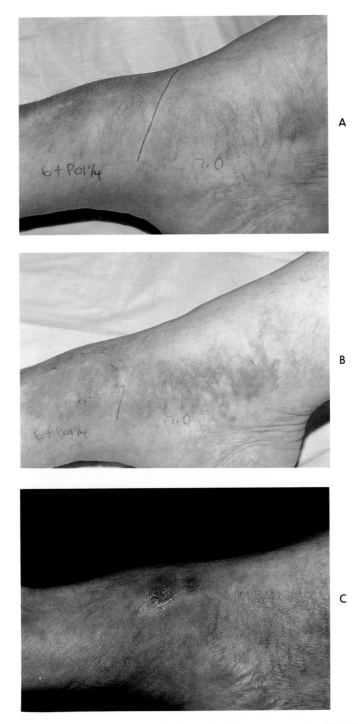

**Fig. 12-18**   Essential telangiectasia on the feet. Distal aspect treated with PDL 6 $J/cm^2$, 114 pulses, immediately followed by sclerotherapy with POL 0.25%, 1 ml. Proximal aspect treated with PDL 7 $J/cm^2$, 100 pulses. **A**, Immediately before treatment. **B**, Immediately after treatment. **C**, Four months after treatment. Note superficial ulceration at the PDL/SCL-treated site.

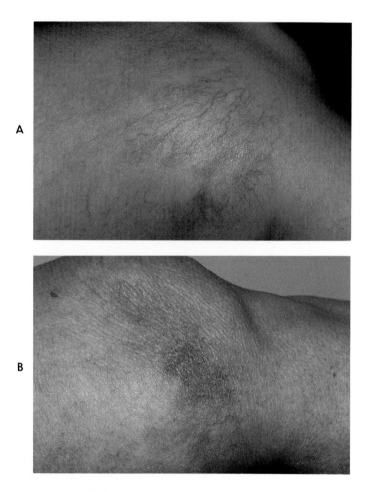

**Fig. 12-19**   Treatment of telangiectatic matting 7 months after sclerotherapy treatment of telangiectasia on the medial knee. **A,** Immediately before initial sclerotherapy treatment. **B,** Development of persistent telangiectatic matting 7 months after initial treatment.

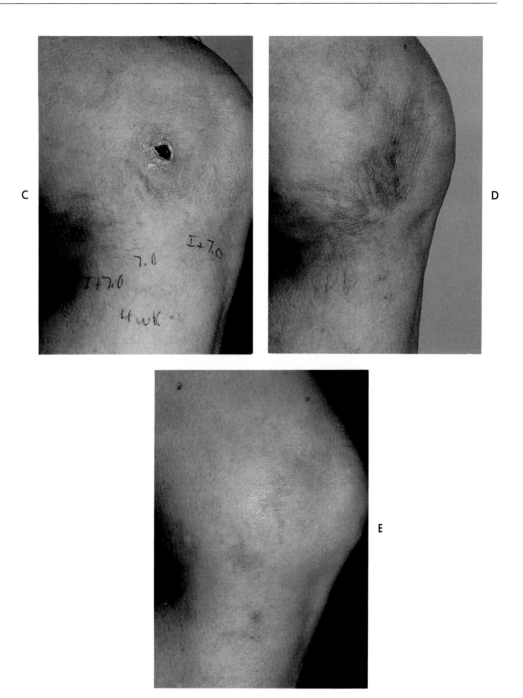

**Fig. 12-19, cont'd.** **C,** Three months after PDL and PDL/SCL treatment showing the development of a persistent superficial ulceration in the two PDL/SCL treatment sites. Anterior site treated with PDL 7 $J/cm^2$, 31 pulses, before sclerotherapy with POL 0.5%, 1 ml; medial site treated with PDL alone at 7 $J/cm^2$, 27 pulses; posterior site treated with PDL 7 $J/cm^2$, 31 pulses, before sclerotherapy with POL 0.75%, 1 ml. **D,** Seven months after initial PDL and PDL/SCL treatment showing persistent telangiectatic matting and healing of the ulceration. **E,** Six months after treatment with chromated glycerin solution (diluted 1:1 with lidocaine 1%), 2 ml. Resolution of the telangiectatic matting has occurred.

---

### PULSED DYE LASER TREATMENT OF LEG TELANGIECTASIA

Posttreatment pigmentation cleared within 2 to 6 months

No episodes of telangiectatic matting were noted (101 treatment sites)

Optimal laser energy: 7.0 to 8.0 J/cm$^2$

Must treat feeding reticular veins first

Results not affected by treatment location

Compression not necessary

---

### PULSED DYE LASER/SCLEROTHERAPY TREATMENT OF LEG TELANGIECTASIA

Persistent pigmentation developed in 6 of 34 nonulcerated treatment sites

Persistent telangiectatic matting developed in 2 of 38 sites

Superficial ulceration developed in 4 of 38 sites (Laser energies above 6.5 J/cm$^2$, Polidocanol >0.5%)

Optimal laser energy: 5.5 to 6.0 J/cm$^2$

Optimal Polidocanol concentration: 0.25% to 0.5%

Must treat feeding reticular veins first

Results not affected by treatment location

---

**Table 12-13** Results of PDL/SCL versus PDL alone

| Treatment modality | No. of sites treated | No change | <90% faded | Total fade | Ulceration/matting |
|---|---|---|---|---|---|
| PDL | 91 | 19% | 25% | 56% | |
| PDL* | 78 | 15% | 20% | 65% | |
| PDL/SCL† | 27 | 11% | 33% | 44% | 11% |

Modified from Goldman MP and Fitzpatrick RE: Pulsed dye laser treatment of telangiectasia: with and without simultaneous sclerotherapy, J Dermatol Surg Oncol 16:338, 1990.
*Less patients with untreated feeding reticular veins.
†All POL concentrations.

## Conclusions

PDL/SCL treatment appears to offer no advantage over PDL treatment alone and appears to have a significant degree of complications when treatment is limited to red telangiectasia less than 0.2 mm in diameter. The important points cited for each treatment modality are listed in the boxes above.

There is theoretical evidence to suggest that PDL/SCL treatment may be more efficacious than either PDL or SCL alone in the rabbit ear vein model. However, this was not demonstrated in human leg telangiectasia less than 0.2 mm in diameter. Future studies on the use of PDL/SCL treatment for larger-diameter blood vessels appear to be necessary.

A comparison of the results of both treatment modalities appears in Table 12-13.

## REFERENCES

1. Absten GT: Laser biophysics for the physician. In Ratz JL, editor: Lasers in cutaneous medicine and surgery, Chicago, 1986, Year Book Medical Publishers Inc.
2. Kaplan I and Peled I: The carbon dioxide laser in the treatment of superficial telangiectasias, Br J Plast Surg 28:214, 1975.
3. Apfelberg DB et al: Use of the argon and carbon dioxide lasers for treatment of superficial venous varicosities of the lower extremity, Lasers Surg Med 4:221, 1984.
4. Apfelberg DB et al: Study of three laser systems for treatment of superficial varicosities of the lower extremity, Lasers Surg Med 7:219, 1987.
5. Pfeifer JR and Hawtof GD: Injection sclerotherapy and $CO_2$ laser sclerotherapy in the ablation of cutaneous spider veins of the lower extremity, Phlebolosie 4:231, 1989.
6. Landthaler M et al: Laser therapy of venous lakes (Bean-Walsh) and telangiectasias, Plast Recontr Surg 73:78, 1984.
7. Dolsky RL: Argon laser skin surgery, Surg Clin North Am 64:861, 1984.
8. van Gemert MJC and Henning JPH: A model approach to laser coagulation of dermal vascular lesions, Arch Dermatol Res 270:429, 1981.
9. Greenwald J et al: Comparative histological studies of the tunable dye (577 nm) laser and argon laser: the specific vascular effects of the dye laser, J Invest Dermatol 77:305, 1981.
10. Haina D et al: Comparison of maximum coagulation depth in human skin for different types of medical lasers, Lasers Surg Med 7:355, 1987.
11. Finley JL et al: Argon laser port-wine stain interaction: immediate effects, Arch Dermatol 120:613, 1984.
12. Arndt KA: Treatment technics in argon laser therapy: comparison of pulsed and continuous exposures, J Am Acad Dermatol 11:90, 1984.
13. Apfelberg DB, Maser MR, and Lash H: Argon laser management of cutaneous vascular deformities: a preliminary report, West J Med 124:99, 1976.
14. Apfelberg DB et al: Analysis of complications of argon laser treatment for port-wine hemangiomas with reference to striped technique, Lasers Surg Med 2:357, 1983.
15. Apfelberg DB, Maser MR, and Lash H: Treatment of nevi aranei by means of an argon laser, J Dermatol Surg Oncol 4:172, 1978.
16. Lyons GD, Owens RE, and Mouney DF: Argon laser destruction of cutaneous telangiectatic lesions, Laryngoscope 91:1322, 1981.
17. Remington BK: Argon laser therapy — rosacea, telangiectasia (Letter to the editor), J Dermatol Surg Oncol 9:424, 1983.
18. Goldman L: Application of laser therapy. Paper presented at the Noah Worcester Dermatologic Society, Hilton Head, April, 1984.
19. Arndt IA: Argon laser therapy of small cutaneous vascular lesions, Arch Dermatol 118:219, 1982.
20. Dixon JA, Huether S, and Rotering RH: Hypertrophic scarring in argon laser treatment of port-wine stains, Plast Reconstr Surg 73:771, 1984.
21. Ratz JL, Goldman L, and Bauman WE: Post treatment complications of the argon laser, Arch Dermatol 121:714, 1985.
22. Landthaler M et al: Argon laser treatment of naevi flammei, Hautarzt 38:652, 1987.
23. Olbricht SM et al: Complications of cutaneous laser surgery: a survey, Arch Dermatol 123:345, 1987.
24. Bonafe JL et al: Hyperpigmentation induced by argon laser therapy of hemangiomas: optimal and electron microscope studies, Dermatologica 170:225, 1985.
25. Gilchrest B, Rosen S, and Noe J: Chilling port-wine stains improves the response to argon laser therapy, Plast Reconstr Surg 69:278, 1982.
26. Welch AJ, Motamedi M, and Gonzales A: Evaluation of cooling techniques for the protection of the epidermis during Nd:Yag laser radiation of the skin. In Joeffe SN, editor: Neodymium-YAG laser in medicine and surgery, New York, 1983, Elsevier.
27. Yanai A et al: Argon laser therapy of port-wine stains: effects and limitations, Plast Reconstr Surg 75:520, 1985.
28. Ginsbach G: New aspects in the management of benign cutaneous tumors. Laser 79 H Opto-Electronics, Conference Proc, Munich, West Germany, 1979, International Optical Society.
29. Rotteleur G et al: Robotized scanning laser handpiece for the treatment of port-wine stains and other angiodysplasias, Lasers Surg Med 8:283, 1988.
30. Apfelberg DB et al: Dot or pointillistic method for improvement in results of hypertrophic scarring in the argon laser treatment of port-wine hemangiomas, Lasers Surg Med 6:552, 1987.
31. Apfelberg DB and McBurney E: Use of the argon laser in dermatologic surgery. In Ratz JL, editor: Lasers in cutaneous medicine and surgery, Chicago, 1986, Year Book Medical Publishers Inc.
32. Craig RDP et al: Argon laser therapy for cutaneous lesions, Br J Plast Surg 38:148, 1985.

33. Apfelberg DB et al: Use of the argon and carbon dioxide lasers for treatment of superficial venous varicosities of the lower extremity, Lasers Surg Med 4:221, 1984.

34. Dixon JA, Rotering RH, and Huether SE: Patient's evaluation of argon laser therapy of port-wine stain, decorative tattoo, and essential telangiectasia, Lasers Surg Med 4:181, 1984.

35. Dixon JA and Gilbertson JJ: Cutaneous laser therapy. In Hightech Medicine (Special Issue), West J Med 143:758, 1985.

36. Bruck LB: Micro-contact argon laser probe may enhance therapy, Dermatol Times, p 15, October, 1988.

37. Fitzpatrick RE: Unpublished observations, 1988.

38. Anderson RR and Parrish JA: Microvasculature can be selectively damaged using dye lasers: a basic theory and experimental evidence in human skin, Lasers Surg Med 1:263, 1981.

39. van Gemert MJC, Welch AJ, and Amin AP: Is there an optimal laser treatment for port-wine stains, Lasers Surg Med 6:76, 1986.

40. Hulsbergen Henning JP, van Gemert MJC, and Lahaye CTW: Clinical and histological evaluation of port-wine stain treatment with a microsecond-pulsed dye-laser at 577 nm, Lasers Surg Med 4:375, 1984.

41. Tan OT, Kerschmann R, and Parrish JA: The effect of epidermal pigmentation on selective vascular effects of pulsed laser, Lasers Surg Med 4:365, 1985.

42. Tong AKF et al: Ultrastructure: effects of melanin pigment on target specificity using a pulsed-dye laser (577 nm), J Invest Dermatol 88:747, 1987.

43. Nakagawa H, Tan OT, and Parrish JA: Ultrastructural changes in human skin after exposure to a pulsed laser, J Invest Dermatol 84:396, 1985.

44. Tan OT, Murray S, and Kurban AK: Action spectrum of vascular specific injury using pulsed irradiation, J Invest Dermatol 92:868, 1989.

45. Anderson R and Parrish JA: The optics of human skin, J Invest Dermatol 77:13, 1981.

46. Kurban AK, Sherwood KA, and Tan OT: What are the optimal wavelengths for selective vascular injury? Lasers Surg Med 8:190, 1988.

47. Gange RW et al: Effect of preirradiation tissue target temperature upon selective vascular damage induced by 577-nm tunable dye laser pulses, Microvasc Res 28:125, 1980.

48. Glassberg E et al: Cellular effects of the pulsed tunable dye laser at 577 nanometers on human endothelial cells, fibroblasts, and erythrocytes: an in vitro study, Lasers Surg Med 8:567, 1988.

49. Glassberg E et al: The flashlamp-pumped 577-nm pulsed tunable dye laser: clonical efficacy and in vitro studies, J Dermatol Surg Oncol 14:1200, 1988.

50. Anderson RR and Parrish JA: Selective photothermolysis: precise microsurgery by selective absorption of pulsed radiation, Science 220:524, 1983.

51. Garden JM et al: Effect of dye laser pulse duration on selective cutaneous vascular injury, J Invest Dermatol 87:653, 1986.

52. Tan TT et al: Histologic responses of port-wine stains treated by argon, carbon dioxide, and tunable dye lasers: a preliminary report, Arch Dermatol 122:1016, 1986.

53. Anderson RR, Jaenicke KF, and Parrish JA: Mechanisms of selective vascular changes caused by dye lasers, Lasers Surg Med 3:211, 1983.

54. Morelli JG et al: Tunable dye laser (577 nm) treatment of port-wine stains, Lasers Surg Med 6:94, 1986.

55. Garden JM, Polla LL, and Tan OT: The treatment of port-wine stains by the pulsed-dye laser: analysis of pulse duration and long-term therapy, Arch Dermatol 124:889, 1988.

56. Garden JM et al: The pulsed-dye laser for the treatment of port-wine stains, J Dermatol Surg Oncol 12:757, 1986.

57. Garden JM et al: The pulsed-dye laser as a modality for treating cutaneous small blood vessel disease processes, Lasers Surg Med 6:259, 1986.

58. Garden JM, Tan OT, and Parrish JA: The pulsed-dye laser: its use at 577-nm wavelength, J Dermatol Surg Oncol 13:134, 1987.

59. Polla LL et al: Tunable pulsed dye laser for the treatment of benign cutaneous vascular ectasia, Dermatologica 174:11, 1987.

60. Smith T et al: 532-nanometer green laser beam treatment of superficial varicosities of the lower extremities, Lasers Surg Med 8:130, 1988.

61. Goldman MP et al: Sclerosing agents in the treatment of telangiectasia: comparison of the clinical and histologic effects of intravascular polidocanol, sodium tetradecyl sulfate, hypertonic saline in the dorsal rabbit ear vein model, Arch Dermatol 123:1196, 1987.

62. Goldman MP et al: Pulsed-dye laser treatment of telangiectases with and without sub-therapeutic sclerotherapy: clinical and histologic examination of the rabbit ear vein model, J Am Acad Dermatol 23:23, 1990.

63. Goldman MP and Fitzpatrick RE: Pulsed-dye laser treatment of leg telangiectasia: with and without simultaneous sclerotherapy, J Dermatol Surg Oncol 16:338, 1990.

64. Biegeleisen K: Primary lower extremity telangiectasias: relationship of size to color, Angiology 38:760, 1987.

65. Ashton N: Corneal vascularization. In Duke-Elder S and Perkins ES: The transparency of the cornea, Oxford, 1960, Blackwell.

66. Duffy DM: Small vessel sclerotherapy: an overview. In Callen JP et al, editors: Advances in dermatology, vol 3, Chicago, 1988, Year Book Medical Publishers Inc.

67. Green D: Compression sclerotherapy techniques, Dermatol Clin 7:137, 1989.

68. Ouvry PA: Telangiectasia and sclerotherapy, J Dermatol Surg Oncol 15:177, 1989.

69. Goldman MP: Compression in the treatment of leg telangiectasia: theoretical considerations, J Dermatol Surg Oncol 15:184, 1989.

70. Goldman MP et al: Compression in the treatment of leg telangiectasia: a preliminary report, J Dermatol Surg Oncol 16:322, 1990.

# 13 Setting up a Sclerotherapy Practice

## DECIDING WHO WILL DELIVER PATIENT CARE

Before proceeding with the practical aspects of establishing a practice, one must decide who will deliver patient care. Most physicians agree that the sclerotherapy procedure should be performed by a physician. However, there are some clinics that employ nurses to treat "spider" telangiectasias. A survey of the membership of the North American Society of Phlebology (NASP) found that approximately 25% of the members would allow a registered nurse and 20% would allow a nurse practitioner to perform sclerotherapy on spider veins.[1] And of NASP members surveyed, 10% would allow a registered nurse to perform sclerotherapy on varicose veins versus 7% who would allow nurse practitioners to perform this procedure.

Employing registered nurses to perform intravenous therapeutic injections is legal in the state of California. Recently, a resolution was submitted to the California Medical Association that would limit the practice of sclerotherapy to licensed physicians. Action on the resolution is pending at this time.

The arguments for allowing nurses to render such care are both economic and procedural. An economic benefit is realized for both the patient and physician if a lower-salaried person performs the sclerotherapy procedure, and in these days of cost containment, this issue does assume importance. Since the injection of spider veins is primarily cosmetic and is rarely fully reimbursable under most insurance plans, cost containment is translated into economic marketing.

Because the cannulation of a blood vessel is relatively easy to perform and there are relatively few serious or life-threatening complications that can arise from sclerotherapy treatment of spider telangiectasias, an argument can be made for employing nonphysicians as sclerotherapists. On the other hand, although rare, serious complications can occur as a result of injection of spider telangiectasias. Anaphylactic allergic reactions do occur with the use of many sclerosing agents; a fatality was recently reported that occurred as a result of a "trial" injection of sodium tetradecyl sulfate.[2] Pulmonary emboli also have been reported to occur from the injection of a leg telangiectasia (see Chapter 8). Injection into an arteriovenous anastomosis will usually produce a cutaneous ulceration. Injection into a superficial artery, especially around the malleoli, can theoretically lead to arterial embolism and pedal gangrene. Thus, as with most of medicine, sclerotherapy is not entirely risk free.

In addition to being skilled at sclerotherapy technique, the sclerotherapist must also have a thorough knowledge of the anatomy and pathophysiology of venous disease, as well as knowledge of the mechanism of action of the procedure including potential complications. Being able to appreciate these mechanisms and immediately recognize potential complications and render preventive treatment is critical if one is to maintain optimal patient care.

356

## EQUIPMENT

Relatively little specialized equipment is required to perform successful sclerotherapy. In the future certain types of lasers may be available for treating specific types of leg veins (see Chapter 12). For now all that is required is a needle, syringe, sclerosing solution, binocular loupe, foam pads, tape, graduated support stockings, and camera. (See Appendix F for information on manufacturers.)

### Needles

The injection of telangiectasias requires a fine-gauge needle. Although some physicians prefer a 32-to-33 gauge or 26-to-27 gauge needle, I prefer the 30-gauge needle. There are two types of 30-gauge needles. The Becton-Dickinson (B-D) Precision Glide needle has an elongated bevel on a ½-inch needle with a 45-degree angle at the tip. The needle can be easily bent at varying angles to penetrate telangiectasias. In addition, it is relatively sharp and holds up well when used for multiple punctures of the skin. The second type is a tri-bevel tipped needle. The Acuderm and Delasco 30-gauge needles have a ½-inch metal hub and a silicone-coated tri-bevel point. This type is preferred because its silicone coating and more acute angle at the tip allows it to pierce the skin with less pain. Also the length of the bevel is shorter than that of the B-D needle. Accordingly, extravasation of solution perivascularly while the needle is in the vessel lumen is less likely. And finally, it costs less. An illustration comparing the bevels of all of the recommended needles is shown in Fig. 13-1. However, even with this magnified comparison, one cannot fully appreciate the differences between the needle tips. Clinical trials using each needle type are necessary to discern the subtle differences.

One objection to the use of a 30-gauge needle has been the perception that it dulls after multiple insertions into the skin. Microscopic examination of a needle used to pierce the skin up to 15 times did not show the needle tip to be dulled.

Some sclerotherapists advise the use of a 33-gauge needle to cannulate the smallest diameter telangiectasia. Recently, a Delasco 32-to-33 gauge ½-inch needle has become available (Fig. 13-2). These needles have several drawbacks. They are not disposable and need to be cleaned and sterilized between patients. Repetitive sterilization will dull the needle point. Also, they are sold for animal use only and are not approved for use in humans. In addition, the tips of these needles bend and dull more quickly than the 30-gauge needles, and the needle shafts are thinner and thus less stable when injecting through tough skin. John

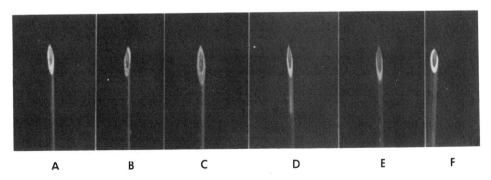

**Fig. 13-1** A comparison of bevels of recommended needles. **A**, Acuderm needle, 30-gauge. **B**, Becton-Dickinson (B-D) needle, 30-gauge. **C**, 27-gauge Yale needle (B-D) **D**, Yale needle (B-D) 26-gauge. **E**, Butterfly needle (Abbott), 25-gauge. **F**, Butterfly needle (Abbott), 23-gauge.

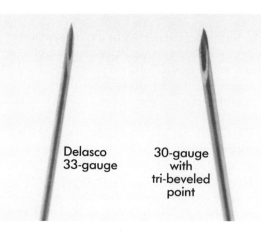

**Fig. 13-2** Comparison of 33-gauge Delasco needle tip with a 30-gauge tri-bevel point. (Courtesy Dermatologic Lab and Supply, Inc.)

Phiffer, M.D., reported recently on the construction of a rigid shaft used to support the 32-gauge needle tip to help stabilize it. However, as mentioned previously (Chapter 11), I find these needles to be of little use.

Finally, some physicians prefer 26- or 27-gauge needles for injecting telangiectasias. Again, the preference arises from a perceived sharpness of the bevel allowing for easier, more painless insertion. The 27-gauge needle comes separately on a ½-inch length as either a Yale hypodermic needle or as an Allergy needle-syringe combination fixed to a 1-mm syringe. The benefit of using the 1-mm syringe is the ease of handling perceived by some sclerotherapists. The Yale 26-gauge needle also comes in a ½-inch length and has the advantage of a sturdy, nonbendable shaft. In short, all types have their advantages and disadvantages. The best needle is the one the physician is most comfortable with.

Larger needles are most often used to inject varicose veins. When injecting varicose veins, it is critical to determine the proper placement of the needle. Therefore, the smallest recommended needle size is 25-gauge (23-gauge if there is any doubt as to whether the vessel to be cannulated is an artery or vein or if one is using a highly caustic sclerosing solution such as Variglobin). Larger-bore needles offer no additional advantage. A 25-gauge easily allows retrograde blood flow through the inserted needle, which aids in determining if placement is intravenous or intraarterial.

The surest method of determining proper needle placement is to insert an open needle into the vein. With this technique blood flow from the needle serves as the indicator of arterial versus venous injection. In an effort to avoid blood exposure, some sclerotherapists attach a syringe to the needle and withdraw to determine flow. Still others combine the needle with a glass syringe to "feel" for proper intravascular placement.

To take advantage of the safety of a large-gauge needle without incurring the risk of blood contamination, one may use a 21-, 23-, or 25-gauge butterfly needle. The needle length is ¾-inch, and the tubing is 30 cm. The plastic tubing on the proximal end of the needle allows for visualization of arterial versus venous flow without risking blood exposure. The tubing takes up 0.41 ml of fluid. Some physicians fill the needle tubing with sclerosing solution to prevent blood clotting within the needle tubing. However, if the injection is performed within a few minutes of blood aspiration, this is not necessary.

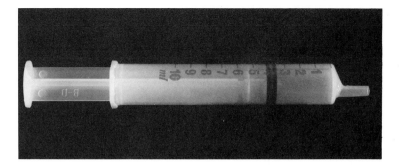

**Fig. 13-3**   Plastipak eccentric syringe by Becton-Dickinson. Note eccentrically placed hub.

## Syringes

Although glass syringes have been used in the past to allow early detection of an arterial puncture, modern plastic syringes have a feel comparative to that of glass syringes. The disadvantage of the glass syringe is that it requires practice both to fill and to use smoothly and, obviously, needs to be cleaned and sterilized between patients.

The 3-ml plastic syringe Luer Lok, or nonLuer Lok, is used exclusively in my practice. This syringe allows an ideal quantity of solution to be used, and when filled to a 2-ml capacity, fits easily in the palm of the hand. If one does not bend the needle to facilitate penetration of the vein, the Plastipak eccentric syringe (Fig. 13-3) is useful. With this syringe, the hub is eccentrically placed at the syringe tip so that it abuts the skin surface. It is available in 1-ml, 2-ml, 5-ml, and 10-ml sizes.

## Sclerosing Solutions

The various sclerosing solutions available are discussed in detail in Chapter 7. The addresses of the manufacturers and distributors of these solutions are listed in Appendix B.

## Binocular Loupes

Protective eyeglasses are necessary equipment for the physician who performs any surgical procedure. These glasses should be constructed so as to prevent the splatter or spray of body fluids (blood) from coming in contact with the orbital tissues. This will help prevent the physician being contaminated with infectious, blood-borne viral or bacterial disease. For this reason, it is recommended that protective glasses be worn when performing sclerotherapy.

The injection treatment of varicose veins does not require magnification of the surgical field. However, when one is cannulating venulectases or telangiectasias, magnification of the treatment site is important. The enhanced detail that magnification affords allows for more accurate placement of the needle within the vessel lumen, which prevents extravasation of the sclerosing solution into extravascular spaces.

To magnify the field of vision, one moves closer to the viewed object to enlarge its field on the retina. Moving closer to an object requires the eyes to refocus and converge more. The consequences of maintaining this close focusing distance are eye strain and back muscle stress. Eye tension and muscle fatigue may then occur, which tends to reduce one's efficiency. Optical magnification offers an alternative to such strain and allows a more comfortable working distance to be maintained.

**Table 13-1** Comparison of loupe magnification

| Measurement | Refractive power | | |
| --- | --- | --- | --- |
| | 3 diopters | 5 diopters | 8 diopters |
| Magnification | ×1.75 | ×2.25 | ×3 |
| Lens-to-object distance | 8-34 cm | 13-20 cm | 10 cm |
| Eye-to-object distance | 17-45 cm | 22-36 cm | 20-25 cm |
| Field of view | 8 cm | 4 cm | 2 cm |
| Depth of field | 25 cm | 8 cm | 1 cm |

The magnifying loupe allows the focusing and converging systems of the eye to relax. The loupe also allows one to switch back and forth between normal vision and magnified vision as necessary. This versatility is relaxing to the eyes. Viewing through magnification for long periods is not harmful and cannot damage vision. The only question is how much magnification is necessary?

The ideal magnifier provides a wide field of view with distortion-free magnification within a reasonably long working distance. Unfortunately, with presently available optics, the higher the magnification, the smaller the field of view and depth of field. Complex, multilens binocular magnifiers overcome some of the limitation of short working distances. Some of these are detailed on p. 362. An independent evaluation of magnifiers for use in dermatology appears in another source.[3]

When choosing the proper magnification, five factors need to be addressed: magnification, lens-to-object distance, eye-to-object distance, field of view, and depth of field. Table 13-1 shows a comparison of these factors in regard to a person with normal focusing-converging ability. Note that magnifications above 5 diopters decrease the field of view and depth of focusing sufficiently to make its use impractical for sclerotherapy. In my experience, lenses with 2.25 to 3 diopters provide the ideal combination of focal distance and magnification.

**Magnifying glasses.** Half-frame clip-on lens are available in multiple powers. The most useful is a 5-diopter, 2.25×-power lens with a 19-cm focal distance. These lenses produce marked peripheral distortion but have a usable field of view of 7 cm for the 3-diopter and 5 cm for the 5-diopter lens. The working distance from lens to object is 17 cm for the 3-diopter and 12 cm for the 5-diopter lens (Fig. 13-4). This type of magnification aid is available from most opticians and department stores.

**Headband-mounted simple binocular magnifiers.** Headband magnifiers are available equipped with interchangeable lens plates that provide a range of magnification from 1.5× to 3.5× (Fig. 13-5). These can be comfortably worn over prescription eyeglasses. The most widely used magnifications with the least peripheral distortion and best working distance are the 2× and 2.5×. An optional Optiloupe attachment lens adds 2.5× magnification to any base lens but has a very small field of view without distortion. These magnifiers are available from many manufacturers and vary in price, type of headgear padding, and adjustibility; Optivisor and Mark II Magni-focuser are two examples.

**Simple binocular loupes.** The Precision binocular loupe comes with varying diopter loupes fitted on a double-hinged telescoping rod so that one can ad-

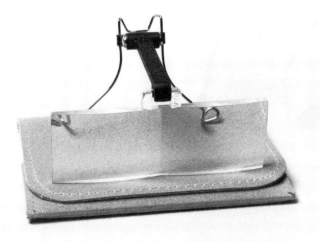

**Fig. 13-4**    Almore Clip-On Loupe. (Courtesy Almore International.)

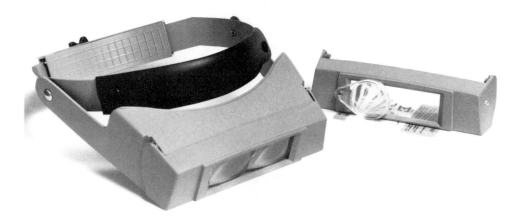

**Fig. 13-5**    Mark II Magni-Focuser. (Courtesy Edroy Products Co., Inc.)

just the eye-to-object distance. Also, it comes with an adjustable bridge-of-nose-to-lens distance of 9 to 21 cm, thus increasing the eye-to-object distance from 19 to 44 cm depending on the diopter used. The 3-diopter lens has a 13-cm usable field of view and a working distance of 16 cm from lens to object. The 5-diopter lens has a 10-cm field of usable view and a working distance of 13 cm from lens to object. It is available with 3-, 5-, or 8-diopter lenses [4] (Fig. 13-6) and is also available as a multidistance headband loupe. Available powers include 1.5×, 1.75×, 2.25×, and 2.75× with working distances from 50 to 15 cm respectively.

**Binocular loupes.** Multilens binocular magnifiers are referred to as binocular loupes, telescopic magnifiers, and surgical telescopes. They are available in magnifications ranging from 2× to 8× and are designed to provide a working distance of between 25 and 40 cm. Their drawback is their limited field of view; however, the entire field is usually not distorted, and thus the nondistorted portion of the field of view approaches that of lesser-quality magnifiers. Some high-quality binocular loupes have a field of view larger than other brand models; therefore, one should compare many loupes.

Epstein[3] has found the Designs for Vision loupe to be best suited for dermatologic examination. The working distance of this loupe is 35 cm for the 3.5× and 40 cm for the 2.5× magnifier.

Other less expensive models include the N1064 Oculus loupe (Fig. 13-7, *A*). Another, the Westco 2-to-2.5× adjustable loupe, is used by myself, and I find it of excellent quality. The lens-to-object working distance is 13 cm with a 3-cm field of view at 2.5×.

Recently a new type of loupe has become available, the Keeler Panoramic Surgical Loupes. This optical system has the following advantages: optics that can flip up out of view when not needed, lightweight frames, and optics with an antireflection coating. The 2.5× magnification loupe (Fig. 13-7, *B*) has a field size of 9.4 cm and a working distance of 42 cm. A 3× magnifier is available with a working distance of 34 cm and a field size of 6.2 cm or with a working distance of 50 cm and a field size of 7.6 cm.

Finally, the lowest-priced loupe of high quality is the See Better Loupe. The magnification is 2.5× with a field of view of 9 cm and an eye-to-working distance of 35 cm.

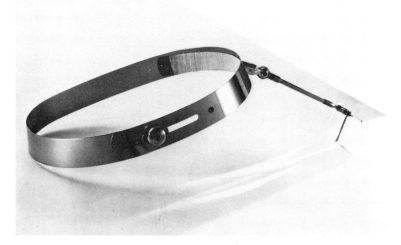

**Fig. 13-6**  Almore +3-diopter Loupe. (Courtesy Almore International.)

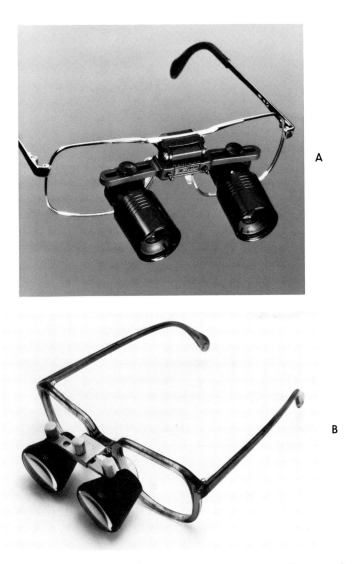

**Fig. 13-7** **A,** N1064 Oculus Loupe. (Courtesy Storz Instrument Company.) **B,** Keeler 2.5× panoramic loupes. (Courtesy Keeler Instruments, Inc.)

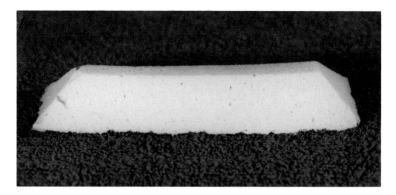

**Fig. 13-8**    Foam compression pad.

### Foam Pads

Foam compression pads (Fig. 13-8) are manufactured from white latex rubber. They are beveled to produce maximum compression along the line of the injected vein segment. STD Pharmaceutical distributes two sizes of pads that are useful for providing additional compression over varicose veins (see Chapter 6). They are:

D pad (5 cm × 13 cm × 2.5 cm high)
E pad (4 cm × 13 cm × 1.75 cm high)

### Tape Dressings

To support the placement of foam pads with minimal pressure, three sizes of microfoam surgical tape is recommended:

Size D: 7.5-cm diameter (for legs)
Size E: 8.75-cm diameter (for legs or small thighs)
Size F: 10-cm diameter (for thighs)

To support the placement of pads and/or apply additional localized pressure, Coban tape or Medi-Rip Bandages are recommended. Medi-Rip Bandage is a cohesive, tearable, elastic bandage rolled in 1-inch tubes. It is available in 1-, 2-, 3-, 4-, and 6-inch widths. It is composed of 99.2% cotton and 0.8% polyurethane and has a latex cohesive finish. The cotton-covered rubber threads minimize constriction and control elasticity. The microfine cohesive cover allows it to stick to itself instead of hair or skin and eliminates slippage.

### Graduated Compression Stockings

Information regarding graduated compression stockings can be found in Chapter 6 and Appendix A.

One useful aid for helping support the thigh stocking on the leg in proper position is a body adhesive called "It Stays!" This body adhesive comes in a roll-on bottle. It does not dry on the skin and remains tacky until it comes in contact with water. The product has been proven to be nontoxic, nonflammable, and only rarely causes skin irritation.

### Antiseptic

Alcohol-soaked cotton balls are liberally applied to the telangiectatic area before injection to cleanse the area of bacteria and applied oils and grime. In addition, it improves the refraction of light to enhance the appearance of the vessels.

# PHOTOGRAPHY

Photographic documentation is recommended when treating any patient with varicose or telangiectatic leg veins. Not only do many insurance companies require photographic documentation before approving reimbursement, but also patients often cannot remember later exactly how their leg veins appeared initially. In addition, because varicose and telangiectatic leg veins may continue to appear throughout a patient's lifetime, documentation of treated areas will help distinguish between new veins and recurrent veins. And finally, some patients with long-standing varicose veins have hyperpigmentation around the varicosity. Preoperative photographic documentation is thus important.

Ideally, all photographs should be taken with the same camera, same type of film and processing, same lighting, same F-stop and shutter speed, and same distance and angle of exposure from the camera to the patient. I recommend a Nikon 2020 fully automatic camera fitted with a Nikon 105-mm macro lens and Sunpak auto 444D Thyrister flash. It is beneficial to replace the factory "split-image" internal lens with a clear lens to aid in close-up focusing. All photographs are taken at standard F-stops: F16 for close up, F11 for half-leg view photos, and F8 for full-leg view photos. Photographs are taken at an automatic "through-the-lens" (TTL) setting. Kodachrome ASA 25 film gives the highest quality reproductions.

# PATIENT INFORMATIONAL BROCHURES

To educate patients concerning sclerotherapy, it is best for the physician to produce a brochure or information sheet that incorporates his or her unique and personalized approach to such treatment. Indeed, there is no totally right way to perform sclerotherapy, and there are relatively few absolutes regarding preoperative preparation, treatment, and postoperative instructions. However, to produce personalized brochures is expensive. As an alternative, a number of ready-made commercial brochures are available (see Appendix G).

# INSURANCE REIMBURSEMENT

Many physicians have expressed frustration in regard to obtaining insurance reimbursement for the treatment of varicose veins with compression sclerotherapy, despite those veins being symptomatic. It appears from a limited review of insurance reimbursement in my practice that there is a marked variability in the amount of reimbursement not only among different insurance companies, but also within the same insurance company from patient to patient.

Table 13-2 is a random selection of cases from my practice showing insurance reimbursements for sclerotherapy treatment of symptomatic varicose (not spider) veins billed using RVS code 36471 (Injection sclerotherapy of varicose vein) plus RVS code 99070 for a surgical tray during 1986. The wide-ranging variations reflect the enigma of insurance reimbursement for sclerotherapy of varicose veins. Reimbursement of primarily cosmetic or symptomatic spider telangiectasias or venulectases is even more of an enigma. Unfortunately, spider vein reimbursement is made worse by the actions of many physicians.

Most physicians will not submit for insurance reimbursement charges for treating purely cosmetic veins. However, some of our colleagues correctly point out that what is perceived as cosmetic by the patient is in reality a normalization of cutaneous blood flow and thus not, strictly speaking, cosmetic. In addition, many of our colleagues use RVS codes in the 17000 series that indicate destruction of benign lesions for this treatment. Although one may be able to defend this

**Table  13-2**  Insurance reimbursements for sclerotherapy treatment

| Insurance co | Amount billed* | Amount paid† |
|---|---|---|
| Cigna | $210 | $114 |
| Medicare | $200 | $34.20 |
|  | $150 | $54.70 |
| Aetna | $125 | $108 |
| Blue Cross of California | $100 | $56 |
|  | $150 | $82 |
|  | $100 | $80 |
| Greater San Diego Health Plan | $125 | $28.34 |
| Admar | $125 | $50 |
| New York Life | $150 | $37 |
| Champus | $150 | $108 |
| Principal Mutual Life | $145 | $145 |
|  | $130 | $51 |
|  | $175 | $60.50 |
|  | $195 | $95 |
| Insurnational Insurance | $160 | $149 |
|  | $250 | $250 |
|  | $210 | $210 |

*Represents a charge of $125 for 15 minutes, $225 for 30 minutes plus surgical tray charge of either $15, $25, or $30 depending on the quantity of solution, number of compression pads, and number of syringes and butterfly needles used.
†Represents the amount allowed by the insurance company without reflecting the patient's deductible or co-payment fees.

practice, I believe that to use the 17000 codes only serves to confuse the insurance companies further and may result in furthering a distrust between the insurance carrier and the sclerotherapist. It is my belief that those who perform sclerotherapy should use the sclerotherapy code, and when reimbursement is less than adequate, the insurance claim should be petitioned, and the company should be properly educated as to the cost effectiveness of sclerotherapy.

Many methods have been used by our colleagues to educate insurance companies on the technique of compression sclerotherapy. Some of us send the insurance companies detailed operative reports with or without summaries on the history of compression sclerotherapy and the cost-effective nature of this treatment versus surgical ligation and stripings (see Appendix H). However, this education process, despite being time-consuming for the physician is often met with unresponsiveness on the part of insurance companies. In the future, it is hoped that organizations like the North American Society of Phlebology will succeed in properly educating the insurance industry, physicians, and the general public regarding sclerotherapy treatment for varicose and telangiectatic leg veins.

**REFERENCES**

1. Butie A and Goldman MP: Preliminary results from the North American Society of Phlebology membership questionnaire. Newsletter North Am Soc Phlebol 2(3):3, 1988.
2. Food and Drug Administration: Communication under the Freedom of Information Act, 1990.
3. Epstein E: Magnifiers in dermatology: a personal survey, J Am Acad Dermatol 13:687, 1985.
4. Siegel DM: The precision binocular loupe, J Dermatol Surg Oncol 15:388, 1989.

# Appendices

# Manufacturers and Suppliers of Compression Hosiery, Compression Bandages, and Pressure Pads

## COMPRESSION HOSIERY
### Camp

Camp is a relatively new manufacturer of compression stockings. Three types of stockings are available: the 1800, 1600 L.C. (light compression), and 1600 Classic. All are produced by a circular knitting process and are seamless. Two knitted yarns provide the required longitudinal elasticity, or vertical stretch. A laid-in yarn builds up the necessary lateral compression. This combination of lateral and vertical elasticity provides a two-way stretch fabric. Yarns used in Camp stockings are double wrapped for improved comfort and greater durability. The double wrapping protects the yarn so there is less fraying.

The advantages of the Camp stocking, stated by the manufacturer, are that they have an increased number of stitches per inch to provide greater elasticity, easier application, and increased durability. They also claim to use a low-modulus, high-elongated yarn that allows greater elasticity without change in compression. The knitting process begins in the toe, so it will not unravel or run.

These support stockings are available in six styles: below-knee stocking, half-thigh stocking, thigh stocking, thigh stocking with waist attachment, panty stocking, and maternity panty. The L.C. series is available only in the 20-to-30 mm Hg compression class and only in the below-knee, panty, and maternity panty styles. The 1800 series is available in the 30-to-40 mm Hg compression class for all six styles. The 1600 Classic is available in 3 compression classes, 30-to-40 mm Hg, 40-to-50 mm Hg, and 50-to-60 mm Hg, for the calf and thigh length styles only. The panty and maternity stockings are only available in the 30-to-40 mm Hg compression class.

All panty and maternity stockings have a ventilated cotton crotch piece. All maternity panty stockings have a single seam in back and two in front for greater comfort as the abdomen expands.

Available from:
Camp International, Inc.
P.O. Box 89
Jackson, MI 49204-0089

### Haines Alive

Haines Alive is a readily available support panty hose that provides a nongraduated compression of 8 mm Hg.

### Jobst

Arising from a desire to treat his own venous insufficiency, which resulted in stasis ulceration, Conrad Jobst, inventor and engineer, designed and patented the graduated compression stocking in the 1940s and 1950s in the United States. The original stocking was custom-made from a template-cut bobbinet fabric. The template consisted of a vertical strip of paper to which horizontal strips of paper were attached and then cut to the size of the leg. Graduation was achieved by reducing the length of the horizontal template strips by the appropriate percentage.

Jobst manufactures several types of graduated medical compression stockings. The Jobst Custom Support conforms to the original design concept of Conrad Jobst. Jobst Custom Supports are made with a unique Bobbinette fabric. This fabric is composed of either natural rubber or Lycra, cotton, and dacron. Each stocking is engineered individually to design a garment with precise measurements taken every 1½ inches along the leg. Counterpressures are prescribed according to the severity of the condition as described by the physician. Five classes of compression are most often used, 25, 30, 35, 40, or 50 mm Hg, commencing at the ankle and decreasing proximally. However, higher or lower compression can be engineered into the supports.

Vairox graduated compression stockings are moderate-weight ready-to-wear seamless support stockings available in four styles: knee-length, with or without a zipper; thigh length; thigh length with waist attachment; and waist-high length. They are available in 12 sizes and in two compression ranges: 30-to-40 mm Hg and 40-to-50 mm Hg. Depending on the style, a maximum of five measurements are needed to fit a patient. (Knee-length requires only three measurements.)

Fast-Fit graduated compression stockings are ready-made and lightweight. They can be obtained without a prescription. The stockings are constructed of a seamless blend of nylon and Lycra. Fast-Fit stockings are available in four styles: knee, thigh, waist, and maternity. Also, they are available as closed- or open-toe stockings in small, medium, and large sizes in a mild, 18-to-25 mm Hg, or moderate, 25-to-35 mm Hg, compression range at the ankle. Only one leg and foot length is available, limiting its use for some patients.

Ultimate Sheer is the newest ready-made graduated compression stocking from Jobst. It is composed of uncovered Lycra and nylon. This style is available as either a closed-toe knee high or panty hose with compression of 30-40 mm Hg.

Available from:
The Jobst Institute, Inc.
P.O. Box 652
Toledo, OH 43694

## JuZo

JuZo medical two-way stretch compression stockings have been manufactured for over 75 years in Germany by Julius Zorn, Inc. They are manufactured and distributed by Julius Zorn, Inc. in the United States. These support stockings are available in seven styles: below-knee stocking, half-thigh stocking, thigh stocking, thigh stocking with hip attachment, thigh stocking with panty part, compression leotard, and compression leotard for maternity. These styles are available in both closed-toe and open-toe designs and are all seamless. They are also available in four compression classes: 25 mm Hg, 35 mm Hg, 45 mm Hg, and 60 mm Hg. As with most large stocking manufacturers, the stocking can also be made to custom fit each patient.

One unique advantage of the JuZo line is the availability of different textile coatings over the compression threads. Standard compression threads are covered with cotton on the inner layer, which comes in contact with the skin (JuZo-Varin cotton style). For an easier and smoother fit, the compression threads of the inner stocking layer are covered with silk in the JuZo-Varin soft-in style. A style with a woolen lining in the knee area is also available to help prevent chaffing.

Another unique aspect of this stocking line is a relative increase in the elastic knit in the upper thigh area of the Varilastic model. This allows for proper compression to be maintained in patients with large diameter thighs and also helps prevent slippage as the patient moves.

Available from:
Julius Zorn, Inc. (JuZo)
80 Chart Road, Northhampton
P.O. Box 1088
Cuyahoga Falls, OH 44223

## Legato

The Legato lightweight, sheer support stockings are available as a panty hose and knee high. They are distributed by Freeman Manufacturing Co. These two-way stretch therapeutic medical compression stockings have a stated gradient compression of 20-to-30 mm Hg at the ankle and are composed of 35% Lycra and 65% nylon.

The available sizes, small, medium, large, and extra large, are determined by the height and either weight or calf circumference. Therefore, these stockings may be a true graduated compression stocking for only a select standard population. Indeed, they have a much less compressive feel when compared to other graduated 30-to-40 mm Hg compression stockings, such as Camp, Jobst, JuZo, Medi, Sigvaris, or Venosan.

Because of their sheer appearance, these stockings will probably be most useful for everyday wear for patients after completion of sclerotherapy treatment. However, it is unknown whether venous flow studies with this stocking can demonstrate any improvement in circulation.

Available from:
Freeman Manufacturing Co. (Venosan and Legatto)
900 W. Chicago Rd.
Sturgis, Michigan 49091-9756

## Medi

In 1962 Medi developed and patented a new knitting technology for the production of a seamless, ultra-shear product. The Medi stocking is differentiated from other compression stockings by its use of uncoated spandex threads. Medi uses five leg circumference sizes. The company claims that using a larger number of ankle sizes allows a more accurate fit. In addition, Medi's processing technique uses a spandex thread inlaid into every woven row in its Medi Plus and Medi 75 lines. This technique is said to impart a finer quality to a sheerer stocking. Most other compression stockings use spandex threads in every other row. Finally, Medi offers a size VII stocking to fit legs with a thigh circumference over 33 inches. This allows very large people to use ready-made stockings in lieu of made-to-measure stockings.

Medi stockings are all produced with white threads. The final product is then dyed to impart the desired color. It is therefore available in many colors; nude, off-white, black, and gray are presently available in the United States.

One study found that after 6 weeks, 36% of 226 patients with venous outflow disorders treated by 82 practitioners in various specialties discontinued treatment with the Medi stocking as compared to 53% of patients who discontinued treatment in a previous study with another brand of graduated compression stocking.[1]

Medi compression stockings are available in seven styles: below-knee stocking, half-thigh stocking, thigh stocking, thigh stocking with waist attachment, compression leotard, and compression leotard for maternity. And Medi is the only company that offers a ready-made full-length leotard, with a fly, for men. These styles are available as closed-toe or open-toe, come in two foot and leg lengths, and are all seamless. They are also available in three compression classes for all styles: 20-to-30 mm Hg, 30-to-40 mm Hg, and 40-to-50 mm Hg. The stockings can also be made to custom fit each patient.

Available from:
Medi USA (American Weco)
76 W. Seegers Rd.
Arlington Hts., IL 60005

## Sigvaris

Sigvaris support stockings are available in six styles: below-knee stocking, half-thigh stocking, thigh stocking, thigh stocking with waist attachment, panty stocking, and maternity panty stocking. These styles are available in both closed-toe and open-toe and are all seamless. The four available compression classes are 20-to-30 mm Hg, 30-to-40 mm Hg, 40-to-50 mm Hg, and 50-to-60 mm Hg.

The 500 series is composed of natural rubber threads and nylon and is available in various graduated compression ranges:

503: 30-to-40 mm Hg, available in all styles
504: 40-to-50 mm Hg, available in all but panty styles
505: 50-to-60 mm Hg, available in calf and thigh only

A 601 line is available as a 20-to-30 mm Hg graduated compression calf stocking with synthetic rubber threads covered with nylon.

An 801 line is available as a 20-to-30 mm Hg graduated compression panty hose and maternity panty stocking composed of synthetic rubber with nylon.

An 802 line is available as a calf-length, closed-toe graduated compression stocking in beige or black. The compression is 30-to-40 mm Hg at the ankle. The stocking is composed of synthetic rubber and nylon.

A 902 line is available in calf, thigh, and panty styles in a 30-to-40 mm Hg compression class composed of synthetic rubber threads covered with nylon.

Recently, a 202 line with 30-to-40 mm Hg compression was introduced as a graduated calf-length stocking made of a cotton blend. The synthetic Lycra threads are covered with cotton. This line is softer and easier to put on than the other Sigvaris lines by virtue of its cotton-coated thread lining.

Available from:
Sigvaris
P.O. Box 570
Branford, CT 06405

## Venosan

Venosan Medical Therapeutic Compression Stockings and panty hose are distributed in the United States by Freeman Manufacturing Co. These support stockings are available in 10 basic ready-to-wear models including below-knee stocking, over-knee (half-thigh) stocking, thigh stocking, thigh stocking with hip attachment, compression panty hose, and maternity compression panty hose. These stockings are available in closed-toe and open-toe and with short or long foot lengths and are all seamless. In all there are 60 different styles: 12 sizing options, and 4 compression classes. Each small, medium, and large size has an additional "normal" or "extra" sizing measurement at the midcalf and midthigh levels to optimize fit. The four compression classes include 20-to-30 mm Hg, 30-to-40 mm Hg, 40-to-50 mm Hg, and 50-to-60 mm Hg.

The stockings are manufactured on circular knitting machines. Venosan 2000 stockings have a material content of 60% nylon, 25% Lycra, and 15% cotton. Venosan 1000 are lighter in weight with a material content of 72% nylon and 28% Lycra. The inner lining of cotton, unique to the Venosan 2000 series, adds to the porous nature of the stocking.

## COMPRESSION BANDAGES
## Medi-Rip

The Medi-Rip compression bandage is particularly useful in applying localized pressure to a segment of the leg. Since the bandage only sticks to itself, it must be applied circumferentially around the limb. Thus it can only be applied in an approximate graduated manner by the nurse or physician. Graduation in support is achieved by wrapping the bandage either more or less tightly around the leg. In addition, support padding underneath the bandage can provide a localized increase in compression pressure.

It is recommended that this bandage be used when compressing lateral thigh varicosities. A graduated compression stocking will apply a limited compression in this proximal location, and even less compression will be applied to the lateral aspect of the limb by virtue of its oval configuration. Therefore, applying pads or cotton balls on the lateral thigh and compressing them locally with a bandage will increase the compression strength without unduly compromising the advantage of graduation in compression.

The composition of the bandage fabric is 99% cotton and 1% polyurethane (spandex). The warp is constructed with longitudinal threads of alternating cotton, twisted spandex thread, and twisted cotton threads in a 3:1 ratio. Threads are twisted 1950 times per meter in an alternate clockwise and counterclockwise manner. An equal number of clockwise and counterclockwise twisted threads maintain proper stability. Fill threads of the weft are woven with 100% cotton for strength and porosity.

A fine latex spray is then applied to the fabric. The unique application of the spray in Medi-Rip adheres only to the surface of the yarn and does not occlude the openings between, which maintains the porosity, breathability, and absorption qualities of the cotton fabric.

Available from:
Conco Medical Company
Bridgeport, CT 06610

## Tubigrip

Tubigrip is an elasticated surgical tubular bandage knitted from either 100% cotton (flesh shade) or 67% cotton and 33% rayon (natural shade). Covered elastic threads are laid into the material to form continuous spirals. When applied to the affected area, the elastic moves within the bandage, evening out pressure over the contours of the body.

Tubigrip is best used as a cover or support bandage for compression pads in patients who are allergic to adhesive tape or Medi-Rip tape. In these circumstances, the compression pad can be held in place before application of the graduated support stocking by a layer of Tubigrip. Using Tubigrip as a support bandage is cumbersome and of doubtful validity as a graduated support stocking because of the ease with which the bandage can migrate with movement of the leg.

The amount of pressure to be applied can be selected by choosing the appropriate size of Tubigrip with the aid of the Tubigrip Tension Guide. Because the tension guide measures only the widest diameter of the limb, true graduated compression cannot be obtained. It is recommended that Tubigrip be applied as a double layer with the cut edges uppermost. The second layer should overlap the first by 2 to 3 cm to prevent occlusion.

Tubigrip Shaped Support Bandage is an anatomically shaped compression bandage available in a range of full leg and below-the-knee sizes that provide a degree of graduated compression to the limbs. The material only stretches in a radial direction, thus providing firm support without slipping. One chooses the size by measuring the widest diameter of the limb; therefore a "true" graduation in pressure with the greatest pressure being at the ankle cannot be obtained.

Available from:
Se Pro Healthcare, Inc.
Montgomery, PA 18936

## PRESSURE PADS

At times, additional pressure is required in a localized area. The use of foam rubber padding or cotton balls, as previously mentioned, can provide this additional compression. Foam rubber padding may also be required to more evenly distribute compression around the leg. The ankle area (where the greatest degree of compression is applied by a stocking) is the most irregularly contoured part of the leg. Here the medial and lateral malleoli jut out of the smooth plane of the leg resulting in a concavity posteriorly (see Fig. 6-3). When patients complain about compression stockings, they usually complain about pain in this area. Various pads have been constructed to fill this concavity and more evenly distribute the compression.

Such padding fills the pocket formed by the bridging of elastic material from the malleolus to the Achilles tendon. The padding will also create additional pressure in this area to prevent pooling of fluids (Fig. A-1).

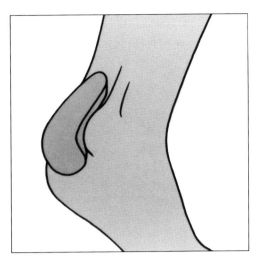

**Fig. A-1**   Foam pad placed to fill in the concavity behind the lateral malleolus. (Courtesy Julius Zorn, Inc.)

## Jobst Stasis Pads

Three types and sizes of Jobst Stasis Pads are available to properly fit the concavity: small crescent, large crescent, and oval. Pads are made of a layer of foam rubber and a layer of polyurethane foam. They are washable and reusable.

Available from:
The Jobst Institute, Inc.
P.O. Box 652
Toledo, OH 43694

## JuZo-Helastic

The JuZo-Helastic model 3022 compression stocking is composed with a specially designed pressure pad at the lateral malleolar area. The pressure pads are sewn into elastic knitted pockets and connected to the two-way stretch stocking to preserve the two-way stretch properties of the fabric. The pads are composed of silicon.

Available from:
Julius Zorn, Inc. (JuZo)
80 Chart Road, Northhampton
P.O. Box 1088
Cuyahoga Falls, OH 44223

### REFERENCE

1. von Beratung U: Die therapie venoser Beinleiden Kompressionstherapie, medikamentos kombiniert? Der Bayerische Internist 1:46, 1987.

# B Manufacturers and Distributors of Sclerosing Solutions

**ETHANOLAMINE OLEATE**

Available from:
Block Drug Company
1 New England Avenue
Piscataway, NJ 08855

**HYPERTONIC SALINE 23.4%**

Available from:
Invenex
Gibcol Invenex Division
The Dexter Corporation
Chagrin Falls, OH 44022

American Regent Laboratories, Inc.
Shirley, NY 11967

Omega
Montreal, Canada H3M3A2

**POLIDOCANOL**

Available from:
Globopharm AQ
P.O. Box 1187
8700 Kusnacht, Switzerland

Chemische Fabrik
Kreussler & Co. GmbH
D-6200 Wiesbaden-Biebrich
West Germany

Laboratoiries Pharmaceutiques DEXO, S.A.
31 Rue D'Arras
92000 Nanterre, France

## POLYIODINATED IODINE

*Variglobin* from:
Globopharm AQ
P.O. Box 1187
8700 Kusnacht, Switzerland

*Sclerodine* from:
Omega
Montreal, Canada H3M3A2

## SCLEREMO

Available from:
Laboratories E. Bouteille
7, Rue des Belges
87100 Limoges, France

Omega
Montreal, Canada H3M3A2

## SCLERODEX

Available from:
Omega
Montreal, Canada H3M3A2

## SODIUM MORRHUATE

Available from:
American Regent Laboratories, Inc.
1 Lutipold Dr.
Shirley, NY 11967

Palisades Pharmaceuticals, Inc.
219 Country Road
Tenafly, NJ 07670

## SODIUM TETRADECYL SULFATE

Available from:
Eklins-Sinn, Inc.
A subsidiary of A.H. Robins Company
2 Esterbrook Lane
P.O. Box 5483
Cherry Hill, NJ 08034

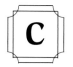

# C   Sample Patient Questionnaire

DATE _____

NAME _____

AGE _____        SEX _____

HEIGHT _____        WEIGHT _____

REFERRED BY: _____

1. How many years have you noticed this problem?

2. Have you ever been previously treated for this problem?         _____

    By whom and when? _____

    With what method?

    |                       |            |
    |-----------------------|------------|
    | Injection             | _____  |
    | Electrocautery        | _____  |
    | Laser                 | _____  |
    | Surgery               | _____  |

3. When did your veins occur?

    |                                      |            |
    |--------------------------------------|------------|
    | Age                                  | _____  |
    | Before pregnancy                     | _____  |
    | After pregnancy                      | _____  |
    | After trauma                         | _____  |
    | After birth control or Premarin therapy | _____  |
    | Other                                | _____  |

4. Is there a family history of varicose or spider veins?

    |            |            |
    |------------|------------|
    | Mother     | _____  |
    | Father     | _____  |
    | Sister     | _____  |
    | Brother    | _____  |
    | Children   | _____  |
    | Aunts      | _____  |
    | Uncles     | _____  |

5. Do you have a history of?

| | |
|---|---|
| Thrombophlebitis | _____ |
| Pulmonary embolus | _____ |
| Deep vein thrombosis | _____ |
| Septicemia | _____ |
| Lupus | _____ |
| Hepatitis | _____ |
| Bleeding disorders | _____ |
| Easy bruisability | _____ |
| Heart disease | _____ |
| Swollen feet/ankles | _____ |
| Migraine headaches | _____ |
| Dark spots after: | |
| Skin injury or surgery | _____ |
| Asthma | _____ |
| Medicines | _____ |
| Local anesthetic | _____ |
| Other | _____ |

6. Are you developing new veins? _____

7. Are your present veins getting bigger? _____

8. After prolonged standing or sitting do your legs ache? _____

9. Do your legs or veins ache before menses? _____

10. Does walking or exercise relieve or aggravate the pain? _____

11. Are you required to be on your feet for long periods? _____

12. Do you jog, run, jump rope, or do aerobics? _____
    How often per week? _____

13. Are you pregnant or planning a pregnancy soon? _____

14. What medicines do you take?
    Birth control pills, Premarin, or hormones? _____
    Other _____

15. Do you smoke cigarettes? _____

# D  Consent Form

---

**SCLEROTHERAPY INFORMED CONSENT FORM**
(Dermatology Associates of San Diego County, Inc.)

This form is designed to provide you with the information you need to make an informed decision about whether to have sclerotherapy performed. If you have any questions or do not understand any potential risks, please do not hesitate to ask us.

**What is Sclerotherapy?**
Sclerotherapy is a popular method of eliminating varicose veins and superficial telangiectasias ("spider veins") in which a solution, called a *sclerosing agent,* is injected into the veins.

**Does Sclerotherapy work for everyone?**
The majority of persons who have sclerotherapy performed will be cleared of their varicosities or at least see good improvement. Unfortunately, however, there is no guarantee that sclerotherapy will be effective in every case. Approximately 10% of patients who undergo sclerotherapy have poor to fair results. ("Poor results" means that the veins have not totally disappeared after six treatments.) In very rare instances, the patient's condition may become worse after sclerotherapy treatment.

**How many treatments will I need?**
The number of treatments needed to clear or improve the condition differs from patient to patient, depending on the extent of varicose and spider veins present. One to six or more treatments may be needed; the average is three to four. Individual veins usually require one to three treatments.

**What are the most common side effects?**
The most common side effects experienced with sclerotherapy treatment are:

1. *Itching*  Depending on the type of solution used, you may experience mild itching along the vein route. This itching normally lasts 1 to 2 days.

2. *Transient hyperpigmentation*  Approximately 30% of patients who undergo sclerotherapy notice a discoloration of light brown streaks after treatment. In almost every patient, the veins become darker immediately after the procedure. In rare instances, this darkening of the vein may persist for 4 to 12 months.

3. *Sloughing*  Sloughing occurs in less than 3% of patients who receive sclerotherapy. Sloughing consists of a small ulceration at the injection site that heals slowly. A blister may form, open, and become ulcerated. The scar that follows should return to a normal color.

4. *Allergic reactions*  Very rarely, a patient may have an allergic reaction to the sclerosing agent used. The risk of an allergic reaction is greater in patients who have a history of allergies.

5. *Pain* A few patients may experience moderate to severe pain and some bruising, usually at the site of the injection. The veins may be tender to the touch after treatment, and an uncomfortable sensation may run along the vein route. This pain is usually temporary, in most cases lasting 1 to, at most, 7 days.

### What are the other side effects?
Other side effects include a burning sensation during injection of some solutions, neovascularization (the development—usually temporary—of new tiny blood vessels), transient phlebitic-type reactions (swelling of the vein might cause the ankles to swell), temporary superficial blebs or wheals (similar to hives), and, very rarely, wound infection, poor healing, or scarring.

Phlebitis is a very rare complication, seen in approximately 1 of every 1000 patients treated for varicose veins greater than 3 to 4 mm in diameter. The dangers of phlebitis include the possibility of pulmonary embolus (a blood clot to the lungs) and postphlebitis syndrome, in which the blood clot is not carried out of the legs, resulting in permanent swelling of the legs.

### What are the possible complications if I do not have sclerotherapy?
In cases of large varicose veins (greater than 3 to 4 mm in diameter), spontaneous phlebitis and/or thrombosis may occur with the associated risk of possible pulmonary emboli. Additionally, large skin ulcerations may develop in the ankle region of patients with long-standing varicose veins with underlying venous insufficiency. Rarely, these ulcers may hemorrhage or become cancerous.

### Are there other types of procedures to treat varicose veins and telangiectasias? What are their side effects?
Vein stripping and/or ligation may also be used to treat large varicose veins. This generally requires a 1 to 3 week hospital stay and is performed while the patient is under general anesthesia. Risks of vein stripping or ligation include permanent nerve paralysis in up to 30% of patients and possible pulmonary emboli, infection, and permanent scarring. General anesthesia has some associated serious risks, including the possibility of serious harm, paralysis, brain damage, and death.

### What if I experience a problem after receiving sclerotherapy?
If you notice any type of adverse reaction, please call the doctor immediately.

Comments: _____

_____

BY MY INITIALS, I ACKNOWLEDGE THAT I HAVE RECEIVED A COPY OF THIS SCLEROTHERAPY INFORMED CONSENT FORM. _____

BY SIGNING BELOW, I ACKNOWLEDGE THAT I HAVE READ THE FOREGOING INFORMED CONSENT FORM AND THAT THE DOCTOR HAS ADEQUATELY INFORMED ME OF THE RISKS OF SCLEROTHERAPY TREATMENT, ALTERNATIVE METHODS OF TREATMENT, AND THE RISKS OF NOT TREATING MY CONDITION, AND I HEREBY CONSENT TO SCLEROTHERAPY TREATMENT PERFORMED BY DR. _____

DATE: _____ , 19 _____     TIME: _____ AM/PM

PATIENT'S SIGNATURE     PATIENT'S REPRESENTATIVE (IF PATIENT IS A MINOR OR IS MENTALLY INCOMPETENT, SIGNATURE OF PARENT OR LEGAL GUARDIAN IS REQUIRED)

WITNESS     RELATIONSHIP TO PATIENT

# E  Diagrammatic Chart Notes and Follow-Up Notes

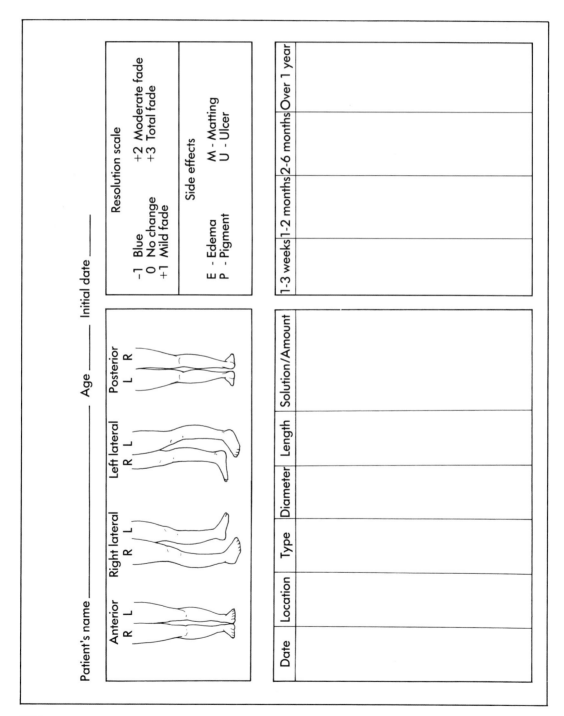

Patient's name _____  Age _____  Initial date _____

**Resolution scale**

-1  Blue        +2  Moderate fade
0  No change   +3  Total fade
+1  Mild fade

**Side effects**

E - Edema      M - Matting
P - Pigment    U - Ulcer

Anterior / Right lateral / Left lateral / Posterior

| Date | Location | Type | Diameter | Length | Solution/Amount |
|------|----------|------|----------|--------|-----------------|
|      |          |      |          |        |                 |
|      |          |      |          |        |                 |
|      |          |      |          |        |                 |

| 1-3 weeks | 1-2 months | 2-6 months | Over 1 year |
|-----------|------------|------------|-------------|
|           |            |            |             |
|           |            |            |             |
|           |            |            |             |

# Equipment Sources

**NEEDLES**
**30-Gauge**

> Precision Glide
>> Becton-Dickinson & Company
>> Rutherford, NJ 07070
>> Cost*: $0.30 each
>
> Acuderm
>> Acuderm, Inc.
>> Ft. Lauderdale, FL 33314
>> Cost: $0.07 each
>
> Delasco
>> Dermatologic Lab and Supply, Inc.
>> Council Bluffs, IA 51503
>> Cost: $0.21 each

**33-Gauge**

> Hamilton
>> Hamilton Company
>> Reno, Nevada
>> 800/648-5950
>> Cost: $9.00 each 2-inch length
>> $11.00 each ½-inch length
>
> Delasco
>> Dermatologic Lab and Supply, Inc.
>> Council Bluffs, IA 51503
>> Cost: $4.58 each ½-inch length

**26- or 27-Gauge**

> Yale
>> Becton-Dickinson & Company
>> Ft. Lauderdale, FL 33314
>> Cost: $0.10 each 27-gauge, ½-inch length
>> $0.10 each 26-gauge, ½-inch length
>
> Allergy
>> Becton-Dickinson & Company
>> Cost: $0.14 each, fixed to a 1-ml syringe

**21-, 23-, or 25-Gauge Butterfly**

> Abbott Hospitals, Inc.
> North Chicago, IL 60064
> Cost: $0.62 each
>
> Surflo Winged Infusion Set
>> Terumo Corporation
>> Tokyo, Japan
>> Cost: $0.48 each

---

*Prices are included for comparison only. More up-to-date information is available from the manufacturers.

## SYRINGES

Luer Lok or non-Luer Lok
Becton-Dickinson & Company
Rutherford, NJ 07070
Cost: $0.09 each
Plastipak eccentric syringe
Becton-Dickinson & Company
Rutherford, NJ 07070
Cost: $0.25 each

## MAGNIFYING GLASSES

Clip-on Loupes
Almore International
Portland, OR 97225
Cost: $37.00 each
Opticaid
Edroy Products Co., Inc.
Nyack, NY 10960
Cost: $16.00 each

## HEADBAND-MOUNTED SIMPLE BINOCULAR MAGNIFIERS

Optivisor
Donegan Optical Company
15549 West 108th St.
Lenexa, KS 66219
Cost: $24.00 each
Mark II Magni-Focuser
Edroy Products Co., Inc.
Nyack, NY 10960
Cost: $18.00 each

## SIMPLE BINOCULAR LOUPES

Precision Binocular Loupe
Almore International
Portland, OR 97225
Cost: $100.00
Multidistance Headband Loupe
Edroy Products Co., Inc.
Nyack, NY 10960
Cost: $16.00

## BINOCULAR LOUPES

Designs for Vision
New York, NY 10010
Cost: $1000.00 (3.5× expanded field model)
$ 600.00 (2.5× model)

N1064 Oculus
    Storz Instrument Company
    St. Louis, MO 63122
    Cost: $200.00 each

    Westco Medical Corporation
    San Diego, CA 92138
    Cost: $300.00 (2-2.5× adjustable)
    See Better Loupe
        Edroy Products Co., Inc.
        Nyack, NY 10960
        Cost: $70.00 (2.5×)

## FOAM PADS

    STD Pharmaceutical
    Fields Yard, Plough Lane
    Hereford, England HR4 0EL
    Cost: $0.70 each

## TAPE DRESSINGS
## With Minimal Pressure

    3-M Microfoam Surgical Tape
        Medical Surgical Division/3-M
        St. Paul, MN 55144
        Cost: $6.33/roll (4 inches wide)
    Tubigrip Tubular Support Bandage
        Seaton Products, Inc.
        Montgomeryville, PA
        Cost: $4.00/roll

### Additional Localized Pressure

    Coban tape
        Medical Surgical Division/3-M
        St. Paul, MN 55144
        Cost: $2.50/5-yard roll (4 inches wide)
    Medi-Rip Bandage
        Conco Medical Company
        Bridgeport, CT 06610
        Cost: $2.00/5-yard roll (4 inches wide)

## BODY ADHESIVE

    It Stays!
        New Horizons Diversified Interests
        Grants Pass, OR 97526

**Patient Brochures**

1. *Spider Vein, Varicose Vein Therapy*

This excellent eight-panel brochure accurately describes the pathogenesis and treatment of both varicose and telangiectatic leg veins (with a heavy concentration on "spider veins"). Operative and before and after color photographs are reproduced with excellent quality. The common patient questions are addressed and the common side effects are given.

Source:

> American Academy of Dermatology
> 1567 Maple Ave.
> P.O. Box 3116
> Evanston, IL 60204-3116

2. *Sclerotherapy: Treatment of Leg Veins*

This simple six-panel brochure describes the treatment of spider veins only. There are no color photographs. This brochure can be personalized with your name, address, and some individualized information on the rear panel.

Source:

> Contemporary Communications
> 494 Greystone Trace
> Marietta, GA 30068
> $50.00/125 brochures

3. *Treatment of Unwanted Leg Veins (Spider Veins)** 

This brochure was developed by my practice, Dermatology Associates of San Diego County, Inc. It is copyright-protected, and the following text from the brochure is reproduced here only as an aid to those who wish to produce their own individualized products.

*Unwanted leg veins (spider veins),* known medically as telangiectasias or superficial varicosities, are dilated skin capillaries. These may become unsightly with time and may also lead to a dull aching of the legs after prolonged standing.

*Sclerotherapy* is the technique of instilling a specific solution into these vessels (tiny capillaries or larger varicose veins), using a small needle. The solution irritates and destroys the inner lining of the blood vessel so it ceases to carry blood. The body then replaces this damaged vessel with an imperceptible scar tissue. *This does not harm the circulation — it improves it by eliminating the abnormal, unnecessary vessel.* Several injections may be needed for a specific *area* of telangiectasia. The procedure is virtually painless. Fading of the vessels is a slow process which takes 1 to 6 months. The goal is to produce a 75% to 90% improvement.

*Charges* relate to the amount of time spent by the doctor. Actual injection is done only by the doctor, rather than by a nurse or assistant. There is also a one-time purchase charge for compression stockings. The stockings cost from $25 to $75 depending on the type required. These stockings are washable and last years.

*Insurance* may cover the procedure in full or in part depending on the type of vessel treated and the type of insurance coverage you have.

---

*Copyright © 1987 by Dermatology Associates of San Diego County, Inc.

**384**

*Appointments* are required in advance. Payment is required at the time of the procedure.

*Results* of treatment cannot be guaranteed, but most patients are very pleased with the cosmetic and functional improvement.

1. *What causes spider veins?*

    No one is totally sure. Certain families are predisposed to this condition, particularly female relatives. Certain things make spider veins worse: estrogens, pregnancy, and birth control pills, tight girdles and garter belts, prolonged standing or sitting, and trauma.

2. *How does it work?*

    The solution destroys the tiny cells which line the blood vessels, without damage to the surrounding tissues.

3. *How soon will the vessels disappear?*

    Each vessel usually requires one to three treatments. The vessels disappear over a period of 2 weeks to 3 months. Recurrences may rarely occur over a period of 1 to 5 years. This treatment does not prevent new telangiectasias from developing.

4. *Are there certain vessels which tend to recur more commonly?*

    Yes. They are the type of vessels which occur in a mat of very fine radiating vessels.

5. *How often can I be treated?*

    The same area should not be injected for 3 to 4 weeks to allow for complete healing. Additional different areas may be treated every week.

6. *How many times does it have to be done?*

    This varies with the number of areas that have to be injected, as well as the response to each injection. It usually takes one to three injections to obliterate any vessel, and 10 to 40 vessels may be treated in any one session.

7. *Are there certain kinds of spider veins that can't be treated?*

    Certain types of large varicose veins may not respond readily to sclerotherapy alone. These vessels may require a minor surgical procedure followed later with sclerotherapy. You may be referred to a vascular surgeon for complete or partial treatment of these specific types of large varicose veins. Some of the extremely small vessels (less than $1/1000$ of a millimeter) may require treatment with a Pulsed Dye Laser.

8. *Are there other methods of treating these vessels?*

    Three other methods are used:

    a. Laser surgery

       To date, this method has only been effective for tiny facial blood vessels. The present laser systems tend to produce a greater risk of scarring. The laser is an expensive devise and treatment is thus more costly. We have recently evaluated the use of a new type of laser (Candela Pulsed Dye Laser) for vessels which do not respond to injection treatment or are too small to be injected. Although more expensive than conventional sclerotherapy, this new laser system is quite effective for treating the tiniest of red blood vessels that may remain after successful treatment of other varicose and telangiectatic leg veins.

    b. Electrodesiccation

       This method produces a non-specific destruction of both the vessel and overlying skin, thus resulting in a greater incidence of scarring.

    c. Surgical ligation or circumsuture

       This operative procedure always results in a scar and is best reserved for large varicose veins.

9. *Is there any way to prevent them?*

    The use of support hose may be helpful. Reducing your weight and regular exercise may also be of help.

10. *What are the side effects?*

    a. Slight blistering may occur around the injected vessels and resolves in a day or so.

    b. Ten to 30% of patients develop a small freckle-like tan to brown spot around the injected vessel. This usually resolves in 80% of these patients within 3 to 6 months. A few patients will have a persistent freckle for up to a year.

c. Slight stinging or burning may occur with injection of certain types and concentrations of solutions in certain areas.

d. Sometimes a clot develops at the injection site (especially if the recommended pressure stockings are not worn for the proper amount of time). This clot will never cause internal problems, but its removal within 2 weeks of the injection will speed the healing process and decrease the incidence of "freckling."

e. Swelling over the injection site may rarely occur. It is particularly common when patients have jobs in which they stand for long periods of time or when vessels in the ankles are injected. The swelling is never dangerous but occasionally must be treated with elevation and compression dressings.

f. A small superficial ulceration of the skin overlying the injected vessel may occur. This does not usually leave a scar but needs to be seen as soon as possible by your doctor.

g. Superficial thrombophlebitis, an irritation of the injected vessel, occurs in less than 1 per 1000 patients. It may have to be treated with antiinflammatory agents and compression stockings.

11. *What should I do before my appointment for treatment?*
    a. Discontinue aspirin and so-called blood thinning drugs 1 week prior to your appointment. Consult your prescribing physician.
    b. Do *not* shave your legs for 2 days prior to your appointment.
    c. Eat a light breakfast or lunch an hour or so prior to your appointment.
    d. Bring shorts to wear during the procedure and slacks to wear out of the office.

12. *What should I do after the procedure?*
    a. Walk for 30 minutes immediately following the injections.
    b. If possible, do not drive home yourself; if you have to drive, keep the legs moving and make frequent stops for walking (every 20 minutes).
    c. Maintain normal daytime activities; walk at least an hour a day — the more the better.
    d. No hot baths for 2 weeks.
    e. Avoid standing without moving about. If you must stay in one place, move your feet and toes frequently.
    f. If the legs become painful after the injection, walk.
    g. Do *not* remove the stockings for _____ days. Cover them with a plastic bag when showering.
    h. Avoid strenuous physical activity (aerobics) for the first 48 to 72 hours.

# Sample Letter to Insurance Company to Accompany Operative Report

Date line

Insurance Company
Street Address
City, State ZIP Code

Department of Claim Reimbursement:

The method of sclerotherapy we practice is a combination of the Swiss (Dr. Sigg) and Irish (Dr. Fegan) schools for the treatment of varicose veins. We have been using this method for over 8 years with very good results. In contrast to the older type of treatment, which is still practiced in some places, our approach is based on a concentrated effort to obliterate the diseased vessels in a very limited number of sessions. Depending on the number and extent of varicose veins, the treatment is usually completed in 2 to 4 sessions. The treatment of extensive telangiectatic vessels may take a little longer.

Compression sclerotherapy makes it possible to successfully treat even large varicosities, which would otherwise require surgical removal (ligation, vein stripping), except in those patients for whom we recommend surgical treatment. As you are aware, the cost incurred with surgical treatment is extensive: charges for hospitalization, surgeon's fee, anesthesiologist's fee, and operating room, not to mention the loss of work time for the patient as a result of the treatment. In contrast, sclerotherapy, as performed in our clinic, requires only the time needed to perform the examination and treatment. The patient can immediately resume his or her normal everyday activities and is able to return to work the same day. Also, the absence of anesthesia and postincision scars associated with this procedure is not to be underestimated.

As already pointed out, we inject as many varicose veins in one session as is medically indicated (limited only by the amount of injected sclerosing agent), thus further economizing the treatment (limited number of visits). Obviously, if only one or two injections are performed in one session, the time spent with the patient is significantly shorter. We spend an average of 15 to 45 minutes with each patient (including Doppler examination).

Before the therapeutic procedure is initiated, a complete medical history and physical examination is required to rule out possible contraindications. This is followed by a series of special tests (including Doppler ultrasound) to determine the status of the deep venous system, the presence and location of perforator veins, and the sufficiency of the superficial and deep venous systems.

After mapping out the most suitable injection sites, a small amount of the sclerosing substance is injected to test the patient's sensitivity. Equipment and drugs to be used in case of allergic responses must be on hand. Each injection is followed by a special bandaging procedure. After completion of the injection session, in which up to about 20 injections can be performed in each leg, the patient is instructed to walk and then report back in 30 minutes, at which time the condition is reassessed.

Sincerely,
Doctor's signature

# OPERATIVE REPORT
## Compression Sclerotherapy of Superficial Varicosities


PATIENT:


DATE:


PHYSICIAN:


TREATED VESSELS:
(- Location - Size - Color - Arborization)


SCLEROSING AGENT:
(- Type - Concentration - Quantity)


PROCEDURE:
After signing detailed informed consent and posing for complete photographic documentation of the condition, the patient was examined using venous Doppler and placed in a reverse Trendelenburg position. The area to be injected was prepped with alcohol. Butterfly needles, 23- or 25-gauge, were then inserted into the most appropriate points along the varicose veins beginning with areas of reflux. The leg was then elevated above 180 degrees, and the vein was emptied of blood. An appropriate quantity of sclerosing solution was injected (usually 0.5 ml), and the vessel was immediately compressed using foam rubber pads under a 3-to-4 inch  microfoam-tape dressing. The procedure was then repeated using a 26-to-30 gauge needle with the patient supine in a proximal to distal direction, proceeding from larger to smaller vessels. Repeat injections into the same vessel were made at approximately 3-to-5 cm intervals along its path.

Telangiectatic veins were treated after all reticular and varicose veins were sclerosed. Under appropriate magnification using operative loupes, the abnormal vessels were cannulated with a 30-gauge needle fitted to a 3-ml syringe containing 2 ml of the appropriate sclerosing solution.

After the vessels were injected along their entire length, the entire limb was wrapped in a 30-to-40 mm graduated compression stocking.

The compression stocking is to be left in place for _____ days.

The patient was instructed to return to this office in 2 weeks for examination and treatment of any thrombi that may have occurred in the injected vessels.


COMPLICATIONS:

# Index

*Page numbers in *italics* indicate illustrations.
Page numbers followed by a *t* indicate tables.

Blood flow in lower leg, during walking, 12, *12*
Blood pressure, venous
  exerted by blood column from heart to measurement location, *66*
  factors determining, 64, *65*
Brodie-Trendelenburg test, *114,* 114-116
  Bracey variation of, 116, *118*
  interpretation of, *115*
Bronchospasm after sclerotherapy
  incidence of, 247
  treatment of, 247
Brown, William, 158

**C**

Calf muscle pump, *11, 12*
Camper's fascia, 20
Capillaritis, telangiectasia associated with, 99
Carbon dioxide laser
  disadvantages of, 326
  for telangiectasia treatment, 325
Carcinoma
  as complication of venous ulceration, 48, *49*
  pancreatic, Maffucci's syndrome associated with, 95
Celsus, varicose treatment by, 1
Cherry hemangioma, case history of, 322
Children
  telangiectasias in, 38
  varicose veins in, 37-38
Chondrosarcoma, Maffucci's syndrome associated with, 95
Chromated glycerin
  advantages of, 209
  allergic reactions to, 251
  clinical use of, 206, 208-209
  disadvantages of, 209
  dorsal ear vein injection/biopsy before and after injection of, *200*
  experimental evaluation of, 198
  ocular effects of, 251
  vessel patency over time after injection of, *199*
  vessel visibility over time after injection of, *199*
Chronotherapy, 227
Cirrhosis, telangiectasias associated with, 100
Claudication, venous, 118
Coagula after sclerotherapy, and incidence of pigmentation, 225
Cockett perforating veins, 19, *19*
  distribution of, 17t
Collagen
  in varicose veins, 61-62

Collagen — cont'd
  in vein walls, function of, 25
Collagen vascular disease, telangiectasias as component of, 97
Compression bandages
  compared with compression stockings, 162-163
  drawbacks of, 163
  versus graduated compression stockings, 162-164
  indications for, 163
  manufacturers and suppliers of, 371-372
Compression hosiery
  available stretch of, 165
  care of, 178-179
  external pressure provided by, 160-162
  graduated, 160-161, 364
    advantages of, 163-164
    characteristics of, 164-170
    charactersitics and care of, by brand name, 166t
    conversion chart for, *167*
    lengths of, 168-169
    measurement for, 167-168, *168*
    proper fit and position of, 169-170
    stretch resistance of, 164
    types of, *169*
  holding power of, 165
  made-to-measure, 165, 167
  manufacturers and suppliers of, 368-371
  methods for donning, 175-178, *176, 177, 178*
  modulus of, 165
  ready-made, 165
  schematized cross section of midcalf after application of, *161*
  stretch recovery of, 165
  symptom relief from, 171
Compression therapy, 1, 3
  after microsclerotherapy, 314-315
  after sclerotherapy, 276
  ancient use of, 158
  combined with laser therapy, 345, 345t
  duration of, 172-173
  excessive, cutaneous necrosis caused by, 245
  historical developments in, 158
  historical references to, 4
  idealized, schematic diagram for, *170*
  Laplace's law and, 160
  mechanism of action, 158-159
  versus pharmacologic therapy, 159
  postsclerosis, 4
  practical considerations in, 173
  during pregnancy, 162
  preventive use of, 159-164
  pulmonary embolism and, 257

Compression therapy — cont'd
  rationale for
    in telangiectasia management,
      173-175
    in varicose vein management,
      170-173
    for telangiectasias
      amount of, 174
      duration of, 174-175
      inadequacies of, 175, 175t
Consent form, 378-379
Constipation, varicose veins and, 69
Contraceptives, oral; *see* Oral
    contraceptives
Contusions, telangiectasias associated with,
    101
Corona phlebectasia, *35*
Corticosteroids, topical, telangiectasias
    associated with, 100
Cough test, 111, *112,* 113
  sources of error in, 113
Cutaneous necrosis; *see also* Ulceration
  after polidocanol injection, *246*
  after sclerotherapy
    etiology of, 239, 241-243, 245
    with STS, *239, 240*
    superficial, *239*
    treatment of, 245-246
  arterial injection and, 255
  from lymphatic injection, 243, 245
  from polyiodide iodine, 251-252
Cutis marmorata telangiectatica congenita,
    characteristics of, 96

**D**

Deep vein thrombosis
  and absence of iliofemoral valves, 75
  history of, as contraindication to
    sclerotherapy, 277
  increased incidence of, in patients with
    varicose veins, 188
  oral contraceptives and, 257
  patient evaluation for, 108-109
  photoplethysmography in diagnosis of,
    *137,* 137-138, *138*
  superficial thrombophlebitis and, 50
  symptoms of, 108
  varicose veins as risk factor for, 50, *51,*
    52
  venous hypertension and, 32
Deep venous pressure, increased, 67-74
  distal, 70-74
  proximal, 68-70
Degos' disease, telangiectasia associated
    with, 99
Dermatitis, venous (stasis), 42, *44, 45*
Diet, low-fiber, varicose veins and, 69

Diffuse neonatal hemangiomatosis,
    characteristics of, 96-97, *97*
Dihydroergotamine
  varicose vein constriction caused by, 61
  venous constriction produced by, 159
Disodium ethylenediamine tetraacetic acid,
    hyperpigmentation treatment with,
    227
Distal angioplasia; *see* Telangiectatic
    matting
Disulfiram
  as contraindication to certain sclerosing
    solutions, 277
  interaction with Aethoxysklerol forte,
    213
Dodd's perforating veins, 19
Doppler ultrasound
  bidirectional tracing, *121*
  chart for recording venous examination,
    *130*
  compared with Duplex scanning, 129t
  differential diagnosis with, 132-133, *134*
  for evaluating venous disease, 119-120,
    *121, 122, 123,* 124-129
  examination technique, 124-129
    femoral vein, 124-126
    perforating veins, 128-129
    popliteal vein, 126-127, *127*
    posterior tibial vein, 127
    superficial veins, 127-128
  for examining deep veins, 147-148
  method of producing flow augmentation,
    *123, 124*
  pitfalls and supplemental methods, 147t
  preceding surgery, 294
  principles of, 120
  sound interpretation in, 122t
  venous tracings of, *125*
  waveform characteristics, 120, 122, 124
Drug therapy, versus compression therapy,
    159
Drugs, venoconstriction caused by, 29
Duffy classification of varicose veins, 52,
    *53, 54, 55*
Duplex scanning, 129, 132-135
  advantages of, 134
  as aid to sclerotherapy, 132
  anatomic images from, *131*
  anomaly visualization with, *133*
  characteristics of, 129
  compared with Doppler ultrasound, 129t
  deep vein thrombosis imaging with, *132*
  flow images from, *131*
  posttreatment evaluation with, 132-135
  preceding surgery for recurrent
    varicosities, 299
DVT; *see* Deep vein thrombosis

Progesterone, venous dilation and, 77, 78
Protein C, deficiency of, pulmonary
    embolism and, 257-258
Protein S, deficiency of, pulmonary
    embolism and, 257-258
Pulmonary embolism
    after sclerotherapy, 256-258
    cause of, 256-258
    as complication of superficial
        thrombophlebitis, 50
    incidence of, 256
    prevention and treatment of, 258
    proteins C and S deficiency and, 257-258
Pulsed dye laser
    advantages and disadvantages of, 331t
    alone versus PDL/SCL, 352t
    combined with sclerotherapy, 346, 348
        complications of, 348
        endothelial damage caused by, 346t
        results of, 347t, 348t
    effects after 48 hours, 333t
    endothelial damage caused by, 346t
    histologic effects of, 333
    immediate effects of, 333t
    for telangiectasia treatment, 329-333
        clinical studies of, 335-345
        complications of, 335
        effective energy levels in, 335, 339
        photographic follow-up of, 337-338,
            340, 341
        resolution of, 336
        results by vessel location, 339t
        results without reticular veins, 339t
        for telangiectatic matting, 342-343
    vessel after treatment with, 332, 334
    vessel location and, 339
Purpura annularis telangiectodes,
    telangiectasia associated with, 99

**R**

Radiodermatitis, telangiectasias associated
    with, 103-104
Reflex vasospasm, 227
Reflux
    deep and superficial, differentiating
        relative contribution of, 151-152
    from saphenofemoral junction,
        treatment of, 268-269
Renal failure, acute, from ethanolamine
    oleate, 249
Retinoic acid, pigmentation treatment with,
    227
Rheography, light reflection, 137, 137-138
Rosacea, telangiectasia associated with,
    100
Rothmund-Thomson syndrome,
    characteristics of, 96

**S**

Saline, hypertonic; see Hypertonic saline
Saphena varix, 110, 111
Saphenofemoral junction
    incompetent, treatment with air-bolus
        technique, 284
    reflux from, treatment of, 268-269
Saphenous system, varicose veins and, 4
Scarpa's fascia, 20
Schwartz test, 113, 113
Scleremo; see also Chromated glycerin
    active ingredient and complications of,
        259t
    manufacturers and distributors of, 375
Sclerodex; see also Hypertonic
        glucose/saline
    active ingredient and complications of,
        259t
    manufacturers and distributors of, 375
Sclerosing solutions, 359
    allergic reactions to, 248-253
        chromated glycerin, 251
        ethanolamine oleate, 248-249
        heparin in hypertonic saline, 252
        lidocaine in hypertonic saline, 253
        polidocanol, 250-251
        polyiodide iodine, 251-252
        sodium morrhuate, 248
        sodium tetradecyl sulfate, 249-250
    animal models in evaluation of, 189-190
    categories of, 183, 185-187
    chemical, mechanism of action of,
        186-187, 187
    clinical use and relative potency of,
        190t
    clinical use of, 206-215
        chemical irritants, 208-210
        detergents, 210-215
        hypertonic glucose/saline, 207-208
        osmotic agents, 206-207
    comparative efficacy in animal models,
        203
    comparative efficacy in human models,
        204
    concentration and strength of, for
        microsclerotherapy, 313
    detergent, 185-186
        mechanism of action of, 185
        probable molecular orientation of, into
            aggregates, 185
        toxic effects on formed elements of
            blood, 186
    disulfiram as contraindication to, 277
    effects on arteries, 189
    experimental evaluation of, 189-205
    extravasation method, 239, 241, 241
    FDA-approved, 206

Venous hypertension — cont'd
  chronic, effects of, 64
  cutaneous
    correction of, 1
    etiology of, *33, 34*
  hemorrhage as complication of, 49
  histologic examination of patient with,
    *46*
  lymphostasis verrucose cutis and, *35*
  pathogenesis of, 32, 34, 36-37
  secondary complications of, 48-52
  signs of, 110
  superficial thrombophlebitis as
    complication of, 49-50
Venous insufficiency
  with atrophie blanche, *47*
  chronic
    with cutaneous ulceration, *47*
    edema as manifestations of, 40-41
    telangiectasia with, 34, *35*
  defined, 32
  varicose veins as cutaneous marker of, 40
Venous obstruction, proximal or distal to
    varicose veins, 71
Venous outflow, assessment of, 111, *112*
Venous pressure
  ambulatory, measurement of, 135, 136
  deep; *see* Deep venous pressure
  increased, arteriovenous anastomosis
    and, 71-74, *72-73*
Venous refilling time, 135-136
Venous stasis
  events following onset of, 37
  pigmentation in, 42, *42, 43*
  signs of, 41
Venous system
  components of, 61

Venous system — cont'd
  effect of temperature on, 67
  evaluation of, purpose of, 110
  hormonal influence on, 78
  of legs
    anatomy of, 7, *8-11,* 12-21
    histology of, 21-25
    muscle pump of, *11,* 12
  during menstrual cycle, 78
  peripheral, blood volume percentage in,
    63
  saphenous, *267*
  valvular
    anatomy of, 12-20, *13, 15*
    normal and abnormal function of, 13,
      *13*
Venule
  anatomy and function of, 21, *21*
  telangiectasia arising from, *28*
Venulectases
  with Klippel-Trenaunay syndrome, 90
  magnetic resonance image of, *93*
Venules, histology of, 25-26, *26*
Vitamin E, varicose veins and, 69
Volumetry, foot; *see* Foot volumetry
VRT; *see* Venous refilling time
Vulvar varices
  determining origins of, *152*
  evaluation of, 153
  preferred examination methods, 147t

# W

World Health Organization, varicose veins
    defined by, 61

# Z

Zollikofer, D., 3